Poverty and Sickness in Modern Europe

Poverty and Sickness in Modern Europe

Narratives of the Sick Poor, 1780–1938

Edited by
Andreas Gestrich, Elizabeth Hurren
and Steven King

continuum

Continuum International Publishing Group

The Tower Building	80 Maiden Lane
11 York Road	Suite 704
London	New York
SE1 7NX	NY 10038

www.continuumbooks.com

British Library Cataloguing-in-Publication Data
A catalogue record for this book is available from the British Library.

ISBN 978-1441-18481-8 (HB)
ISBN 978-1441-11081-7 (PB)

Typeset by Deanta Global Publishing Services, Chennai, India
Printed and bound in India

CONTENTS

LIST OF FIGURES AND TABLES

1

Narratives of poverty and sickness in Europe 1780–1938: Sources, methods and experiences

Andreas Gestrich, Elizabeth Hurren and Steven King[1]

Introduction

In the context of a rapidly expanding literature on the histories of European welfare states, and of wider attempts to discern and spatially locate differently configured European welfare systems or regimes,[2] one of the most important empirical advances has been a renewed focus on the experiences of the poor themselves. Historians of poor relief, clothing, medicine, housing, begging, urbanization, language, nutrition, demography, work, migration and politics have increasingly sought to balance representations of the poor in pamphlets, official literature, pictures and popular polemic, with an understanding of the detailed words, lives, feelings, strategies and experiences of the dependent poor.[3] Such work has involved the consideration, re-reading and reconstruction of a set of sources that stray beyond the confines of much earlier welfare history. Some of these sources – emigrant letters, autobiographies, witness statements in court cases, newspaper stories, advertisements for runaway fathers, or begging letters – are familiar even if sometimes read and deployed in unfamiliar ways.[4] Other sources – public petitions, popular ballads, applications for citizenship, the statements of tramping labourers preserved in local guild archives, patient case notes, suicide letters, pauper letters, or forced narratives arising out of pan-European attempts to constrain the spread of venereal disease and to control prostitution – are less well-known.[5] Yet it is clear that across Europe such sources exist in considerable numbers, particularly from the late eighteenth century as the print marketplace grew and both postal services and the underlying base of popular literacy improved. Nowhere is this more apparent than in the proliferation of letters written by paupers themselves or on their behalf. Once thought to have been largely unique to England and Wales, generated by the particularities of the statutory national Poor Law system there, it is increasingly clear that such letters exist in considerable numbers elsewhere in Europe too.[6]

Analysis of these types of source has led welfare and other historians to balance their questions about the administration and organization of welfare, the supply of resources and the political, religious and philosophical rationale for particular welfare structures, with wider consideration of issues such as: the agency and political participation of the poor; the rhetorical and linguistic register that the poor might use to frame and understand their condition; everyday experiences of the economy of makeshifts; concepts of the life-cycle; and the moral and customary spaces within which the European poor operated in the eighteenth and nineteenth centuries. It is not the intention of this introduction to provide an extensive overview of the development of European welfare historiography.[7] Three particular areas might, however, be taken to exemplify these developments and simultaneously highlight the importance of narrative sources for the understanding of welfare histories. Thus, the analysis of posters, speeches, ballads, chapbooks and formalized petitions have been used to illustrate the fact that the poor (a vaguely defined 'labouring poor' and the more 'explicitly poor' identified by the receipt of different forms of charity or communal relief) had both a political consciousness and will, and participated in local, regional or even national politics. This observation might extend from the participation of poor people in the politics of sixteenth-century Henrician England, through the semi-political manoeuvrings of the mobile poor to obtain citizenship status and rights in Switzerland, and to the highly politicized and class-based resistance of poor people to compulsory smallpox vaccination in various nineteenth-century European states.[8] Periodically at least, the poor, even the dependent poor, seem to have been politically aware and to have participated in the political process.

A second example of the new directions in which narrative evidence has taken us is the increasingly lively debate over the character, execution and limits of pauper agency. Studies of pauper letters have begun to reveal that the poor adopted complex rhetorical and strategic devices in their engagement with officials and welfare donors, garnering power and de facto rights to relief where there might otherwise be none. For some commentators at least, pauper letters embody the appropriation and subversion of official language and of the conventional linguistic register – encompassing deference, humility, gratitude, modest demands and a desire for independence – that underpinned the structure of eighteenth- and nineteenth-century social relations.[9] Historians have also pointed to the adoption by the poor of powerful customary, rhetorical, religious and philosophical reference points – dignity, the obligations associated with wealth, yardsticks of human rights such as the right not to be naked, and the Christian duty of officials and donors – in their narrative dealings with those controlling access to resources.[10] Others have sought forcefully to assert the limits of pauper agency.[11] A related, and third, strand of the historiography has used narrative evidence to refine understanding of the process of begging. Tim Hitchcock, for instance, employed stories from the Old Bailey in London to emphasize that beggars had an understood and accepted place in the urban fabric, such that responding to the pleas of beggars on the streets of eighteenth-century London was crucial to the idea of middling masculinity. He also highlights the difficulties that both communities and beggars themselves had in distinguishing begging from work in the eighteenth century.[12] Sigrid Wadauer, both in this volume and elsewhere, observes similar experiences in early twentieth-century Vienna. More widely, these perspectives have been explored across Europe in the context of begging letters, with historians suggesting a widespread culture of writing pleading letters which might reach the very highest levels of European society.[13]

These are interesting and important perspectives, symbolic of a wider change in the focus and tenor of debate about the European poor, whether they be the disordered and disorderly, or the respectable and respectful. For the purposes of this volume, however, we shift our attention to narratives by and about a particular group of the European poor, the sick. There are several reasons for this focus. First, while other groups of the life-cycle poor (the aged, widows, children etc.) have attracted increasing historiographical attention, it has become clear that life-cycle conditions were rarely sufficient in their own right as a reason for charity or formal relief to be given. Nowhere is this clearer than in work on the aged poor, where relief in whatever form was invariably tied into progressive disability and inability to labour because of physical or mental weakness.[14] In short, ill-health broadly defined (to include conditions such as pregnancy or lunacy for instance) is a cross-cutting theme in European welfare studies. For England and Wales at least, sickness was at most times the key reason for relief applications, and more widely contributors to this volume demonstrate admirably how even proximate reasons for relief applications such as unemployment often masked underlying sickness. A corollary of this observation, and a second reason for the focus of this volume, is that the sick poor author or are the subject of more narratives than any group of the European poor. Moreover, the range of narratives, running from letters and petitions on the one hand, through inquests, suicide notes and newspaper reportage, to ballads and poems on the other, tends to be rather wider than for any other subset of the poor.[15] This should not, perhaps, surprise us, since the sick poor arguably appeared in the widest (narrative generating) range of institutional and relational contexts. Thus, we can find narratives emerging from hospitals and hospital visiting committees, work and almshouses, the inquiries of medical charities, the activities of individual doctors, the everyday work of poor relief agencies, the sick poor themselves, regional and central government and in response to the threat of epidemic and pandemic disease. The situational context of the sick poor, in other words, makes them a microcosm of the experiences of paupers more widely.

A final reason for focusing on the sick poor is that this group presented the most complex legal, economic, organizational, philosophical, moral and customary dilemmas for those providing welfare resources. This was true whether we consider the sick poor under the English and Welsh Old and New Poor Law systems (which afforded quasi-legal and customary rights to the sick poor) or under the philanthropic and institutionally based charity that we see in many continental countries. Even in Scotland, arguably one of the harshest welfare regimes in eighteenth- and nineteenth-century Europe,[16] how to deal with the sick poor posed acute philosophical, economic, moral and practical dilemmas. Could sickness and an associated inability to labour be seen as value neutral, a hazard that might be faced by all and carrying inevitable consequences for the liabilities of communities? Or was sickness, as Beate Althammer and Sigrid Wadauer both suggest in this volume, seen as a direct reflection of the moral bankruptcy of the poor? Should sickness be treated at least cost or should officials seek to avoid higher long-term bills by paying for more effective treatment? What was the Christian duty of officials and donors in relation to the sick poor, irrespective of the law? In the sense that sickness and its consequences compromised basic human values (the right to clothing and adequate food, the ability to fulfil the obligations of a parent, the ability to be part of a community and neighbourhood), how should communities react? How might customary, legal and moral obligations intersect to provide a moral space in which the sick poor could negotiate? And if doctors, neighbours, other officials, family, religious ministers, friends and employers wrote in support of charitable or communal relief for the poor, how much weight should officials give to these epistolary advocates? Such questions locate sickness, the sick poor and narratives by or about the sick poor at the interface of wider attempts to understand the nature and experience of European poverty and the agency of the European poor. They also, however, pinpoint the multi-layered (implicit and explicit) decision-making that officials would have to engage in when dealing with the sick poor. While the unemployed, single mothers and other groups of the dependent poor could be ignored or were the focus of practices coalescing around control and the avoidance of concerted social protest, the sick poor constituted a rather less soluble problem for the communities and poor relief systems of Europe. And in the sense that ill-health created, as Peter Wessel Hansen points out in his chapter for this volume, a large group of the 'shamefaced' poor who risked falling down the social scale, the consequences of sickness for officials largely drawn from the same class were all too readily apparent.

Against this broad contextual backdrop, the contributions to our volume deal with the representation and self-representation of the sick poor in Austria, Denmark, England, Germany, Ireland, Spain and Sweden between the later eighteenth century (when opportunities for representation and self-representation began to burgeon) and the 1930s (after which the very nature of welfare itself began to be transformed). The definition of the 'sick poor' employed here is a wide one. In typological terms our chapters focus on a spectrum that runs from the 'shamefaced' poor – the respectable independent labouring and lower-middle classes for whom sickness amounted to the threat of permanent downward social mobility, considered by Georgina Laragy and Peter Wessel Hansen – through to what many contemporaries thought of as the 'degraded poor', such as the syphilitic women analysed by Anna Lundberg or the wandering poor that are the subject of Sigrid Wadauer's chapter. The range of ill-health encompassed by the volume is equally wide, running from insanity/melancholy (chapters by Cathy Smith, Georgina Laragy and Peter Wessel Hansen), through infectious diseases (in chapters by Anna Lundberg and Beate Althammer) and to the chronic but usually poorly specified sicknesses often associated with old age, grinding poverty and unemployment (in chapters by Steven King and Alison Stringer, Katrin Marx-Jaskulski and Tamara Stazic-Wendt). This range in-and-of itself gives a sense of the centrality of sickness to the experience of European poverty. By way of further context, the rest of this introduction focuses on three core issues: a discussion of the disparate European relief and settlement systems within which narratives were generated, read and exchanged, and thereby a consideration of potential chronological and typological variations in the source base between different sorts of welfare regimes; a detailed discussion of the contexts within which narrative sources by or about the sick poor were generated (and some of their problems) and a coeval discussion of the way in which the types of 'voices' found in them might be classified so as to facilitate systematic comparative studies; and a brief consideration of where, collectively, the work on narratives explored in our chapters sits within the wider framework of knowledge on the European sick poor.

European welfare contexts

A literature which once saw the English and Welsh Old and New Poor Laws and associated settlement legislation as somehow unique has more recently given way to a sense that most European states had the same welfare building blocks available but simply sequenced them differently and often with bewildering rapidity.[17] The English and Welsh Old Poor Law rarely provided enough for the dependent poor to subsist with, such that they had to explore complex makeshift economies which look little different in terms of range or depth to those on the Continent.[18] While England and Wales can boast the first legally enshrined national settlement system for deciding who could apply for relief and where, in practice the Swiss and Dutch systems were equally comprehensive if more *ad hoc*.[19] The level of philanthropic resources available to combat poverty fell progressively behind the scale of the national poverty problem in eighteenth-century England. However, a philanthropic resurgence from the early nineteenth-century meant that, in many urban areas, private and organized charity came to play a role in welfare not dissimilar to that in Amsterdam and other major European urban centres.[20] Nor should we forget that for the later nineteenth and early twentieth centuries at least there is an emerging consensus about a convergence of European welfare thought, sentiment and range of practice. Partly informed by the transmission of policy debates and the exchange of officials and investigators, this convergence was characterized by the assertion of a greater degree of central control and a corresponding loss of local autonomy, greater use of institutions, the removal of particular groups from the ambit of discretion and the cementing of rights to relief into the sentimental fabric of welfare practice. While welfare structures in countries such as Switzerland or The Netherlands remained highly fractured even in the 1930s, other bastions of localism, such as France, increasingly saw the encoding of a recognizably 'national' welfare state.[21]

How to make sense of these differently sequenced building blocks within and between states has proved problematic. Distinctions between a broadly conceived 'Catholic Europe' where religiously based philanthropy underpinned the welfare system, and an equally broadly conceived Protestant Europe where lay philanthropy entwined with municipal, Royal or national welfare resources, have many problems. Related mechanisms for characterizing 'national' welfare arrangements – for instance those which draw broad distinctions between northern and southern Europe, central and peripheral Europe, or between welfare systems centred on institutional provision and those not – have also proved problematic.[22] Not least, an increasing number of European studies have drawn attention to the fact that welfare practices within states might vary more strongly than between them, as for instance and most markedly between the different Swiss cantons or between Scotland and England.[23] This said, historians have also drawn attention to persistent regional differences in welfare spending and organization, such that rather than talking in shorthand about the English or Prussian welfare system, we might be better advised to assemble and compare regional typologies that span state boundaries. For this, we need a set of key indicators of welfare sentiment and practice. Part of the value of the current volume is that the issue of how differently constituted local and regional welfare systems treated the sick poor might be one of those key indicators, a point to which we will return below.

In the meantime, historians of poverty and welfare have become increasingly concerned with issues of intra-regional variation and local practice. For the purposes of the current volume, six aspects of this literature are important. First, philanthropic funds were a crucial part of the welfare resource in Europe. Communities and individuals from Ireland to central Austria and beyond raised substantial charitable resources in response to pressing need such as harvest failures, the closure of international markets or spiralling prices. Often allied with specific municipal responses or (in France for instance) central initiatives, these resources were usually situationally-specific and short-lived. In 'normal' times, subscriptions, endowed charities and (crucially for much of Europe outside the temporary reforms of the Napoleonic period) religiously based charities underpinned much day-to-day welfare. While the prize of biographies of the welfare avenues explored by individuals at different stages of their life and family-cycle remains elusive, the importance of philanthropic resources even for a country such as England should not, as we have seen, be underplayed. Equally important for welfare in many European states, was the practice of begging. For England, Tim Hitchcock has emphasized the importance of informal street begging or the door-to-door tour in which begging elided seamlessly into individual charity. Elsewhere, in Austria for instance, begging was more formalized, not to say officially sanctioned, and inscribed into a framework of Christian obligation, custom and mutual expectation of behaviour and sentiment.[24] A further form of begging has, however, largely escaped historiographical attention: just as some Belgian citizens felt that it was within their purview to write begging letters to the Royal Family, so private individuals across Europe received considerable numbers of such narratives. Many were from the 'shamefaced' poor discussed by Peter Wessel Hansen in his chapter for this volume, but considerable numbers also came from ordinary working-class people and paupers who had encountered hard times. In England, Quaker families in particular seem to have attracted or (more likely) preserved such begging letters. Beyond the compass of this book, such begging letters number in the tens of thousands for England alone and provide one future avenue for research on the narratives of the poor.

A second observation is that all systems of makeshift economy, whether focused on resources generated by the state, community or church, struggled with what to do about migration. While it has become increasingly clear that early modern societies were by no means immobile, there is a clear sense across Europe that industrialization, urbanization and proletarianization led to a step-change in the scale if not the distance or type of migration. In England and Wales the response was a set of enabling national 'settlement laws' in which the precise decision on who 'belonged' to a place and could access its resources was decided in tortuous case law at local and regional level. In other countries, whether one belonged and could access resources was a matter of religion, citizenship status, accumulated economic contribution, or birth. No system was as complex as that in Switzerland, but complexity and contradiction was the key characteristic of European settlement systems, which had to sensitively balance the needs of local labour markets against the pockets of local taxpayers, churches and philanthropists. Not until the later nineteenth and early twentieth centuries did European states move decisively towards place-based settlement systems, in which accumulated residence in a place generated entitlement to stay and potentially to draw on local welfare resources. Even then, communities and central authorities might manipulate the length of time that one had to be resident before settlement could be claimed so as to protect communal resources.

It is important to be clear, however, and a third observation of the historiographical literature, that simply belonging to a place did not guarantee access to communal resources. By the same token, failing to gain a legal settlement did not necessarily exclude individuals and families from local resources. In England and Wales, being settled gave individuals a right to apply for tax-funded local welfare payments under the Old and New Poor Laws, rather than any right to receive them. In practice many people were turned down, got less than they asked for or experienced long delays in consideration of their case. Across Europe, officials and others could and did bundle up different types of welfare resources (access to religious charities, other charitable resources, rights of common, begging licenses, food and fuel doles and tax-funded allowances) for those with different types of belonging. Much more detailed work is needed on the way that 'bundles of rights and rights to access' were claimed, granted and lost. We also need to know more about the value of those bundles; without detailed biographies of the poor across the life-cycle it is difficult to unpick what value access to common land, charities, begging and tax-funded doles had in total and relative to each other. In the meantime, if it is clear that in most places and at most times the sentimental watchword of European welfare systems was 'economy', there are also contrary indicators. Under the English Poor Law system, for instance, the sick were often treated with extraordinary generosity whether they had a settlement or not.[25] Even the nineteenth-century workhouse rapidly became a diagnostic and treatment space giving the very poorest access to health care better than in some hospitals.[26]

In turn, and a fourth observation, it is clear that European welfare systems evidence considerable inter-state, inter-regional and intra-regional differences in the emphasis on institutional provision for the poor. Officials under the English and Welsh Old Poor Law had a famously fickle relationship with workhouses, and while most places experimented with them few workhouses had any longevity. The New Poor Law has been yoked closely to the institution of the workhouse, but almost all relief for the poor after 1834 continued to be paid to those outside its walls. Unlike their German counterparts, British officials never got the legal power to forcibly confine the poor, with the result that workhouses rapidly became receptacles for the aged, infirm and mothers of illegitimate children.[27] This was true of both urban and rural areas. In urban France, by contrast, institutionally based relief was throughout the period considered in this volume the symbolic fulcrum of welfare. Of course, much charity was dispensed outside the institutional context (something reinforced by the chapters in this volume), particularly in the European provinces, but the distinction between England and Wales and Continental Europe in these terms is nonetheless marked.

It follows from this, and a fifth observation of the historiographical literature, that within and between states the role, professionalization and hierarchy of officials connected to welfare varied widely. In the sense that such men set the 'tone' of local welfare practice, the fact that there is so little research on them as a group is unfortunate. As Beate Althammer implies in her chapter comparing responses to Cholera in Germany and Spain, the 'attitudes' of officials and the wider class from which they were drawn could have fundamental – life-and-death – consequences both for how the poor were represented and treated. In England and Wales the amateur overseer of the Old Poor Law, appointed for one year and drawn from the general body of the ratepayers according to a rota, has become an accepted part of the historical landscape. This despite the fact that urban areas moved quite quickly to pay more professional people who thus stayed in post for much longer. Paupers living inside and outside their settlement community made their case primarily to this official. Although they had a right of appeal to magistrates, few contested the decisions on their case. Under the New Poor Law of 1834, local overseers remained in place but many of their powers were transferred to relieving officers who worked across groups of parishes. The right of appeal now was either to local guardians (the elected officials representing the parishes) or to the central state. Broadly, then, the English and Welsh system was in hierarchical terms 'flat'. The Scottish Poor Law, by contrast, contained more, and more central, intermediaries. These included religious ministers, investigating committees, inspectors of the poor and magistrates, as well as local officials. The German system, outlined by Katrin Marx-Jaskulski and Tamara Stazic-Wendt in their contributions to this volume, was equally hierarchical and multi-layered, and might involve relief applications to paid or amateur officials, religious ministers, elected politicians, figureheads such as the mayor, and a range of regional and national administrations. Unlike England, Switzerland or Austria, many of these functionaries were paid professionals. In Spain, the system was even more complex, melding together all of these figures (though on a largely amateur basis) plus powerful local elites, guilds and aristocrats determined to have their say in both general welfare policy and specific decisions.[28] While all welfare systems became more professionalized from the mid-nineteenth century, the differences highlighted here prior to this date inevitably feed through into differences of sentiment, on which we need rather more research.

Of course, sentiment was shaped by moral and financial consideration as well as by the character and power of administrators. Another variable was the way in which welfare structures were inscribed into the wider legislative and state-building context, and a final observation of the literature is that this context seems to have varied considerably. The syphilitic patients who stride through Anna Lundberg's chapter for this volume were subject to forced treatment under a repressive national law but this was just one of a suite of national legislative initiatives (on education, registration of residence and settlement, for instance) that sought to control the poorest segments of society. In turn, these laws were based upon one of the most comprehensive, and certainly the earliest, information states in Europe. Similarly the chapters on Germany, Austria and Denmark in this volume point explicitly or implicitly to the treatment of the poor and understanding of their plight being increasingly intertwined with a wider set of legislative imperatives and a wider state-building impetus. By contrast, the British state, at least in so far as it related to England and Wales, adopted largely permissive legislation and for most of the period considered here maintained little effective central control over the dispensation of welfare or the lives of the poor. And while the law of the Poor Laws became intricately connected to other medical and welfare legislation (for instance on medical training and the use of the poor for anatomy purposes after 1832) it was not bundled with wider social legislation on matters like education as was the case in Sweden or Denmark. In France, too, it was not until the early twentieth century that the central state could inscribe treatment of the poor into a wider legislative programme, a project to build a definitive national identity and into a coherent information state underpinned by national statistics.[29]

These observations are at best a partial rendering of the rich secondary literature. Yet they are fundamental to an understanding both of the treatment of the sick poor (a topic revisited below) and the scale, form and typologies of narratives by or about the sick poor that emerge in Europe from the later eighteenth century. Broadly, the nature of the welfare system faced by the poor, whether 'shamefaced' or pauper, shaped how they were depicted, how many narratives were written, in what form and to whom. It also shaped the likelihood of survival of the sorts of evidence that our contributors are interested in. Thus, the balance of philanthropic resources in the local welfare package matters because applying for and obtaining charity generated more narrative material *about* the poor than *by* them. Those who administered charitable resources frequently surveyed the poor, and in places like Scotland or Norway such surveys might involve mediated testimonies of the poor themselves. Charities often had to report to donors, and might do so through publications or newspapers. Equally, as Peter Wessel Hansen shows in his chapter for this volume, stories about the poor might be published so as to elicit support for charities in the first place. Published testimony *about* the poor arising out of the operation of charities thus tends to be relatively rich, at the same time as original documentation collected for and by charities tends to be relatively thin given their often short-term nature. Narratives written by the poor to charities (as opposed to begging letters to individuals) do exist for some countries, particularly for instance in the urban areas of The Netherlands and Belgium,[30] while in others – England and Wales for instance – they are completely missing. Where they are extant, the very act of applying to a charitable body or donor shaped the nature of the communication, with many such narratives taking the form of a petition rather than a plea, request or demand. The philanthropic (religious and lay) basis to the Scottish welfare system prior to the 1830s does much to explain the almost complete absence or letters authored by individual paupers in that country and in contradistinction to England.

Settlement systems matter equally for the generation, survival and structure/content of narratives. Residence-based systems of the sort increasingly adopted in European states after the 1850s tended, given the contentious nature of settlement changes, to generate examinations, reports and inspections, alongside voluminous articles *about* the poor and poverty. They tended to stifle the generation of pauper letters, however. Similarly, systems which encompassed automatic or customary monetary transfers between places, when an individual or family fell into poverty and were out of their 'place', tended to generate official correspondence rather than pauper narratives. When the rules on compensatory payments were opaque, migration was substantial, and settlement rules uncertain (as for instance in Germany or England and Wales) the system tended to generate pauper narratives and more formalized petitions. And where there were simply no rules at all on the entitlements of migrants (as for instance in Ireland), pauper narratives of all sorts also tend to be thin on the ground. It is thus unsurprising that pauper letters are being unearthed in Belgium, Germany, Norway and Denmark but hardly at all in Ireland, Scotland or France.

The way in which resources were bundled and with what expectations also shaped the scale, nature and survival of narratives by or about the poor. Systems in which 'rights' enshrined in law and custom dictated both the generalized access to resources and the specific package of welfare given to the individual (as for instance in Switzerland for the different levels of citizenship) tended to generate fewer narratives by the poor themselves but rather more in terms of second-hand reporting of how those 'rights' were used and abused. Where rights were opaque, rights to appeal enshrined in law or practice (as in England and Wales) and the bundle of resources associated with being granted relief was uncertain, both petitions and letters tended to be more numerous. Equally, where the package of resources granted in consequence of need was variable over the life-cycle or according to the financial position of the community concerned, necessitating multiple approaches to officials, so narratives by the poor were usually correspondingly more frequent. In the sense that these sorts of system relied heavily on precedent, narratives are also much more likely to have been preserved. The picture is no less complex if we shift our attention to the institutional complexion of welfare systems. Though there are exceptions (admittance to venereal disease institutions or voluntary hospitals), the poor rarely wrote to officials seeking entrance to institutions, though they might write frequent and energetic correspondence trying to remain out of the workhouse. Remarkably few of the pauper narratives now located across Europe were written either from or too institutions, in contrast for instance to prisoners in jails who appear to have been prolific writers.[31] Welfare systems dominated by institutional relief are thus likely to have generated fewer pauper narratives than those where institutional relief was less central or more transient. By contrast, such systems appear to have disproportionately generated narratives (inquiries, neglect and negligence cases involving witness statements, newspaper reporting, etc.) *about* the poor, something that is plainly visible in the historiography of the English and Welsh New Poor Law.[32]

Organizational and contextual issues also influenced the number and types of narratives written and preserved. Whether the poor were more or less likely to write to paid and professional administrators is unclear. The rich material uncovered by Tamara Stazic-Wendt suggests that for Germany the development of a multi-layered professional administration was met with a vibrant correspondence culture. In England and Wales the exact opposite is true. Here the development of professional administrations led to more reporting on the poor, more examinations and inquiries, more letters from the epistolary advocates of the poor, more correspondence between officials themselves, but many fewer narratives authored by paupers. Preliminary evidence also suggests that letters written to professional administrators tended towards the more formal end of the letter-writing spectrum, and that places with professional administrations also tended to generate more newspaper reportage than places administered by amateurs.[33] Deeply hierarchical administrative structures also tended to generate more narratives by or about the poor, a reflection of the opportunities for multiple levels of engagement between officialdom and the poor and their advocates. Where welfare law sat in the wider legislative framework and structures of power and state identity is also important in these respects. In countries such as Sweden/Norway, where welfare law was intricately entwined with the criminal law, national moral codes and education structures, the voices of the poor themselves might be found in mediated and unmediated form in other areas of the state archives. Hence, for Norway pauper letters are relatively uncommon but the police archives, held at municipal level, are replete with material on the poor and their reported and direct narratives. Nor should we forget the wider impact of the development of the information state on narrative form, survival and frequency. Centralization was invariably accompanied by the development of pre-printed forms and claims-making procedures which militated against the sending of free-form narratives. Where such letters were written, they often ended up in central archives, merged carelessly with volumes of other correspondence such that finding direct pauper testimony becomes uneconomic. On the other hand the very same information state generated statistics which facilitated comparison between places and associated forms of social investigation, and it became easier to detect and report scandal and innovation. Reporting *on* the poor thus increased exponentially with the development of more rigorous and centralized administrative structures and processes after the 1830s. Convergence of European welfare structures and philosophies after the 1850s simply accentuated these complex trends.

Against this backdrop, uncovering the scale, depth and spectrum of direct pauper narratives is still in its early stages. The nature of reporting *on* the poor, and the numerous ways in which the mediated voices of paupers can be obtained, are more clearly understood. Yet, we lack a clear sense in any European state of the absolute depth of resources for understanding the everyday lives, experiences, feeling and voices of the poor. Even in England and Wales, where the process of discovery has arguably moved furthest, we have barely scratched the surface of the narrative material available. Partly reflecting this observation, the editors have sought to commission for this volume chapters which, collectively, explore the fullest range of narrative material by or about the sick poor, yielding a corpus which runs through pauper letters and petitions, begging letters, newspaper reporting, suicide notes, letters about paupers, lunatic and venereal disease case notes, admission letters and to multi-faceted peddler case files. Nonetheless it seems clear, for the combination of reasons noted above, that in most countries (including England and Wales) the survival of pauper narratives themselves is highly patchy both spatially and chronologically. Whether this reflects an accident of survival or the fact that some places and local welfare regimes generated more narratives than others, as we have suggested above, remains to be seen. For some countries, however, we can point persuasively to an almost complete lack of narrative material directly from paupers themselves. In Scotland, petitions and official request/inspections stand in the stead of pauper narratives given the nature of the welfare system with its focus on philanthropic provision. In Ireland a generally patchy welfare archive is notable for its almost complete absence of pauper narratives. The same is true of France. Whatever the extent of the narrative source base, however, such documents are by no means easy to read, analyse or set in context, and it is to these issues that we now turn.

Narratives of/about the poor: Problems of context, method and analysis

If the organization, financing and institutional context of the underlying welfare system influences the number of pauper narratives generated and kept as well as the scale and nature of reporting on the poor, a complex array of other variables shapes the tone, structure and content of those narratives and reports. They are in other words to some extent contingent. At the most general level stand changes in the perception and representation of self in the Enlightenment and post-Enlightenment periods. Porter reminds us that nineteenth-century Europe was to see an explosion of autobiographical work, a reflection of 'heightened perceptions of individuality, the ego glorying in its own being'.[34] While it would be a chapter in its own right to think about the poor's sense of self, it is unthinkable that the conditions making for a re-evaluation of self – of a new interiority – did not also percolate down the very poorest and shape both whether they wrote but also the standards by which they judged their conditions and thus how and about what they wrote. In this volume, sources such as suicide notes or reporting on letters dealing with the mental condition of the dependent and shamefaced poor clearly reflect and embody changing conceptions of the self. At an equally general level, internal migration and urbanization across much of late eighteenth- and nineteenth-century Europe left many people 'out of their place' when they came to experience poverty. Becoming poor in this context necessitated letters by, about or on behalf of the poor and the very fact that officials had to judge a case at a distance shaped what sort of information ought to be included in a pauper letter and, in turn, what might be left out. It is for this reason that reading the silences of pauper narratives is as important as understanding and interpreting what stands on the page in front of the historian.[35] There is also a sense in which particular aspects of the migratory flow are important. Recent research, for instance, has begun to point to very considerable migration among the already aged, something which might shape the likelihood of writing, the value structures that paupers brought to bear and the sense of entitlement embodied in their narratives.[36] Crudely, and as several of our contributors demonstrate, aged and sick paupers wrote very different letters to the insane, those who were unemployed or bore illegitimate children.

General influences like these on the tone, structure and content of reports and narratives are supplemented by source-specific contextual factors. The newspaper articles and reporting analysed by Beate Althammer, Peter Wessel Hansen and Georgina Laragy must be understood against the backdrop of an extending marketplace for print and particularly the rise of newsprint and wider circulation of popular newspapers across Europe in the later eighteenth and nineteenth centuries.[37] While the march of print culture was uneven within as well as between countries, in almost all places we see a burgeoning of articles about the poor, a reflection of an increasingly voracious appetite among Europeans for tittle-tattle, scandal, sensation and views of the underside of the societies in which they existed.[38] In turn, newspaper reporting on the poor undoubtedly made its way to the poor themselves, in effect extending the subjects appropriate for discussion and action in the public sphere as well as providing an accumulating set of rhetorical devices not open to earlier generations which could then be used in pauper narratives themselves.[39] Meanwhile, the politicization of newspapers and newspaper editors also influenced what came through for public consumption, how stories were pitched and the representativeness of individual cases cited, as was clearly the case when cities across Europe grappled with how to confront the spread of Cholera. Other types of source also have complex interpretative backdrops. The coronial records used by Georgina Laragy and the patient case records and police case files used by Anna Lundberg or Cathy Smith must be read in the context of the increasing reach of the criminal and civil law, changing religious or socio-cultural understandings of suicide, madness and prostitution and the development of the information state across nineteenth-century Europe.[40]

The tone, content and rhetoric of pauper letters, particularly for the sick poor, must be read against an even more complex backdrop, and three variables loom particularly large. The first was the growth of a generalized letter-writing culture between the mid-seventeenth and early nineteenth-centuries.[41] Irrespective of whether ordinary people could turn to scribes or letter-writing manuals as some have suggested, work on the narratives of the English poor in particular has pointed to the percolation of the norms and forms of formal letter writing to the very poorest classes on a previously unimaginable scale by the 1800s.[42] This extension of letter-writing culture was coincident with a definitive nineteenth-century upsurge in popular petitioning and public meetings – or what Charles Tilly has labelled the 'transformation of popular participation in public life' and a radical change in 'popular contention'.[43] Together these experiences necessarily gave pauper letter writers an increasing familiarity both with the genre of letter-writing and with contesting the systems that shaped their lives. It is in part for this reason that pauper letters in England increasingly embody the same linguistic register that officials used in making, justifying and communicating their decisions. A second variable was the rapid proliferation of forums in which the poor were allowed or forced to 'speak'. These include the space of the criminal and civil courts, where they were often called to give evidence, the social surveys under which their detailed life histories were increasingly sought and governmental enquiries where they were often called as witnesses.[44] Pan-European efforts to suppress begging equally involved ordinary people being inspected, called as witnesses and dealing on a routine basis with officials.[45] The poor were, in other words, increasingly likely in nineteenth-century Europe to have gained experience of what we might broadly call 'testimony', something which must have influenced the tone, content and rhetoric of their narratives. For the sick poor in particular, one form of testimony loomed large: the patient case history or illness narrative. While medical historians have disagreed over how far the 'patient narrative' of the eighteenth century remained a central diagnostic tool in the nineteenth and twentieth centuries as medical professionals turned to physical examination, there is emerging evidence that for the poorest classes the narrative did indeed endure.[46] The study of patient case records in particular has revealed extensive first hand and mediated pauper testimony as to the nature of the illnesses for which they were treated.[47] Sick paupers in effect encountered numerous outlets for telling and retelling their health histories and it is unsurprising to see complex and multi-layered sickness narratives increasingly underpinning pauper letter-writing in nineteenth-century Europe. As a variant of this observation, and a third contextual variable, the medicalization of old age in the nineteenth century provided both occasions for writing and a medicalized language with which to write.[48] Certainly by the 1830s many pauper letter writers could quote medical opinion at officials, while Tamara Stazic-Wendt in her chapter for this volume provides persuasive evidence that paupers copied the contents of medical certificates into their appeals. In effect they borrowed the authority of doctors and other medical men to embellish their case and combat what she styles 'a certain speechlessness' in the face of authority.

Reading pauper narratives is not, however, just a matter of understanding the broad context in which they were generated. The letters and petitions analysed by Cathy Smith, Alannah Tomkins, Steven King and Alison Stringer, Tamara Stazic-Wendt, Sigrid Wadauer and Katrin Marx-Jaskulski, also pose very particular problems. Some are technical. Orthographic spelling and a complete lack of punctuation are, for instance, common across Europe in respect of these sources. This makes the understanding of tone and intent somewhat difficult. Other problems coalesce around the issues of honesty and selective reporting. Tamara Stazic-Wendt and Katrin Marx-Jaskulski both suggest that the contents of letters and petitions to German officials were shaped by ingrained perceptions of what the authorities might want to hear or what was most likely to be successful in a relief claim. In English letters too claims that men and women could not fulfil the natural duties of father and mother or son and daughter, or that women and children were naked, probably constitute rhetorical devices to exploit the grey areas of entitlement rather than a persistent reality. By the same token, there were things to which English pauper letter writers rarely referred. Particularly at times of sickness, for instance, writers usually neglected to mention the presence of proximate or co-resident kin given well-known legal liabilities under which English and Welsh families could be compelled to provide support for pauperized relatives. Nor is honesty an issue just for pauper narratives narrowly defined. Peter Wessel Hansen suggests that newspaper editors expected their readers to doubt the veracity of their stories about the shamefaced poor. Moreover, as Sigrid Wadauer shows very well different sources of information contained in case files relating to peddlers often conflicted because of oversight, poor memory, misunderstanding or sheer dishonesty. Letters by peddlers themselves were almost standardized, a clear reflection of widespread understanding of what the authorities wanted to hear and in what form. Other potential problems stem from issues of authorship. Crudely, did the person who signed a letter or petition actually write it? While few European countries had a professional group of scribes on a par with urban France,[49] there is compelling evidence that some letters might be constructed by a group of people in the community even if only written by one of them.[50] Diaries and autobiographies from across Europe illustrate the process by which the less literate or illiterate sought out those who could write. For the sick, where sickness itself compromised the ability to write, the issue of authorship looms particularly large and it is no accident that this group disproportionately sought out epistolary advocates to write and appeal on their behalf. Whoever authored pauper narratives, analysing them as part of a large sample also poses basic logistical problems. It is likely, as we have already hinted, that letters or petitions by aged paupers would embody a radically different rhetorical infrastructure and claims-making mechanism compared to those written by the young unemployed. Women were likely to have used different claims-making structures to men. Urban and rural letters might also have been very different.[51] Such dichotomies provide an opportunity for sophisticated analysis but also throw up important questions about the possibility of comparability where the ages of paupers (and sometimes their sex) or the places from which they wrote are not identified.

There is, of course, scope for a more detailed discussion of the specific problems posed by the narrative sources used in this volume. The bigger question though is how historians should read the multiple voices that these sources often embody and the perspectives on experience, sentiment and agency that they seem to offer? More widely, is there a framework which will both allow a systematic comparison of the voices present in different genres of sources *and* the comparative analysis of sources which, while part of the same broad genre, differ subtly in tone, content, rhetoric and range of voices over European time and space. Crudely put, should we read and compare English pauper narratives from the early nineteenth century with German narratives from the early twentieth century and the petitions and letters of Swedish venereal patients or Austrian peddlers? If so, how? Simple conceptual divisions between ego documents and 'others' are not fit for purpose given the complex interweaving of the individual pauper voice in many of the sources used by our contributors. Pauper letters might be ego documents or they might not. Case notes are not generally regarded as ego documents and yet many of them contain significant direct pauper testimony. Even newspaper articles might embody very different narrative forms depending on the subject – some verging on ego documents while others impose the linguistic and behavioural norms of one class on another. There is not the space in this chapter to explore these issues in the depth they deserve. Table 1.1 below, however, suggests a basic matrix by which we might seek to understand and classify the intent, generative framework and the nature and type of voice inherent in each of the main sources underpinning the individual chapters in this volume.

In broad terms we can see that most of the sources embody observation of and advocacy for, the poor. Most too embody some form of codified narrative, where the nature of the forum to which the narrative was angled heavily shaped the form, content and structure of the narrative itself.

Table 1.1 Classifications of narrative documents

Source Type	Advocacy	Free-form ego	Official correspondence	Observation	Mediated testimony	Codified narrative	Imposed narrative
Pauper letters		X			X	X	X
Petitions						X	X
Begging letters		X				X	
Letters about paupers	X		X	X	X		
Letters to newspapers	X	X	X	X			
Letters of admission	X			X		X	X
Lunatic case notes			X	X		X	X
VD case notes			X	X			X
Peddler case files	X	X	X	X	X	X	X
Newspaper reporting of Cholera	X		X	X	X		
Newspaper reporting of shamefaced poor	X			X	X		
Newspaper reporting of suicide	X			X			X
Coroner reports			X	X	X	X	X

Imposed narratives – where the 'voice' of the subject was imposed upon them – are also common. Thus, pauper letters were not, and not meant to be, simply free-form ego documents. They embody mediated testimony (where letters were written by a single person but constructed by a group for instance), codified narratives (because they were often angled to what the pauper thought the overseer might want to hear) and imposed narratives (in the sense that throughout Europe pauper letters appear rapidly and necessarily to have come to share the same linguistic platform as official correspondence). The case notes of lunatic patients embodied official correspondence, observation (of the patient) and codified narrative (in the sense that nineteenth-century Europe saw the gradual coalescing of the 'way' to record case notes around a small number of acceptable models). They also imposed narratives on the lunatics themselves, such that the 'voices' of the lunatic poor have often elided with the 'voices' imposed upon them by case notes.[52] Newspaper reporting of the shamefaced poor combined advocacy, observation and mediated testimony (less often free form voices of the poor themselves) while newspaper reports about cholera embodied advocacy (in the case of Barcelona for instance), observation and mediated testimony, but also an element of official correspondence given the manipulation of newspaper stories by political elites. What Table 1.1 seeks to show, in other words, is a matrix for reading and comparing the multiple voices inherent in our narrative sources and which stands over and above the particular strengths and weaknesses of the individual sources themselves. Some of the implicit conclusions of the matrix (that one cannot really compare the voice in pauper letters with that in petitions for example) are obvious and a commonplace in the secondary literature. Others – that one can and should compare the voices in newspaper reports about paupers with letters written by the epistolary advocates of the poor – offer considerable analytical possibilities.[53]

There are, of course, a variety of other ways in which one might choose to classify narrative sources, and to develop this framework would be an essay in its own right. Only when we have such a classification, however, is it genuinely possible to assess the potential of narrative forms for transforming our understanding of welfare systems in Europe between the eighteenth and twentieth centuries. In the meantime, it is important not to overplay the potential problems with individual narrative sources. Letters, petitions, court cases and even case records can and do provide a window onto the agency if not always the objective feelings of the poor. While the 'truthfulness' of narratives of all sorts should be questioned, many of our contributors suggest that resources were rarely given without some form of surveillance. Even the newspaper editors in eighteenth-century Copenhagen invited their readers to go and view the shamefaced poor for themselves. The scope for untruths or radical embellishments was thus probably relatively slim. And while many of the sources used by our contributors are, directly or indirectly, mediated we should not automatically assume that they thus fail to reflect either the lived realities of the poor or even their own sentiments or words. The multiple sources brought to bear to investigate suicide cases (Georgina Laragy), the activities of peddlers (Sigrid Wadauer) and the lives of women with venereal disease (Anna Lundberg) sometimes contain the directly quoted words of the individual, and always provide multiple interlocking perspectives on their thoughts, feelings, standing in the community and basic characteristics such as honesty. They also contain physical descriptions of the poor, something rarely obtained from the administrative and financial sources which have dominated the writing of the history of poverty and welfare across Europe. The multi-functionality of narratives – newspaper articles served political, personal and philanthropic causes; pauper letters were simultaneously a vehicle for reporting and supplication and the assertion and assumption of rights; case notes were at once a record of a disease/treatment and a personal history but also documents in which silences and elaboration were inscribed in complex ways according to social norms, the desire of the subject to retain agency and the desire of the state to control particular groups of people – make them difficult to 'read'. Yet this complexity also generates important insight. Thus, many of our contributors suggest that their sources provide a way into the question of pauper agency. The same sources often reflect and embody the sentiments of communities – seen most clearly in Beate Althammer's discussion of the ways in which newspapers report and colour the impact of cholera on the poor – and provide a yardstick against which we can understand the nature of entitlement, structures of power relations, the operation of the law and perceptions of state and communal duties. Employed in large numbers, as surely they will be with various European initiatives underway to identify and collect them, pauper narratives in particular provide a way, though corpus linguistics and large-scale consideration of intertextuality, to understand the very genealogy of the language of the poor. Detailed engagement with narrative sources by or about the poor can, in other words, offer important new perspectives on the operation of European welfare systems. They offer even greater scope for enriching and reconsidering the particular experiences and claims of subgroups of the poor such as the aged and sick, alongside and partly informing wider attempts to classify narrative sources. And it is to these experiences that the chapter now turns.

Thinking about the sick poor

The broad patchwork of avenues through which the sick poor might seek specific (medicine, hospital care or treatment by doctors) or generalized (cash doles, extra food etc) relief have become increasingly clear both for our period as a whole and within individual countries. Religiously inspired charities survived Reformation, Counter-Reformation and Napoleonic invasion and continued to provide resources for medical institutions, nursing care and supplementary relief for the sick and their families. Such funding was rarely generous and often fell behind the level of inflation in welfare budgets in general and medical welfare costs in particular. Its importance in the overall welfare package also varied considerably, both within and between countries. There was a heavy dependence upon such religious medical charities in Ireland, Scotland and Italian states at the opening of the nineteenth century while it was relatively unimportant in England and Wales at the same date. Similar observations might be made of individual and endowed charity from the elites, which remained an important if ultimately unquantifiable contribution to medical welfare across eighteenth and nineteenth-century Europe. Such charity had rich roots in France[54] and was inscribed into the very fabric of many tenancy arrangements in continental Europe. Even in the highly proletarianized environment of early nineteenth-century England, estate owners in rural areas and factory owners, sojourning aristocrats and the middling sorts in urban areas retained a deeply embedded sense of obligation to medical charity.[55] We see this enduring commitment played out in the burgeoning number and range of physical institutions catering for the sick that proliferated across nineteenth- and early twentieth-century Europe. In England and Wales, where the Old Poor Law had generally provided small and short-lived workhouses in which medical care might be dispensed, the 1834 New Poor Law ushered in much larger workhouses. While infirmary provision in such places was often poor or non-existent, by the 1860s officials across the country had embarked on a fundamental programme of infirmary building and associated staff professionalization. Such provision was increasingly supplemented with or even eclipsed by the building of 'voluntary hospitals' established and run through subscription charities, a national Dispensary movement for out-patient treatment and a network of county asylums for the insane poor. Here, as elsewhere in Europe, self-help institutions such as friendly societies, guilds and companies also provided medical care as of right. Certainly by the later nineteenth century the network of institutions was providing medical care for the poor and labouring poor of at least the same quality as could have been afforded by the lower middling classes at the same period. In other European states, the provision of medical care and wider forms of welfare had taken on institutional forms at much earlier dates, but even in these contexts it is possible to trace both an increase in the scale and number of institutions and in the range of medical options that they provided.[56] The emergence of specialist hospitals – dealing with everything from eye complaints to venereal disease – is also especially notable and can be traced in some of the narrative sources used by our contributors.

Yet if institutions have been the focus of much of the historiographical writing on medical relief for the poor, it is also clear that the role of institutional medical care in the life-cycles of illness and treatment for the poor is inadequately understood. Patient case records often do not survive. Where they do, a lack of research on their content across Europe hinders our ability to see whether going to a hospital or workhouse was a regular part of the medical welfare spectrum of the sick and infirm of the labouring classes, or whether attendance at such institutions was highly infrequent, something that happened only at time of sudden accident or emergency or near the end of an illness cycle that would result in death. Micro-studies suggest that even within individual cities the answer to these questions could be highly variegated, with some patients having long histories of attendance at hospitals while others with equally long and complex ill health histories had never attended. Equally, some hospitals seem to have had a patient body that was highly engaged with institutional medicine while others did not.[57] Perhaps one should not be surprised by this patchwork; the rich historiography of European lunacy points to the often tortuous path that individuals took to the asylum, and has traced with considerable certainty the limited role that institutions usually played in the life-cycle of a lunatic compared to family care.[58] Cathy Smith, in her contribution to this volume, shows this process in operation for the Northampton General Lunatic Asylum.

It is for these reasons that those with interests in the sick poor have usually pointed to a complex array of strategies and resources that served to keep people outside of institutions. Doctors would sometimes provide medical care free of charge, or they might be engaged where paupers could borrow money or were part of self-help schemes. When they were not available or could not be afforded, self-dosing, quack remedies and recourse to herbal remedies administered by wise men and women were often the first response to illness. Indeed medical historians across Europe have provided a rich picture of this informal medical marketplace for the sick poor.[59] Increasingly too the local, regional and national 'state' became involved in the provision of direct and indirect medical relief outside of institutions. England and Wales had the only 'national' system of welfare prior to the nineteenth century, and recent work on the Old Poor Law has begun to suggest that an increasing proportion of tax-funded welfare was spent on recognizable medical relief spanning treatment by doctors in the homes of the poor, nursing, extra food, cash relief and consequential payments such as rent.[60] Most European states, however, saw periods of epidemic and crisis stimulating municipal or central action in addition to resources provided by charities and institutions. Moreover, for the 'settled poor', medical relief in countries such as Switzerland could be as comprehensive and extra-institutional as in England and Wales.[61] Over the course of the nineteenth century and into the early twentieth, as we have seen, the gradual extension of municipal intervention on the one hand and central state codification of welfare structures on the other resulted in a convergence of European welfare thinking and practice. Initially this generated a range of new extra-institutional welfare avenues for the poor, and, by the early twentieth century, had fed into tax-funded or insurance-based schemes specifically aimed at generating hypothecated resources for poverty occasioned by sickness or accident.[62]

If this broad pattern is now well established, however, there remains much that we simply do not know. Thus, while Peter Lindert and others have established the broad dimensions of change in welfare spending between the eighteenth and twentieth centuries, there is very little sense of what component of this spending was hypothecated to medical welfare either narrowly or widely defined.[63] Nor is it clear what sort of medical care the resources that were spent actually purchased and what impact it had on the life-chances of the poor themselves.[64] As with the operation of the welfare system more generally, micro-studies that touch upon the sick poor seem to point to a complex patchwork of inter and intra-regional and inter-state practices and experiences, notwithstanding the common moral, practical and philosophical dilemmas that the claims of the sick poor posed. Different areas and states spent radically different proportions of their welfare resources on the alleviation of sickness and had varying expectations of when the sick poor would engage with charities and municipal or state funding. The consequences of seeking and accepting medical welfare also varied markedly, and might run on a spectrum from incarceration and forced treatment through to liberty and active engagement with treatment. Moreover, it is also clear that other potential predictors of official attitudes towards welfare – religion and theology, landholding, the nature and scale of philanthropic or tax resources or the nature of appeal processes under the law – simply do not work as yardsticks by which to categorize local, regional and national attitudes to and experiences of medical welfare. Crudely, it was perfectly possible for well-resourced parishes, communes, cantons and towns in the 1850s to restrict medical welfare at the same time as poorer places were alive to a moral responsibility for the sick poor and treated them with considerable generosity.

This said, micro-studies focusing or even touching on the sick poor remain relatively uncommon across Europe as a whole and across the period considered here. Moreover, there is a tendency to concentrate on the end-product – the amount spent on medical relief, the nature of medical care given, the range of drugs employed – of what was actually an uncertain process of establishing entitlement, being offered relief in a certain form, and accepting such relief. In this sense a range of very important questions – important for understanding the variety of attitudes towards the sick poor within and between European states but also for locating the agency and experiences of the poor themselves – remain to be answered: was medical welfare given willingly and constructively or was it dragged out of charities and taxpayers? How did paupers access medical welfare and what did they do if turned down? How many people were turned down? Were the rules and processes for applying to officials predictable or opaque? What was the attitude of paupers to their sickness and to the welfare and medical officials with whom they interacted? Were paupers subject to medical care, or could they shape its frequency and form? How did the poor rhetoricize sickness and how did claims-making related to sickness differ from that related to other causes of poverty? What impact did advocates for the sick poor have on the likelihood of gaining medical welfare? How did the construction of the poor and sick poor in newspapers and other public sources influence the treatment of such groups? What was the nature of family care for the sick poor, and how did welfare regimes expect families to act? What did officials and philanthropic donors do about those whose sickness resulted not just in poverty but also downward social mobility, and how did this differ from their attitudes towards a more definitively poor underclass? How did welfare systems, however financed and organized, treat subgroups of the poor such as the aged where sickness was just one cause of poverty? How did such systems cope with the sickness of those who might in other circumstances be considered disreputable, such as beggars, peddlers or the unemployed? How did welfare systems strike a balance between treatment of the sick and control of them? And did certain sorts of communities have empathy and an accepted duty to the sick, melancholy and suicidal poor?

No single volume could hope to answer all of these questions or provide a model for classifying European welfare regimes according to how they treated the sick poor.[65] Nonetheless, individually and collectively our contributors use narrative sources to offer important new insights about the inter-linkages between sickness and poverty, the process of obtaining medical welfare broadly defined and about the feelings, strategies and rhetoric of the poor and their advocates that led up to welfare resources being granted or denied. Georgina Laragy, Alannah Tomkins, Peter Wessel Hansen and Tamara Stazic-Wendt turn the conventional idea that sickness caused poverty on its head, demonstrating that in many cases it was poverty or the threat of it that caused sickness. All of our contributors point to a limited role for institutional care in the relief of the sick poor. Even the Swedish patients with venereal disease considered by Anna Lundberg spent limited time in carcereal or medical spaces. Indeed, it is clear that sick paupers invested considerable rhetorical and emotional energy in garnering the cash resources that would keep them out of institutional care. Failure in this respect, as Georgina Laragy suggests, could lead to suicide. The study of narrative material also reveals that medical welfare was seen, by paupers, their advocates and officials, as contestable. Those whose initial appeals were turned down – and there were many – came back again and again seeking support in different forms. In some cases, as Steven King and Alison Stringer and Katrin Marx-Jaskulski show, eligibility might be fought out with officials over a series of narratives in which the poor showed a considerable capacity both to develop their rhetorical position and to 'borrow' the linguistic registers of officials, doctors and their own advocates. Paupers met an unwillingness to grant medical welfare with a spectrum of appeal and claims-making that ran from abject begging through (as King and Stringer show) to angry assertions of the duties of officials and the communities that they represented. Yet 'the poor' were not a monolithic group in this respect. The shamefaced poor analysed by Peter Wessel Hansen approached sickness and poverty with a wall of silence, unwilling to write petitions or begging letters or to apply for charitable/municipal welfare given that the very act of doing so would confirm their ultimate descent into destitution. For this group, medical and other welfare was a function of garnering charitable donations from others of the same class and for this it was essential that they be represented, in this case in the late eighteenth-century Copenhagen newspapers, rather than representing themselves.

A further striking commonplace of our chapters is the remarkably clear knowledge of the welfare system, its hierarchies and the grey areas of practice and local or national law that the dependent and shamefaced poor demonstrated. The families of lunatics applying for free or subsidized places in the asylum were, as Cathy Smith demonstrates, keenly aware of the possibilities and limits of such support. Moreover, they were able to exploit the fact that for the shamefaced poor at least, the shadow of insanity occasioned sympathy and support from fellow citizens. At the opposite end of the deserving spectrum, the unemployed men analysed by Tamara Stazic-Wendt elided sickness with their unemployment, knowing that unemployment itself was an insufficient cause for welfare benefits to be paid. The venereal patients of late nineteenth-century Sweden were subject to apparently strong national legislation enforcing treatment and social control, but as Anna Lundberg points out, many of them knew the limits of the law, law enforcement and local practice, managing to evade ongoing treatment and surveillance. This ingrained sense that paupers needed constantly to navigate the vagaries of the welfare system and stay one step ahead of the law and officials perhaps explains why even as the European states established legal rights to relief at times of sickness (local or national, tax or insurance funded) the poor continued for many decades to use a language and rhetoric of sickness in their narratives that was orientated towards establishing and maintaining entitlement.

Yet, if the sick poor understood the broad codes and rules that ought to shape their applications for relief, officials did not always react to such conventions in predictable ways. This was true even of places such as England and Wales, where national laws established the broad ground rules of entitlement and obligation. It is in this context that some groups of the sick poor struggled to navigate the relief system. Alannah Tomkins deals with one such group, the depressed working-class male, demonstrating how claims of compromised working-class masculinity were entwined with the reporting of fact, imagery of abject need and helplessness and the rhetoric of depression and hopelessness to press a case for access to relief. She suggests that letters from this group represented 'a semi-public discussion of health and illness . . . tantamount to an evaluation of [the author's] claim to manhood'. In this sense, some pauper letters were more than simply appeals, and instead represented a claim to the very humanity of the official who received them. Such claims, however, betray the liminal status of this particular group of paupers and the opaque conventions that determined how they should apply for relief. Tamara Stazic-Wendt suggests that a similar set of conclusions might be applied to the sick unemployed of early twentieth-century Germany. On the other hand, and as Peter Wessel Hansen and Georgina Laragy both show, the plight of other theoretically liminal groups could attract both empathy and sympathy. The Copenhagen newspaper editors, for instance, felt that the shamefaced poor had a right, grounded in class identity, to call on their peers and that readers had an analogous moral and pragmatic duty to respond.

Such observations emphasize that individual pauper narratives cannot, as is often the case at present, be taken out of context. This is a common theme across all of our contributions. Ego documents were inscribed in a broad framework of positive advocacy (through newspaper reporting, official reports and the letters of epistolary advocates) on the one hand and negative commentary on the other. The poor and their letters were, in other words, to some extent constructed by a wider set of public comment and perception which might in turn have positive or negative feedback loops into how narratives were received and what relief was deemed appropriate. Beate Althammer illustrates this very well, demonstrating how the poor of the nineteenth-century Rhine Province were constructed in newspapers as morally and physically suspect, a weak link in the fight against cholera, while their counterparts in Barcelona had their claims to welfare resources buttressed by public narratives emphasizing solidarity and the need for cooperation between the classes against a disease that did not respect social boundaries. In England and Wales, series of letters from a single individual or family were peppered with addenda written by doctors, neighbours or employers, and letters written by epistolary advocates. They were also often inscribed into a much wider set of official correspondence about the same family and individual. In some places paupers were even able to claim that their struggles were the subject of public comment and the occasional newspaper article. Ego documents necessarily drew on this wider set of narratives, which also influenced the perceived obligations of communities and the rights and deservingness of pauper writers.

Finally, several of our contributors suggest that the actual or rhetorical sickness of those who might, in other circumstances, be considered disreputable – such as beggars or peddlers – posed considerable problems for officials. Sigrid Wadauer shows that officials worried that sickness or disability might simply be made up, and they resented the way that malingerers could construct a case for deservingness. Yet their ability to control such people was ultimately limited because of the powerful claims of sickness on the moral framework of the community. These experiences were not limited to Austria. In England and Wales it is striking how often the most morally suspect paupers manage to make a compelling case for generous relief at times of sickness. Even the unemployed, long typified as among the most dubious subgroups of the poor, could construct themselves or be constructed (in newspaper articles for instance) as deserving where sickness of the individual or family could be placed at the centre of claims-making. This possibility for sickness to rewrite conventional moral and policy boundaries is something that we see time and again in the individual chapters that make up this volume, pointing once again to the importance of more detailed empirical work on European sickness narratives.

Conclusion

The chapters assembled here use a range of narrative material to move behind the analytical façade – 'How much was spent?', 'What was it spent on?', 'What was the role of medial institutions?' – that currently drives our understanding of attitudes towards and the experiences of the poor in general and the sick poor in particular. Collectively they establish sickness as perhaps the key grey area of European welfare regimes, however they were organized, administered and financed. This is not to say that the claims-making of the sick poor was always successful or that the medical facilities and resources afforded the poor were always effective or adequate. It is, though, to suggest that sickness posed a range of potentially insoluble problems for officials. These ranged from issues of moral hazard – how to treat those whose sickness was fully or partly self-inflicted, when not treating them might lead to death or higher future bills – through what to do about paupers who obtained advocacy from others in a specific (via letters to officials) or a general (via newspaper articles) sense, and to the moral dilemmas posed by illness. In the latter sense, paupers or those writing for them could point to the fact that sickness compromised dignity, the integrity of the family and even the very essence of masculinity and femininity. The poor were alive to the possibilities afforded by a welfare and community system bisected by these considerations and were remarkably adept at forming their claims-making to exploit the grey areas thus created. The Danish shamefaced poor stayed silent and let others make their case for them. Their English counterparts wrote long letters calling on officials to demonstrate fellow feeling in a situation that might afflict them were circumstances different. Where pauper letters have been discovered, and as several of our contributors show, the rhetorical and claims-making strategies employed varied relatively little between, say, England or Germany. For pauper writers, newspaper readers reflecting on the causes and consequences of suicides, those who authored newspaper stories about the shamefaced poor or wrote in support of individual paupers, families seeking subsidized asylum places and even individuals seeking treatment for venereal disease, there seems to have been a clear assumption that sickness ought to elicit fellow feeling and trigger the moral, customary and humanitarian rights which stood in place of legal rights to welfare in most countries before the very late nineteenth century. Whether assumed rights became actual rights is often unclear, though evidence is accumulating that the sick poor were often well, not to say generously, treated. In this sense, there may be considerable mileage in the idea that how national, regional and intra-regional welfare regimes dealt with the thorny problem of the sick poor provides a key yardstick by which we might seek to identify and classify ingrained welfare mentalities.

Notes

1 This chapter draws on research conducted under the auspices of grants awarded by the AHRC/DFG (Gestrich and King) and the Wellcome Trust (King, Hurren et al.).

2 For a survey, see King, S. (2011), 'Welfare regimes and welfare regions in Britain and Europe, c.1750–1860', *Journal of Modern European History*, 9, 42–66.

3 For broad surveys, see Snell, K. (2006), *Parish and Belonging: Community, Identity and Welfare in England and Wales 1700–1950*. Cambridge: Cambridge University Press; Jütte, R. (2000), *Arme, Bettler, Beutelschneider. Eine Sozialgeschichte der Armut in der Frühen Neuzeit*. Weimar: Böhlau; Bräuer, H. (2008), *Armenmentalität in Sachsen 1500 bis 1800*. Leipzig: Leipziger Universitätsverlag.

4 See, as examples, Gerber, D. (2006), *Authors of Their Lives: The Personal Correspondence of British Immigrants*. New York: New York University Press; Lyons, M. (ed.) (2007), *Ordinary Writings, Personal Narratives: Writing Practice in 19th and early 20th Century Europe*. Frankfurt: Peter Lang; Mayer, T. and Woolf, D. (eds) (1995), *The Rhetorics of Life-Writing in Early Modern Europe. Forms of Biography from Cassandra Fedele to Louis XIV*. Ann Arbor: University of Michigan Press.

5 See van Voss, L.-H. (ed.) (2001), *Petitions in Social History*. Cambridge: Cambridge University Press; Fabre, D. (1993), *Ecritures Ordinaires*. Paris: POL; Fumerton, P. and Guerrini, A. (eds) (2010), *Ballads and Broadsides in Britain, 1500–1800*. Farnham: Ashgate; and Tabili, L. (2005), '"Having lived close beside them all the time": Negotiating national identities through personal networks', *Journal of Social History*, 35, 369–87.

6 See Sokoll, T. (2001), *Essex Pauper Letters 1731–1837*. Oxford: Oxford University Press; and Furger, C. (2010), *Briefsteller. Das Medium 'Brief' im 17. und 18. Jahrhundert*. Weimar: Böhlau.

7 For this, see Lindert, P. (2004), *Growing Public: Social Spending and Economic Growth since the Eighteenth Century*. Cambridge: Cambridge University Press; or Baldwin, P. (1990), *The Politics of Social Solidarity and the Bourgeois Basis of the European Welfare State, 1875–1975*. Cambridge: Cambridge University Press.

8 On popular politics, see contributions to Harris, T. (ed.) (2001), *The Politics of the Excluded, c.1500–1850*. Basingstoke: Macmillan; while for citizenship in Switzerland, see Head, A.-L., and Schnegg, B. (eds) (1989) *La Pauvreté en Suisse (XVlle–XXe siècles)*. Zurich: Chronos, pp. 1–14. On resistance to vaccination, see Durbach, N. (2000), '"They might as well brand us": Working class resistance to compulsory vaccination in Victorian England', *Social History of Medicine*, 13, 45–62.

9 King, S. (2011), '"In these you may trust". Numerical information, accounting practices and the poor law, c.1790 to 1840', in Crook, T. and O'Hara, G. (eds), *Statistics and the Public Sphere: Numbers and the People in Modern Britain, c.1750–2000*. London: Routledge, pp. 51–66.

10 Bräuer, *Armenmentalität*.

11 See King, P. (2004), 'The summary courts and social relations in eighteenth century England', *Past and Present*, 183, 125–72.

12 Hitchcock, T. (2005), 'Tricksters, lords and servants: Begging, friendship and masculinity in eighteenth century England', in Gowing, L., Hunter, M. and Rubin, M. (eds), *Love, Friendship and Faith in Europe 1300–1800*. Basingstoke: Macmillan, pp. 177–96; and Hitchcock, T. (2007), *Down and Out in Eighteenth Century London*. London: Hambledon.

13 See the intriguing van Ginderachter, M. (2007), '"If your Majesty would only send me a little money to help buy an elephant": Letters to the Belgian Royal Family (1880–1940)', in Lyons, *Ordinary Writings*, pp. 69–84.

14 See Thane, P. (2005), *A History of Old Age*. London: Getty Trust; and contributions to Campbell, E. (ed.) (2006), *Growing Old in Early Modern Europe: Cultural Representations*. Aldershot: Ashgate.

15 The term 'narratives' is used widely in framing this volume, eschewing sometimes unhelpful distinctions between ego and other documents, or between letters and petitions. Table 1.1 offers some justification for this approach, but on the problems raised by adopting narrow categorizations, see also Earle, R. (ed.) (1999), *Epistolary Selves: Letters and Letter Writers 1600–1945*. Aldershot: Ashgate; and Hopkin, D. (2004), 'Storytelling, fairytales and autobiography: Some observations on eighteenth and nineteenth century French soldiers' and sailors' memoirs', *Social History*, 29, 186–98.

16 See Mitchison, R. (2000), *The Old Poor Law in Scotland: The Experience of Poverty 1574–1845*. Edinburgh: Edinburgh University Press.

17 Innes, J. (1999), 'The state and the poor: Eighteenth century England in European perspective', in Brewer, J. and Hellmuth, E. (eds), *Rethinking Leviathan: The Eighteenth Century State in Britain and Germany*. Oxford: Oxford University Press, pp. 225–80; Lindert, *Growing Public*; Mommsen, W. (1981), *The Emergence of the Welfare State in Britain and Germany 1850–1950*. Newton Abbott: Croom Helm.

18 Lis, C. and Soly, H. (1979), *Poverty and Capitalism in Pre-Industrial Europe*. Brighton: Harvester; Fontaine, L. and Schlumbohm, J. (eds) (2000), *Household Strategies for Survival 1600–2000*. Cambridge: Cambridge University Press.

19 Winter A. (2008), 'Caught between law and practice: Migrants and settlement legislation in the southern Low Countries in a comparative perspective, c.1700–1900', *Rural History*, 19, 137–62; Flückiger-Strebel, E. (2002), *Zwischen Wohlfahrt und Staatsökonomie. Armenfürsorge auf der bernischen Landschaft im 18. Jahrhundert*. Zürich: Chronos.

20 On the urban charitable resurgence in England, see King, S. (2010), *Women, Welfare and Local Politics 1880–1920: 'We Might be Trusted'*. Brighton: Sussex Academic Press. For comparative context, see van Leeuwen, M. H. D. (2000), *The Logic of Charity: Amsterdam 1800–50*. Aldershot: Ashgate.

21 See contributions to King, S. and Stewart, J. (eds) (2007), *Welfare Peripheries*. Frankfurt: Peter Lang; and Leimgruber, M. (2008), *Solidarity Without the*

State? Business and the Shaping of the Swiss Welfare State, 1890–2000. Cambridge: Cambridge University Press.

22 For a review, see King, 'Welfare regimes'.

23 For an excellent set of discussions of the variability in Swiss welfare practice, see contributions to Head and Schnegg, La Pauvreté en Suisse.

24 Scheutz, M. (2003), Ausgesperrt und gejagt, geduldet und versteckt: Bettlervisitationonen im Niederösterreich des 18. Jahrhunderts. St Pölten: NÖ Institut für Landeskunde.

25 King, S. (2007), 'Regional patterns in the experiences and treatment of the sick poor, 1800–40: Rights, obligations and duties in the rhetoric of paupers', Family and Community History, 10, 61–75.

26 See, for instance, Green, D. (2002), 'Medical relief and the New Poor Law in London', in Grell, O., Cunningham, A. and Jütte, R. (eds), Health Care and Poor Relief in Eighteenth and Nineteenth Century Northern Europe. Aldershot: Ashgate, pp. 220–45.

27 Goose, N. (2005), 'Poverty, old age and gender in nineteenth-century England: The case of Hertfordshire', Continuity and Change, 20, 351–84.

28 Martz, L. (1983), Poverty and Welfare in Habsburg Spain: The Example of Toledo. Cambridge: Cambridge University Press.

29 Smith, T. (2003), Creating the Welfare State in France 1880–1940. Montreal: McGill-Queen's University Press.

30 van Leeuwen, The Logic of Charity.

31 Palk, D. (2007), Prisoners' Letters to the Bank of England 1781–1827. London: London Record Society.

32 Price, K. (2008), 'A regional, quantitative and qualitative study of the employment, disciplining and discharging of workhouse medical officers of the New Poor Law throughout nineteenth-century England and Wales', Unpublished PhD, Oxford Brookes University.

33 This conclusion flows from ongoing work collecting and comparing British and German pauper letters and conducted under the auspices of an AHRC/DFG grant held by Professors Gestrich and King.

34 Porter, R. (1997), 'Introduction', in R. Porter (ed.), Rewriting the Self: Histories from the Renaissance to the Present. London: Routledge, p. 3. Also Gagnier, R. (1991), Subjectivities: A History of Self-Representation in Britain, 1832–1920. Oxford: Oxford University Press; and Martin, L., Gutman, H. and Hutton, P. (eds) (1988), Technologies of the Self: A Seminar with Michel Foucault. London: University of Massachusetts Press.

35 On the general issue of how to approach silence, see Poland, B. and Pedersen, A. (1998), 'Reading between the lines: Interpreting silences in qualitative research', Qualitative Enquiry, 4, 293–312.

36 Neven, M. (2003), 'Terra incognita: migration of the elderly and the nuclear hardship hypothesis', History of the Family, 8, 267–95; Rosental, P.-A. (2000), Les sentiers invisibles. Espace, familles et migrations dans la France du 19ᵉ siècle. Paris: EHESS.

37 Though we should note the comparative absence of provincial newspapers in places such as eighteenth- and nineteenth-century France, which may have held back the sorts of social investigations (and consequent reporting on the poor) that we see in Ireland, England or Denmark.

38 See Koven, S. (2006), *Slumming: Sexual and Social Politics in Victorian London*. Princeton: Princeton University Press; and Sachße, C. and Tennstedt, F. (1988), *Geschichte der Armenfürsorge in Deutschland, Fürsorge und Wohlfahrtspflege 1871 bis 1929*. Stuttgart: Kohlhammer.

39 See Halasz, A. (1997), *The Marketplace of Print: Pamphlets and the Public Sphere in Early Modern England*. Cambridge: Cambridge University Press; Zaret, D. (2000), *The Origins of Democratic Culture. Printing, Petitions and the Public Sphere in Early Modern England*. Princeton: Princeton University Press.

40 For an important discussion of this broad point, see Jütte, R. (1996), 'Syphilis and confinement: Hospitals in early modern Germany', in Finzsch, N. and Jütte, R. (eds), *Institutions of Confinement*. New York: Cambridge University Press, pp. 97–116.

41 Gray, L. (2002), 'The experience of old age in the narratives of the rural poor in early modern Germany', in Ottaway, S., Botelho, L. and Kittredge, K. (eds), *Power and Poverty: Old Age in the Pre-Industrial Past*. Westport: Greenwood Press, pp.107–23; Vandenbussche, W. (2007), 'Lower class language in 19th century Flanders', *Multilingua*, 26, 279–90; and Whyman, S. (2009), *The Pen and the People: English Letter Writers 1660–1800*. Oxford: Oxford University Press.

42 Sokoll, *Essex Pauper Letters*, pp. 1–70. Also Dauphin, C. (2000), *Prête moi ta Plume . . . Les manuels épistolaires au XIXe siècle*. Paris: Kimé.

43 Tilly, C. (2010), 'The rise of the public meeting in Great Britain, 1758–1834', *Social Science History*, 34, 291–9, p. 292.

44 Suzuki, A. (2007), 'Lunacy and labouring men: Narratives of male vulnerability in mid-Victorian London', in Bivins, R. and Pickstone, J. (eds), *Medicine, Madness and Social History. Essays in Honour of Roy Porter*. Basingstoke: Palgrave, p. 119; Green, D. (2006), 'Pauper protests: power and resistance in early nineteenth-century London workhouses', *Social History*, 31, 137–59.

45 For some examples, see Jütte, *Arme, Bettler, Beutelschneider*, and contributions to Althammer, B. (2007), *Bettler in der europäischen Stadt der Moderne: Zwischen Barmherzigkeit, Repression und Sozialreform*. Frankfurt: Peter Lang.

46 On the disappearance of the patient narrative, see Fissell, M. (1991), 'The disappearance of the patient narrative and the invention of hospital medicine', in French, R. and Wear, A. (eds), *British Medicine in an Age of Reform*. London: Routledge, pp. 92–109. For alternative views, see Stolberg, G. (2002), 'Health and illness in German workers' autobiographies from the nineteenth and early twentieth centuries', *Social History of Medicine*, 6, 261–76; and Stolberg, M. (2011), *Experiencing illness and the Sick Body in Early Modern Europe*. Abingdon: Palgrave. Also Lachmund, J. and Stollberg, G. (1995), *Patientenwelten: Krankheit und Medizin vom späten 18. bis zum frühen 20. Jahrhundert im Spiegel von Autobiographien*. Opladen: Leske and Budrich.

47 Brändil, S., Lüthi, B. and Spuhler, G. (eds) (2009), *Zum Fall machen, zum Fall werden. Wissensproduktion und Patientenerfahrung in Medizin und Psychiatrie des 19. und 20 Jahrhunderts*. Frankfurt: Campus; Pethes, N. (2008), *Medizinische Schreibweisen. Ausdifferenzierung und Transfer zwischen Medizin und Literatur (1600–1900)*. Tübingen: Niemeyer; Vrettos, A. (1995), *Somatic Fictions: Imagining Illness in Victorian Culture*. Stanford: Stanford University Press.

48 Von Kondratowitz, H-J. (1991), 'The medicalization of old age: continuity and change in Germany from the late eighteenth to the early twentieth century',

in Pelling, M. and Smith, R. (eds), *Life, Death and the Elderly. Historical Perspectives*. London: Routledge, pp. 134–64.

49 Métayer, C. (2000), *Au Tombeau des Secrets: Les écrivains Publics du Paris Populaire, Cimetière des Saints-Innocents XVIe–XVIIIe siècle*. Paris: Albin Michel.

50 This conclusion flows from ongoing work collecting and comparing British and German pauper letters and conducted under the auspices of an AHRC/DFG grant held by Professors Gestrich and King.

51 King, S. (2008), 'Friendship, kinship and belonging in the letters of urban paupers 1800–40' *Historical Social Research*, 33, 249–77.

52 See for instance, Bartlett, P. (1998), 'The asylum, the workhouse and the voice of the insane poor in 19th-century England', *International Journal of Law and Psychiatry*, 21, 421–32.

53 We are currently exploring frameworks of comparison for different narrative forms.

54 Dinan, S. (2006), *Women and Poor Relief in Seventeenth-Century France: The Early History of the Daughters of Charity*. Aldershot: Ashgate.

55 Waddington, K. (2000), *Charity and the London Hospitals*. Woodbridge: Boydell; Loudon, I. (1981), 'The origins and growth of the dispensary movement in England', *Bulletin of the History of Medicine*, 16, 322–42.

56 Gillis, J. (2006), 'The history of the patient since 1850', *Bulletin of the History of Medicine*, 80, 490–512.

57 See Cullen, L. (2011), 'Patient Case Records of the Royal Free Hospital, 1902–12', Unpublished PhD, Oxford Brookes University.

58 Suzuki, A. (1998), 'The household and the care of lunatics in eighteenth century London', in Horden, P. and Smith, R. (eds), *The Locus of Care: Families, Communities Institutions and the Provision of Welfare since Antiquity*. London: Routledge, pp. 153–75; and Scull, A. (1993), *The Most Solitary of Afflictions: Madness and Society in Britain, 1700–1900*. New Haven: Yale University Press.

59 As one example of the very broad medical market, see Dinges, M. (2002), 'Men's bodies "explained" on a daily basis in letters from patients to Samual Hahnemann (1830–35)', in Dinges, M. (ed.), *Patients in the History of Homeopathy*. Sheffield: European Association for the History of Medicine and Health Publications, pp. 85–118.

60 King, S. (2005), '"Stop this overwhelming torment of destiny": Negotiating financial aid at times of sickness under the English Old Poor Law, 1800–40', *Bulletin of the History of Medicine*, 79, 228–60.

61 Head-König, A.-L. (forthcoming, 2012), 'Citizens but nevertheless not belonging: the difficulties in obtaining entitlement to relief for migrants in Switzerland from the 1550s to the early twentieth century', in King, S. and Winter, A. (eds), *Settlement and Belonging in Europe 1600s to 1900s*. Oxford: Berghahn.

62 See Hennock, E. P. (1987), *British Social Reform and German Precedents: The Case of Social Insurance 1880–1914*. Oxford: Clarendon; Hennock, E. P. (2007), *The Origin of the Welfare State in England and Germany: 1850–1914: Social Policies Compared*. Cambridge: Cambridge University Press; Frohman, L. (2008), *Poor Relief and Welfare in Germany from the Reformation to World War I*. Cambridge: Cambridge University Press.

63 Lindert, *Growing Public*.

64 Though see King, S. (2006), 'Pauvrete et assistance: La politique locale de la mortalite dans l'Angleterre des XVIII et XIX siecles', *Annales*, 61, 31–62, for the argument that the medical spending of the Old Poor Law preserved infant life.

65 Though a consideration of the broad historiography suggests that it might be possible to talk in terms of a three-strand model incorporating systems which linked medical welfare with control or incarceration (disciplinary regimes), those which actively and expensively sought to treat or prevent sickness (investing regimes) and those which deployed the minimum resources necessary to combat an immediate problem (stable state regimes).

2

Grief, sickness and emotions in the narratives of the shamefaced poor in late eighteenth-century Copenhagen

Peter Wessel Hansen

Introduction

Under the headline 'The News of the Indigent' in the 15 August 1783 issue of the newspaper *The Copenhagen Evening Post* (*Kiøbenhavns Aften-Post*), the Copenhagen public could read the heartbreaking story of the impoverishment of a former official. The story described in detail how this 'active and honest' 60-year-old ended up in deep poverty. The root of all his troubles was the very low wages he was paid in his office, in turn insufficient to support a family of the middle classes.[1] The last straw was when

> Sickness came to his house and resided for good, especially with his wife. What do these guests require? Expenses for pharmacists and physicians. Neglect of the house, grief and sorrow are the consequences of their attendance; miserable consequences, which often lay claim to a man's ability.

Similar sentiments are to be found in the letters of unemployed and sick men analysed elsewhere in this volume by Alannah Tomkins and Tamara Stazic-Wendt. At the same time the official could not downscale his consumer pattern – or cut his coat according to his cloth. Lowering the living standards was inappropriate 'for a man, who held a royal office, and who carried on public business which meant that he on a daily basis had to appear'. Consequently over the years he ended up incurring large debts, and now the extreme of distress threatened.

The story shows how a vicious combination of insufficient wages, sickness and expectations of a certain life-style drove the official to incur debts which by summer 1783 became such a burden that through the columns of *The Copenhagen Evening Post* he asked his equals in the Copenhagen middle classes for help. It also reveals how the material and physical distress caused psychological reactions such as grief and sorrow when the feeling and sensible official considered the better circumstances he had been used to and compared his fate to the that of his equals. The main foci of this chapter, reflecting also that of Alannah Tomkins later in the volume, are the mental conditions such as melancholy and depression caused by sickness and poverty, and the conception of their connection with physical sickness as narrated by, or rather on behalf of, the shamefaced poor in late eighteenth-century Copenhagen.[2] It will suggest that a lack of economic, social and symbolic capital was the root of widespread grief among the poor of the middle classes, and trace how these mental conditions even made them fall physically ill or (reflecting the work of Georgina Laragy later in the volume) end their miseries by committing suicide.

Understandably, the shamefaced poor – the respectable poor of the middle classes – were subject of considerable attention from their middle-class equals. The main source material for this chapter thus originates from *The Copenhagen Evening Post*, a newspaper which both committed much attention to the shamefaced poor and simultaneously styled itself as the newspaper of the middle classes. In the last decades of the eighteenth century, the newspaper carried a series of articles covering the specific life stories of the shamefaced poor. Its editor, Emanuel Balling, was the author of these articles which according to him were based on what the shamefaced poor told him when he visited them. The purpose of telling their stories was to induce readers to donate money for them. Because of this Emanuel Balling made great effort to persuade the readers that the stories were real. 'As I'm very conscientious, I'm taking care not to mention other than those, whom I know or who reliable people bear testimony to deserve our compassion and support,' he vouched.[3] But Balling did not stop at guarantees. He often referred to the addresses of the shamefaced poor either directly or through a middleman and invited potential benefactors to visit them in order to satisfy themselves of the genuine need of individuals. This and the fact that the shamefaced poor of Balling's articles in many cases can be traced in other sources seems to emphasize the relative credibility of these mediated narratives as representations of voices of the poor in late eighteenth-century

Copenhagen. The loudest voice, however, was at all times that of the philanthropist.

The shamefaced poor and the public poor relief system

Considering the story of the impoverished official one may ask the question: why did he not turn to the public poor relief system? The Copenhagen Poor Relief Authority (Københavns Fattigvæsen) was actually growing in scope and resources as it relieved larger and larger numbers of paupers in the course of the eighteenth century. Moreover, for centuries sickness had been one of those criteria signifying the 'deserving poor'. As early as in the medieval period, Danish poor ordinances and the first national Danish Code of 1683 the old, sick and disabled were distinguished from vagrants and other 'undeserving' elements.[4]

The great Copenhagen Poor Law of 1708 was no exception to this tradition. In other respects, however, the 1708 law was a dramatic reform. Before this date the most prevalent kind of poor relief was to permit 'official begging' for beggars wearing pauper badges. Very few of the poor were offered alms from the public poor relief system and even fewer were offered indoor relief in an almshouse apartment. The privileged group who were given alms or housed in the pre-eighteenth-century almshouses was called *husarme* which is the Danish term for shamefaced poor. They were the poor burghers of the city. In many respects, the new law of 1708 turned this system upside down. All begging was prohibited and poor relief was now considered a 'civil right' for all who had lived in Copenhagen for more than three years.[5] This right also included the common people and the many soldiers in the capital, so that the distinction between official beggars and the shamefaced poor disappeared from the legal framework. From being reserved to a small privileged group of burghers, the poor relief system changed to embracing the majority of the Copenhagen population irrespective of estate. As a consequence of this, it seems that after 1708 the shamefaced poor turned their back on the public poor relief system. As privileged persons of estate they opposed being bracketed together with the mob of common people.

The central characteristic of the eighteenth-century shamefaced poor was that they neither begged nor wanted public poor relief because they were ashamed of their poverty. An announcement in a Copenhagen newspaper dated March 1790 described the shamefaced poor as people, whose 'social position, age and frailty exclude them from public workhouses, and modesty forbids them to beg or to open their heart for anyone'.[6] For this group, poverty was a matter strongly connected to societal standing and stood in contradistinction to the central concern of the poor laws which mainly measured the 'deservingness' of the poor in consideration of age, sickness and so on, and with little or no attention to their former rank. Their position had some basis in the reality of Danish society where a strongly hierarchical order dominated most other contexts outside poor relief in the eighteenth century. Denmark was a typical estate society where the population was grouped in relatively separated estates. In many respects the gentry, middle classes and the common people did not mix with each other and had very few shared values. On the other hand, among those of equal estate there is considerable evidence of common cultural values coalescing around shared conceptions of honour, respectability and reputation which were the foundation stones of so-called 'horizontal honour groups'. For example, shared notions of honour existed within the communities of the artisans, the military and the gentry. The broader group of the middle classes also seems to have shared a number of such common ideas. One's belonging to an estate or honour group implied the ability to meet basic expectations concerning the behaviour and lifestyle of one's estate – including, for instance, clothing consistent with one's position. Failing to live up to these expectations could ultimately result in the forfeiture of one's estate honour and sinking into a lower honour group in the vertical system of hierarchical estates. Consequently, members of the estates above the common people made strenuous effort to avoid being identified with the lower estates while they at the same time imitated the lifestyle of the higher strata.[7]

Thus the problem for the shamefaced poor was that they had a 'too great sense of honour' to apply to the public poor relief for help, as one of the most prominent managers of the Copenhagen Poor Relief Authority, Johan Hendrich Bärens, wrote in 1807.[8] Likewise, the local poor relief commission of Trinitatis parish in Copenhagen in 1778 refused to make a list of the 'bashful poor' of the parish because one should only record those who 'have no hope of saving their honour as burghers and their respectable living'.[9] A piece in a 1784 edition of *The Copenhagen Evening Post* explained the discrepancy between the shamefaced poor's ambition of keeping up appearance, their sense of honour and their actual state of poverty:

> The shamefaced poor who have owned something and been somebody in the world are however the most unfortunate. On the one hand they suffer terrible because they feel their need more than others, and on the other hand their ambition doesn't permit them to uncover their grief, and this always makes their need double. What particularly surprises me is that they rather suffer hardships than show their poverty. Yes, you see, it's because of their inborn ambition, their manners, and their many old friends and acquaintances who live in prosperity, for whom they are ashamed to uncover their condition. One knows how man is; the majority regard honour higher than nature. Many a man goes around with a hungry stomach and with his head as high as the one, who panting gets up from his large meal, opens the street window and with a gorged look proclaims to the low starving souls passing by, that he's a mighty man.[10]

The poverty of the shamefaced poor was in some instances rather social or symbolic than economic – or in other words, relative. They did not inevitably need to starve but suffered in other contexts. Yet in many cases they deliberately chose starvation in favour of using their scanty economic capital on conspicuous consumption, aiming in turn to reinforce their social or symbolic capital.[11] The consequence of losing the latter could easily turn out to be disastrous for one's social position. In an 1840 report for the Copenhagen Poor Relief Authority, the consequences of mixing poor people of different estates was described. The workhouse (*Ladegaarden*) primarily housed vagrants, released prisoners and prostitutes, but at the same time temporarily unemployed artisans and workers were offered voluntary work as a mean of self-help in the same buildings. However, because the *Ladegaarden* housed vagrants and released prisoners it had a very bad reputation and every respectable artisan or worker 'lay oneself open to be unappreciated by his fellow citizens who learn that he has been in a place where crimes and vices are the common characteristics of the workers'.[12]

Against this backdrop, and because the poor laws operated without regard to ideas of honour and respectability, the shamefaced poor were, perceived themselves to be and were perceived by others to be constantly in danger of losing their segregation from the lower estates. For this reason they had to make do with alternative survival strategies such as pawning, loaning and applying for work of all sorts. At the same time several private philanthropic or mutual enterprises – almshouses, loan associations, sick-benefit associations, food charities – were founded especially aiming at this group and especially taking into consideration its need for maintenance of honour and respectability.[13] Emanuel Balling's campaign on behalf of the shamefaced poor was such an honour-preserving alternative to public poor relief. The people behind these enterprises whether their aims were charity or self-help were not mainly interested in the deservingness or undeservingness of the shamefaced poor, but rather in helping them to stay respectable and honourable and prevent their definitive social come-down or stigmatization from which there was no way back to their former social standing. The alternative, as Cathy Smith and Georgina Laragy note elsewhere in this volume, might be the asylum or self-harm.

Relief and compassion for the sick shamefaced poor

That sickness was in many cases the direct cause of poverty was a fact for both the middle classes and the common strata. Most people below the wealthiest circles of society were in danger of facing poverty at some point in life. The Copenhagen merchant Abraham Hviid formulated this omnipresent insecurity when in 1788 he took the initiative of establishing a mutual insurance company called *the Friend of the Citizen (Borgervennen)*:

No one can pride himself on success, before he is in the grave, and everyone
no matter how substantial his occupation, can in old age or unfortunate
circumstances become poor and destitute, and how easily becomes
the beggar's staff and finally The House of Correction [*Børnehuset*] the
reward of the respected and honoured man and his wife.[14]

Yet, apart from being in the large group at risk of becoming impoverished,
people of the middle and common classes differed greatly from each other
both in their experience of poverty, how they coped with it and how they were
relieved. For example, the poor institutions formed a hierarchy equivalent to
that of the society with special institutions for the impoverished gentry, the
honourable but poor middle class, the common people and the lowest levels
of society such as beggars and the insane. The shamefaced poor were by
and large favoured with more plentiful relief than the poor of the common
people. Indeed, several hospitals exclusively offered their services to the sick
poor of the middle classes. Thus, the burghers of the city were first in line for
being treated in Frederik's Hospital founded in 1756.[15] Even in the mental
facility St Hans Hospital, members of respectable families were admitted
to special wards called honourable chambers and honourable bedlams.[16]
Another institution with a similar purpose was Abel Cathrine's Almshouse
(*Abel Cathrines Stiftelse*). It was founded in 1675 and provided 24 sick
and bedridden poor women with separate apartments and 52 rixdollars
annually at their disposal.[17] In the will of the founder and noblewoman
Abel Cathrine van der Wisch it was not specified that the apartments were
reserved for sick women of high birth but much points to the fact that it
simply was implied, and in practice this was the outcome. In 1808, Bärens
of the Copenhagen Poor Relief Authority assumed that the residents of the
almshouse were intended to be 'miserable women who besides being poor
also are tormented by the memory of past happy days' and his inquiry into
the selection process of the residents also revealed:

> That ladies above the class of common people were picked out. Many an
> at one time rich but now needy widow of a burgher, many a widow or
> sister of a deserving official would gladly receive accommodation in this
> almshouse.[18]

The founding of almshouses and other institutions for the middle classes
either was, or at least was considered as, a kind of class-conscious act on
behalf of one's own social strata. In 1859 the almshouse was still characterized
as 'an institution for the sick of the middle classes' in *The Doctor's Weekly*
(*Ugeskrift for Læger*).[19] In a number of years short assessments of recently
admitted residents were published in the journal *Penia*, which was dedicated
to matters of industry, medicine, education and especially the poor relief
system. These are illuminating. For example, the 57-year-old widow of a
deceased drysalter, Gunild Marie Hansen, was described as follows:

She's got a bursting, dizziness, and an incurable injured leg because of which infirmities she's been bedridden. In 1795 and 1807 she was a victim of the fire. These misfortunes have been the cause of her poor economic condition.[20]

In these assessments the main qualifications for admission into the almshouse were elaborated in every single case which gives us a good picture of what characteristics made a person deserving of this particular kind of relief. Thus the typical reasons for the approval of the residents were that they were women, sick (and preferably bedridden), a member of the middle classes and blameless in their own misery.

Another initiative to the solace of the sick people of the middle classes was the Sick-Benefit Association (*Sygekassen*), founded in 1765 by the prominent philanthropist and owner of several Copenhagen newpapers Hans Holck. In connection with the launching of a 1777 appeal, Holck painted the following picture of the sick shamefaced poor who were supported by the Association. It is worth quoting at length:

Old shamefaced poor men and women of the middle classes, whose strength doesn't permit them to work anymore, and who suffer so much more, because of their age are stunted by much sickness and grief. Widows in the same circumstances and age, who neither have friend nor kin, no attention, no care by the family, who usually satisfy their hunger with a sea-biscuit and a drop of small-beer, and sleep in a ragged bed, wet, cold, sick, and hungry, and wake up on their beds with sickness, need, and grief. Cripples, maimed, and blind, who either are born with it or became it by accident and by this became unfit to the trade of life and so to obtain their penurious livelihood; and those, who are troubled with the unhappy apoplexy, cancer, horrible excrescences, and other awful cases, which restrain them from being with other people and bind them to both miserable and hidden dwellings. Miserable shamefaced poor, who because of permanent sickness are bedridden, where they often lack the simplest care, feel pain and torment, and no other comfort than death.[21]

The initiative marks the opening of a veritable campaign of appeals and articles in favour of the shamefaced poor published over the next 15 years in *The Copenhagen Evening Post* and other media owned by Holck. This is not to say that the shamefaced poor were the only group of poor people supported by Hans Holck and his close staff member, the reporter and editor of *The Copenhagen Evening Post*, Emanuel Balling. Rather, the considerable positive attention they devoted to the situation of the shamefaced poor by publishing numerous heartbreaking descriptions of their miserable lives between the late 1770s and the beginning of the 1790s points to Holck's and Balling's special devotion to the cause of this particular group. The shamefaced poor had their backgrounds in the same middle class which

Holck and Balling themselves were part of. They empathized with what poverty felt like for the shamefaced poor. They felt compassion and this drove their profound commitment to bringing, with considerable care and empathy, the stories of the shamefaced poor to the Copenhagen middle classes.[22] In turn, these newspaper men wanted their fellow citizens to feel the same kind of empathy and compassion, a compassion which should bring the people of the middle classes to recognize that the shamefaced poor were their equals and in particular needed and deserved financial help. In fact the Copenhagen middle class *was* touched by the emotional stories of the shamefaced poor and the needy families and widows depicted by Holck and Balling received numerous alms in much greater amounts than the ordinary poor or beggars could expect. These alms were specifically directed towards the shamefaced poor. For example, a benefactor in 1778 donated money directly for 'the needy that both bashfulness and other circumstances hold back from asking for help'.[23]

Grief and sickness

The situation of the Copenhagen shamefaced poor was, as we have seen, depicted in emotional terms in order to awake the compassion of their equals in the middle classes. But the shamefaced themselves were also described as particularly emotional and sensitive people. This of course had to do with their shame. In the 1761 edition of the influential Danish journal *The Patriotic Spectator* (*Den Patriotiske Tilskuer*; an imitation of the well-known British journal *The Spectator*), the Danish author and professor of political science J. S. Sneedorff characterized the shamefaced poor:

> The most pitiful of all poor are those who cannot earn their bread in a profession according to their estate. For them, poverty is not only a burden but also a shame. They feel it much more than others because they are used to better circumstances and have finer feelings. These, who we call shamefaced poor have not learned to dig and are ashamed to beg. They would rather suffer the extreme hardship than expose their circumstances for the vain world.[24]

It was often stressed that poverty was worse for those who had previously lived in wealth than for those who had never known it, something expressed eloquently in the frequently quoted Danish proverb: 'Those never wept for gold, who never owned gold.' Thus, in 1786 Emanuel Balling told the readers of *The Copenhagen Evening Post* the story of a widow of high birth, describing her emotional downfall with great empathy:

> Bashfulness hardly allowed this woman to get up from her chair, for she was quite a picture of misery and a repressed soul. About 16 years ago,

this poor mother was a respected young lady in Copenhagen, of good birth and raised to a happy life. What may she feel at this contrast! Those never wept for gold, who never owned gold, but she! Could she have foreseen, would any of her flattering friends have foreseen that she would tempt Providence like that, to be tested on so miserable, and far below poverty awful conditions? This proves how little security a dazzling happiness in adolescence gives us: It proves that nor property, nor high birth deprives us from the persecutions of fate.[25]

The shamefaced poor were depicted as people with 'finer feelings' than common people. Their experience of poverty was not only in the form of economic collapse, it was also an emotional come-down. Due to their upbringing and habits, they were more delicate, and poverty was worse because they knew what it was like to live in prosperity. The common people were more suited for poverty. They were used to a life in poverty and familiar with starvation, they were unfeeling and thus better prepared to tolerate and cope with destitution. Common people by definition were not as sensible as the higher estates. These themes have close resonance with the way that paupers were represented in newspapers at times of crisis, as Beate Althammer suggests in her contribution to this volume.

The narratives of the shamefaced poor in many cases tell the story of emotional responses to the experience of being impoverished. This experience is often portrayed as outright depression, a familiar theme from the chapters by Georgina Laragy and Alannah Tomkins. In a poem dated 1778, Hans Holck gave an evocative description of how the deeply concerned shamefaced poor walked up and down the floor wringing their hands.[26] The most frequently described feelings were the sorrows and grief that struck the shamefaced poor. Poverty and the ensuing grief were outlined as physically disruptive. In two other poems Holck depicted the shamefaced poor as trapped in 'prisons of shortage' where life was destroyed, almost obliterated. He wrote:

> Shamefaced poor are in the prisons of shortage / Here grief, sorrow and many kinds of troubles/Are ruining their lives while they sigh . . . Free from worry? Alas! Only at night/By sorrows and grief they almost will die.[27]

Several narratives of the shamefaced poor in *The Copenhagen Evening Post* picture how shame and grief for lost wealth bred both psychological and physical sickness. Shame, grief and sickness went hand in hand and with this often further impoverishment. In the winter of 1786 the family of a Copenhagen cooper master was afflicted by:

> An unrelenting illness, which has attacked both husband, wife, and their four children. The illness still persists and has cast them under the yoke of poverty. The husband can no longer do his job and the wife's health is

corroded by grief and shortcomings. One misery goes hand in hand with the other and the sad prospects.[28]

The story shows how a family in consequence of 'a unrelenting illness' was thrown into a vicious circle of poverty, grief, further sickness and further poverty. The one misery caused the next to happen. Sickness, poverty and grief were dealt with as one another's followers. A similar case was of the distinguished widow Karen Farenhorst, who once had been the lady of an estate. She witnessed her husband's downfall from being a landowner to a lower civil servant. By his death her fate as one of the shamefaced poor was sealed. In 1783 Balling told her sad life story to his readers:

> This woman once smiled under more fortunate circumstances. There was a time when her husband owned both farms and estate. Back then, she was charitable towards others. Back then she couldn't have imagined that she would end up in a miserable attic, as a widow with two children and with a sickly body, which is the result of the grief of being unable to earn one's own bread. I suppose she feels her need double![29]

Not only did sickness and the ensuing poverty generate grief and depression, often it was the grief of the shamefaced poor that created susceptibility to disease. Thus the father of an impoverished Copenhagen middle-class family 'by grief was thrown to the sickbed; seeing himself too weak to work for him and his family, seeing the wife bowed down with sorrow and cumber about the miserable condition of her house'.[30]

Of course, grief and its disease-inducing effects were not exclusively associated with the shamefaced poor's reactions to poverty. In early modern Europe the phenomenon was widely known. People literally fell ill from grief and grieved themselves to death. An instance of the more fatal effects of grief was that of the farmer Lars Andersen Møller. His son was in 1732 crushed under a sheep pen while Møller was thatching the roof. Møller took this dreadful accident greatly to heart and ended in grieving himself to death.[31] The memories of the Danish writer Charlotta Dorothea Biehl are also instructive. In the 1750s Biehl was in her early twenties and as a daughter of the Copenhagen bourgeois she was 'in play' on the marriage market. Many a young gentleman courted Biehl but her parents had to approve for a good match and make sure that she neither married poor nor below her estate. The pressure of the suitors and the parents was in the long-run too nerve-racking for the young frail Biehl:

> I ate my supper in tears; I left the bed with fear, and lay down with grief ... After having lead this life for somewhat more than a year I was taken very sick, but even though Wolert [the family pshysician] said: that the reason for my sickness was grief, my life and health wasn't spared for long, and I'd hardly left the bed before the chase began again.[32]

The physicians and philosophers of early modern Europe certainly supported the notion of a strong relationship between grief and sickness. It was common knowledge that passions were materialized in matter and physicians routinely treated grief and its physical after-effects.[33] Both the human body and the human emotions were experienced as one concerted flow and the consequence of an imbalance in these flows of bodily fluids and emotions was mental or physical illness: 'Being a social creature meant having feelings, such as grief and sorrow, that could easily become unbalanced and therefore place humans in physical danger'.[34] Accordingly both physical means such as medicine and food, and psychological means such as the comfort of fellow humans, could serve as cure and relief for body and mind. In his essay on friendship, Francis Bacon emphasized the importance of the unburdening of one's worried heart to a trusted friend: 'Because feelings swelled the heart and such swellings, if not relieved, were physically and mentally perilous, openness to exchange was a precondition of human life. As a consequence, a lonely person could neither experience true pleasure nor cope with grief.'[35] In this context it is intriguing that the narratives of the grieving shamefaced poor often depicted them as friendless or isolated people who typically kept themselves to themselves in shame of their poverty and lacking ability to live in accordance with their position in society. Thus the accounts on the shamefaced poor sought to call attention to the existence of a hidden and publicly unknown kind of poverty – or the secrets of the goddess of poverty Penia as Bärens called the shamefaced poor in 1809.[36] For editor Balling this was one of the central motives for publishing their stories:

> You cannot overplead the cause of those, who have no opportunity to speak for themselves; not too much use the tone of lament for the many, who remote from the ears of the happy world groan for the strictly necessary in miserable dwellings.[37]

In the same breath, Balling did not hesitate to recount the story of Johanne Eggert, the poor widow of a journeyman barber-surgeon, who in the summer of 1783 looked up Balling asking for his help. Subsequently he published what she told him:

> I've hesitated to beg and strived to live by the work of my hands as long as possible; that's why I'm unknown. I've for long bemoaned my poverty, but in secrecy. Now it's getting too hard for me – At this point she shed a tear and I was moved. Among the needy, I thought, are however the fate of those who suffer in secrecy the most pitiful, especially when they are strangers to the beneficent of the world.[38]

Sickness, depression and isolation in some cases made the poor resort to extreme measures, as Georgina Laragy has begun to show us elsewhere in this volume. Suicide, and its frequent cause, melancholy, were, like grief, yoked together in the relation between body and mind. Bärens, writing an 1806 account of how to prevent the poor committing suicide, suggested that 'Melancholy which originates in the body is often the cause of suicide. Maybe fewer suicides would take place if the body was healthy, if it was strengthened and inured to withstand sickness earlier.'[39] In the case of the shamefaced poor, however, it was not only the lack of basic necessities which created melancholy and potential suicide, but also 'the sad outlook of being unable to maintain one's former lifestyle and vocation'.[40] Bärens pointed out two methods for preventing suicide among the shamefaced poor. The one was a no-nonsense approach aiming at procuring work, advance payments, tools and sales – in other words, helping them to help themselves. The other method brings us back to Francis Bacon's thoughts on the unburdening of worried hearts. Accordingly Bärens suggested that the patrons should be aiming at gaining the confidence and respect of the shamefaced poor and in that way prevent suicides:

> He should patiently listen to the poor and, when they deserve it, address them with mildness and kindness . . . He encourages and comforts them when they appear to be sad or depressed . . . Then the mournful will not abandon him and the world in despair.[41]

Conclusion: Sickness and emotions as a social marker

The shamefaced poor were characterized by their emotions and sensibility – not only towards the shame but also a variety of other emotions and sicknesses such as grief and melancholy. And they were presented to the broader public as such emotional beings by some of the leading Copenhagen philanthropists. The behaviour of the shamefaced poor was generally approved of by their equals in the Copenhagen middle classes, itself partly a reflection of the often demonstratively sentimental behaviour which dominated the European literature and middle-class culture in the second half of the eighteenth century.[42] They formed what Barbara Rosenwein defines as an emotional community, one which was keen to dissociate from the poor of the common strata and to yoke firmly to the middle classes on which they maintained a de facto claim.[43] This was important in a strongly hierarchical estate society like that of eighteenth-century Denmark. Thus emotional behaviour such as grieving could be used in order to demonstrate the estate connection and social identity of the shamefaced poor. This occurred in correlation with the surrounding society. While beggars and other categories of undesirable poor were confronted by the relief administrators of the upper and middle classes, the sensible shamefaced poor were met with compassion by their equals.

In turn, there is every indication that the shamefaced poor and their sponsors and publicists were inscribed into the emotional community now known as the cult of sensibility, and that both groups used the same emotional vocabulary in order to show their position in the social strata. In all probability, emotional language, codes and behaviours were used consciously or even strategically by the poor in order to demonstrate their social background and to be perceived positively by philanthropists. Yet, the behaviour of the shamefaced poor was hardly sheer strategy and playing to the gallery. Their strong emotional reactions to the experience of social and symbolic poverty were undoubtedly real. And the coincidence between psychologists' description of the emotions of the poor in modern Europe and the emotions in the narratives of the eighteenth-century Copenhagen poor is considerable. Thus, in his 2005 account of *The psychology of poverty. The experience of poverty in modern Norway (Fattigdommens psykologi. Oppleving av fattigdom i det moderne Noreg)*, the Norwegian professor of psychology Kjell Underlid has shown how the long-term unemployed on low social security benefits in the Norwegian welfare state are pinioned by their relative poverty. Emotions such as anxiety, depression, shame and guilt quickly come to be associated with poverty, as do physical and mental sickness.[44] Of course, psychological evaluations of people from the past should only be undertaken with much care: 'Although there are family resemblances between melancholy and what we now term depression, there are also . . . significant discontinuities.'[45] The question would normally be: How could we possibly say anything certain about the psychological emotions of the long dead? On the other hand, newspaper reporting of the attitudes of the shamefaced poor provides compelling evidence that sickness, depression and grief were, in the eighteenth century as now, a direct function of the self-isolation and the pressure of keeping up appearances among those for whom slipping down the social and economic scale, rather than absolute destitution, was the spectre most feared. This theme, as we have seen in chapters elsewhere in this volume, was a core concern for the marginal poor across Europe and across the period from the eighteenth to early twentieth centuries.

Notes

1 In the following chapter, the term middle class/es should be understood in its broader sense: The diverse group which included everybody from artisans to merchants, officials, vicars, officers and their families. In spite of many differences and distinctions between these subgroups they to a certain extent shared views on honour and respectability and not least their superiority to the common people of peasants, day-labourers, soldiers, etc.

2 On shamefaced poor, see Cavallo, S. (1995), *Charity and Power in Early Modern Italy: Benefactors and Their Motives in Turin, 1541–1789*. Cambridge and New York: Cambridge University Press; Trexler, R. C. (1973), 'Charity and the defense of urban elites in the Italian communes', in Jaher, F. C. (ed.), *The Rich, the Well-Born, and the Powerfull: Elites and Upper Classes in History*. New York: Urbana; Ricci, G. (1983), 'Naissance du pauvre honteux. Entre l'histoire des idées et l'histoire sociale', *Annales E.S.C.*, 38, 158–77.

3 *Copenhagen Evening Post*, 24 January 1783.

4 For general accounts of early modern (i.e. 1500–1850) Danish poor relief, see Henningsen, P. (2008), 'Copenhagen poor relief and the problem of poverty, ca. 1500–1800', in Christensen, S. B. and Mikkelsen, J. (eds), *Danish Towns during Absolutism. Urbanisation and Urban Life 1660–1848*. Aarhus: Aarhus University Press, pp. 325–63; Mikkelsen, J. (2008), 'Poor relief in provincial towns in the Kingdom of Denmark and the Duchy of Schleswig, ca. 1700–1850', in Christensen and Mikkelsen, *Danish Towns*, pp. 365–410; Bonderup, G. (2002), 'Health care provision and poor relief in enlightenment and 19th century Denmark', in Grell, O. P., Cunningham, A. and Jütte, R. (eds), *Health Care and Poor Relief in 18th and 19th Century Northern Europe*. Aldershot: Ashgate, pp. 172–88; Vallgårda, S. (1999), 'Who went to a general hospital in the eighteenth and nineteenth centuries in Copenhagen?', *European Journal of Public Health*, 9, 97–102; Vallgårda, S. (1988), 'Hospitals and the Poor in Denmark, 1750–1880, *Scandinavian Journal of History*, 13, 95–105; Løkke, A. (2008), 'Medical law, poor law, health insurance. The long run trends in Danish Health Policy 1672–1973', in Abreu, L. and Bourdelais, P. (eds), *The Price of Life. Welfare Systems, Social Nets and Economic Growth*. Lisboa: Edições Colibri, pp. 285–302.

5 'Forordning om Forhold med Betlere, fattige Børn, rette Almisse-Lemmer og Løsgængere i Kiøbenhavn, saa og om Almisse til deres Underholdning samt Forordning om Betlerne i Dannemark saavel paa Landet, som i Kiøbstæderne, Kiøbenhavn undtagen af 24. september 1708' (1777), in Schou, J. H. (ed.), *Chronologisk Register over de Kongelige Forordninger og Aabne Breve, vol. 2 (1699–1730)*, Copenhagen: Jacob Henric Schou, pp. 157–73.

6 *Copenhagen Directory (Kiøbenhavns Kongelig alene privilegerede Adresse-Contoirs Efterretninger)*, 5 March 1790, p. 51.

7 Henningsen, P. (2006), *I sansernes vold. Bondekultur og kultursammenstød i Enevældens Danmark, vol. 1*. Copenhagen: Landbohistorisk Selskab and Københavns Stadsarkiv, pp. 366–97; Pitt-Rivers, J. (1972), 'Honor', in Sills, D. L. (ed.), *International Encyclopedia of the Social Sciences, vols 5–6*, New York: Macmillian & The Free Press, pp. 503–11; Stewart, F. H. (1994), *Honor*. Chicago: The University of Chicago Press, pp. 54–63.

8 Bärens, J. H. (1807), 'Blandede Efterretninger'. *Penia eller Blade for Skole-Industrie- Medicinal- og Fattigvæsen*, 2, p. 368.

9 Danish National Archives, Danske Kancelli, Kommissionen ang. fattigvæsenet i København 1778–79, F74D, Poor Relief Authority of Trinitatis Parish (1778), *Letter from the Poor Relief Authority of Trinitatis Parish to the commission dated 31 August 1778*.

10 *Copenhagen Evening Post*, 17 May 1784.

11 Bourdieu, P. (1986), 'The Forms of Capital', in Richardson, J. G. (ed.), *Handbook of Theory and Research for the Sociology of Education*. Westport: Greenwood

Press, pp. 241–58; Leeuwen, M. H. D. v. (1994), 'Logic of charity: poor relief in preindustrial Europe', *Journal of Interdisciplinary History*, 24, pp. 596–606; Dinges, M. (2004), 'A history of poverty and poor relief: contributions from research on the early modern period and the late middle ages and examples from more recent history', in Abreu, L. (ed.), *European Health and Social Welfare Policies*. Brno: Compostela Group of Universities, pp. 27–35.

12 Sager, H., Duntzfeldt, W. and Meinert, N. (1840), *Beretning om det kjøbenhavnske Fattigvæsens Stiftelser*. Copenhagen: Schultz, pp. 32–3.

13 Leeuwen, M. H. D. v. (2002), 'Histories of risk and welfare in Europe during the 18th and 19th centuries', in Grell, Cunningham and Jütte, *Health Care and Poor Relief*, pp. 33–40; Dinges, 'A history of poverty and poor relief', pp. 27–34.

14 *Copenhagen Directory*, 13 May 1788.

15 *Fundatz for det i Kjøbenhavn af hans kongel. majestæt allernaadigst oprettende Friderichs Hospital (1756)*. Copenhagen: J.J. Høpffner, section 3; Løkke, A. (2007), Patienternes Rigshospital 1757–2007. Copenhagen: Gad.

16 Zalewski, B. (2008), 'St. Hans Hospital i København 1612–1808', in Kragh, J. V., *Psykiatriens historie i Danmark*. Copenhagen: Hans Reitzel, p. 41.

17 Bergsøe, A. F. (1853), *Den danske Stats Statistik, vol. 4*. Copenhagen: Bianco Luno, p. 222; Hofman, H. (1765), *Samlinger af Publique og Private Stiftelser, Fundationer og Gavebreve, vol. 10*. Copenhagen: Ludolph Henrich Lillies Enke, pp. 368–70.

18 Bärens, J. H. (1808a), 'Hvad udfordres for at kunne komme paa Valg til Abel Katrines Hospital?', Penia eller Blade for Skole- Industrie- Medicinal- og Fattigvæsen, 3, p. 166.

19 'Planen for Sygehjemmet' (1859), *Ugeskrift for Læger*, 14 May 1859, p. 369.

20 Bärens, J. H. (1808b), 'Blandede Efterretninger', *Penia eller Blade for Skole-Industrie- Medicinal- og Fattigvæsen*, 3, p. 160.

21 *Copenhagen Evening Post*, 21 February 1777.

22 On the Danish patriotic and philanthropic movement of the late eighteenth century and Emanuel Balling's role in this, see Engelhardt, J. (2010), *Borgerskab og fællesskab. Patriotiske selskaber i den danske helstat 1769–1814*. Copenhagen: Museum Tusculanum.

23 *Copenhagen Evening Post*, 27 February 1778.

24 Sneedorff, J. S. (1776), *Sneedorffs samtlige Skrivter, vol. 2*. Copenhagen: Gyldendal, pp. 27–8.

25 *Copenhagen Evening Post*, 10 March 1786.

26 *Copenhagen Evening Post*, 12 October and 2 November 1778.

27 *Copenhagen Evening Post*, 7 February and 28 March 1777.

28 *Copenhagen Evening Post*, 5 May 1786.

29 *Copenhagen Evening Post*, 19 December 1783.

30 *Copenhagen Evening Post*, 26 February 1790.

31 Nielsen, O. (1867–68), 'Historiske Efterretninger om Slavs Herred (Ribe Amt)', in Bruun, C., Nielsen, O. and Petersen, A. (eds), *Danske Samlinger for Historie, Topografi, Personal- og Litteraturhistorie, vol. 3*. Copenhagen: Gyldendal, p. 317.

32 Biehl, C. D. (1999), *Mit ubetydelige Levnets Løb*. Copenhagen: Museum Tusculanum, pp. 89–90.

33 Pender, S. (2010), 'Rhetoric, grief, and the imagination in early modern England', *Philosophy and Rhetoric*, 43, 54–7.

34 Rublack, U. (2002), 'Fluxes: the early modern body and the emotions', *History Workshop Journal*, 53, 2.

35 Ibid., p. 3.

36 Bärens, J. H. (1809), 'No. 1', *Penia eller Blade for Skole- Industrie- Medicinal- og Fattigvæsen*, 4, pp. 5–6.

37 *Copenhagen Evening Post*, 20 June 1783.

38 Ibid.

39 Bärens, J. H. (1806), 'Hvad kan, og hvad bør et Steds Fattigvæsen gjøre for at indskrænke Selvmord?', *Penia eller Blade for Skole- Industrie- Medicinal- og Fattigvæsen*, 1, p. 327.

40 Ibid., p. 329.

41 Ibid., pp. 331–2.

42 See, for instance, Todd, J. (1986), *Sensibility. An Introduction*. London: Methuen.

43 'Social groups whose members adhere to the same valuations of emotions and their expression'; Rosenwein, B. H. (2010), 'Problems and methods in the history of emotions', *Passions in Context: Journal of the History and Philosophy of the Emotions*, 1, 1.

44 Underlid, K. (2005), *Fattigdommens psykologi. Oppleving av fattigdom i det moderne Noreg*. Oslo: Det Norske Samlaget.

45 Gowland, A. (2006), 'The Problem of Early Modern Melancholy', *Past & Present*, 191, 80–1.

3

'Labouring on a bed of sickness': The material and rhetorical deployment of ill-health in male pauper letters

Alannah Tomkins

Introduction

Up to the end of the nineteenth century, to quote Grell and Cunningham, 'health care for the poor was inextricably linked with poor relief', and neither they, nor contributors to their volume, really attempt to distinguish or draw a firm line between the two.[1] Nonetheless, historians of health care and poor relief have adopted different positions on the extent to which the two should be regarded as perpetually and unavoidably interrelated, overlapping but not entirely contiguous, or indeed as separate. How far is all poor relief essentially a medical intervention? Certainly in 1991 Mary Fissell did not see any point in separating the two. She was inclined to bracket parish poor relief with the facilities offered by the Bristol infirmary and concluded that the type of assistance sought or dispensed could be predicted by local kinship connectedness. People with family and longevity in the local area went to the parish while incomers or people lacking blood relations went to the infirmary, the implication being that the two avenues of assistance were sufficiently alike to be regarded as meaningful or broadly equivalent alternatives.[2] The poor are always more or less ill, or at least their physical well-being is continually jeopardized by the material privations of poverty, and so welfare ostensibly offered to 'the poor' or 'the sick' comprises such an overlap of experiences and responsibilities that distinctions are at best difficult or at worst futile. Conversely, I, along with Steve King and others, clearly feel that there is much to be learned from trying to distinguish the sick from the total pool of 'the poor' and to examine the provisions of identifiably medical relief.

As historians of the sick poor and their health care options, we have tended to concentrate on the ways in which sickness renders people poor. This is a *relatively* simple concept. Removal from work often prompts a decline in earnings and the burdens of treatment or recuperation entail an increase in costs. Although this sort of explanation might have been contested by contemporary commentators, who preferred to view poverty as a personal failing, these are the sorts of familiar trajectories that are played out in the records of welfare authorities like the English parish or the general infirmary, and are emphasized wherever the individuals concerned leave their own account. They are so familiar that these are the sorts of deprivation that modern governments attempt to combat via basic measures of public provision (such as a health-care service that is entirely or partly free of charge) and that private companies attempt to prevent via personal insurance.

An alternative strand in public-health thinking today concentrates not on how sickness makes you poor but instead on how poverty makes you sick: a concept best summed up by the modern phrase 'health inequalities'. This is not *at all* simple, but instead a very complex interrelationship between housing, diet, lifestyle, culture, education and other factors. Modern interest in health inequalities arises from the political tension between the demand for reliable health care versus its high cost to government and tax-payers. It seems unlikely that historians of any era earlier than the mid-twentieth century will be able to investigate such 'health inequalities' retrospectively in anything other than a fairly broad fashion. Our sources are not calibrated so finely that we can realistically look in detail at the complexity of how poverty made people ill in past times. It is possible, though, in addition to looking at the medical and material needs of the poor, to be attentive to any suggestions of attitudes to illness, both on the parts of the sufferers and their medical practitioners, nurses, charity caseworkers or relieving officers. These are of course notoriously difficult to distinguish, but rare statements of opinion or expression of states of mind should be teamed with considerations about stereotypical expectations for behaviour during illness (from medical personnel but more importantly from kin, friends, neighbours and workmates) and the consequences of living up to (or falling short of) these prescriptions. In what ways was poverty thought to jeopardize people's health?

This is connected to questions about what constituted 'socially appropriate illness behaviour' among the nineteenth-century poor and how that behaviour was modulated by the consequential need to ask for assistance.[3] The medical component of parish poor relief under the Old Poor Law has taken some time to surface as a discrete topic, but recently Steve King has looked in detail at the pathways to relief afforded by sickness and ill-health.[4] I have also looked at medical relief in as much as institutions like workhouses and infirmaries catered for overlapping or separate cohorts of the urban poor, and have considered relief in relation to gender and kinship connectedness.[5] This chapter will look again at gender, but with a rather different emphasis. It will be arguing that, just as gender had a perceptible impact on notions of entitlement among the sick poor (from the perspective of dispensers of welfare), so gender made a fundamental difference to the way illness was experienced and to the positions adopted by the needy and supplicating poor.

In the last ten years the potential of pauper letters to provide direct if problematic insight into the experiences of poverty has been recognized and is now being exploited. Letters can be harvested for histories of the aged poor, the sick poor or other cohorts of the population or aspects of life. Therefore this chapter will explore some of the intersections between ill-health, masculinity, fluency and anger in illustrative case studies drawn mainly from collections of pauper letters in Staffordshire.[6] In so doing it will briefly consider the impact of illness as physical disease or injury, the most usual aspects of ill-health explicitly drawn to the attention of authorities, and at more length the less well-considered issue of mental disturbance (what we would now regard as depression, rather than insanity) and the role of poverty in exacerbating this sort of condition. Contemporary ideologies of working-class masculinity meant that the 'piling up' of both public and domestic consequences of illness prompted responses along a continuum from abject servility via semi-objective representation through to blistering anger. Accounts of men's ill-health, whether of bodily incapacity or mental affliction, could be deployed as a vigorous component of requests for relief and could also give rhetorical justification to outbursts of rage. This is not to say that female writers did not get angry when they were sick; rather I am going to suggest that anger was the last refuge of masculinity for poor sick and depressed men.

Men and ill-health

The gendered roles of the labouring or working-class household economy made a forceful impact on the gendered experiences of ill-health. Male earnings were designedly higher than those of women in the early modern period, and in the early nineteenth century working-class masculinity resided in a combination of skilled employment and family headship.[7] It has been argued that the concept of the male-breadwinner emerged as a 'proletarian ideal' (even if practical experiences were of necessity different).[8] At all times there was apparently an assumption that adult women were responsible for household marketing and budgeting. In this way, the impact of disease on adult men and women was equally devastating but rather different in its character. Reduced or lost male earnings meant the exercise of endless ingenuity and nerve by wives in garnering alternative resources and deploying them wisely. In contrast the loss of female activity in buying or managing necessities could plunge a family into an even worse plight, when men discovered that money alone could not compensate for an absence of canny household management.

As men and women became channelled more firmly into their respective roles (coincidentally over the period when pauper letters are at their most numerous, 1780–1840) a bout of sickness drove an experiential wedge (if not an emotional one[9]) between a married couple; women were perhaps supremely themselves when capable of exercising their utmost creativity in keeping a household afloat, while sick men had been deprived of the chief claim to adult masculinity; sick women were on the face of it little different to well women (both were largely/ideally confined to the home, and they did not lose status through illness, incapacity or dependency; this was merely an exacerbation of the norm), but men learned the hard way that a multitude of domestic tasks had a commercial value that could not be met from the average labouring wage (if indeed they could continue earning and did not need to nurse their wife or care for their children). In the words of one Shropshire widower, writing plaintively in the early nineteenth century, 'I never new the los of a wife Before and I did not think it had been so great for I Can have Nothing don But Wat I most pay throw the nowes for.'[10] This essentially echoes findings about the relative experiences of ageing for men and women. If old age came earlier in the life-cycle for women than for men, it may also be 'that women were actually better equipped than many men to adapt to the challenges of old age' and that women (whether ill or aging) experienced more continuity with previous lives than did men.[11] Shepherd has summarized that 'those blighted by incapacity, particularly if they could no longer support themselves, saw their status as men eclipsed as the negative aspects of ageing became the primary determinants of their identity'. For ageing, one could just as easily read illness.[12] Also the positive attributes of age when applied to manliness in the early modern period, reliance on a long memory for deployment in disputes over property rights or boundary disputes, was no longer part of the customary landscape of most elderly men in the early nineteenth century.[13]

This disparity between the economic impact of sickness for poor men and that for women had its corollary in experiences of bidding for welfare. Poor women who approached parish authorities for help (either because they or their breadwinner was ill) could invoke public discourses about women's role in defending the home to frame their case. Linda Colley argues that in the early nineteenth century British women increasingly made a 'calculated deployment of separate spheres rhetoric . . . to protect their rights such as they were' and this had implications for poor women as well as more prosperous ones. If women were supposed not to intrude on public life, but were compelled to do so by the need to defend their domestic realm, their actions were both legitimized and powerful because they shamed the individual or collective 'men' upon whom they had hoped to depend.[14] The female responsibility for home, childbearing and domesticity could be turned to their advantage, and the addition of ill-health to this potent mix could prove decisive.

Men who asked for relief in illness, particularly when the illness was their own, faced a problem. Even male acknowledgement of illness was problematic given determinants of masculinity that emphasized strength, muscularity, fortitude and reticence in the face of injury.[15] Declining levels of violence in the later eighteenth century have been well documented and associated with changing modes of masculinity that required greater civility and permitted a measure of sensitivity and even emotional outburst.[16] These changes have been associated with the decline of aristocratic and the rise of bourgeois masculinity but it is not clear whether yielding to sickness was an acceptable facet of this sensibility. Furthermore, it seems likely that working men did not enjoy meaningful access to a tradition of romantic sensibility and introspection, where self-examination did not entail effeminacy. The best opportunity for endorsement of emotional reaction was via the evangelical movement; the struggle to recognize personal imperfections and overcome them, self-examination as criticism and (hopefully) improvement. Evangelicalism tended to prize self-restraint but could endorse strong expressions of feeling, particularly when motivated by religious zeal. Yet it may be significant to note that stoicism has remained an element in stereotypical masculinity.[17]

At the same time, admission of illness, and particularly absence from routine employment, ran counter to contemporary men's primary means of asserting their identity (through work). Working-class masculinity has traditionally been delineated in terms of assertions of individual or collective power and identity in the workplace.[18] In institutional settings manliness was defined partly through ritual that entailed the disparagement or derision of female traits or behaviour (e.g., workplace initiation). Defence of specific jobs and broader trades were also important, giving rise to studies of working-class masculinity which essentially treat the rise and significance of trade-union activism.[19] Central to this chapter, the sick man was deprived of identifications with work (possibly temporarily, but the lurking fear must have been of a permanent exclusion from work, either through sickness alone or arising from subsequent unemployment). The loss of physical power conspired to cut away aspirations to breadwinning or even solvency. In doing so, illness arguably reduced men to a state of imitative femininity, dependency on others for material support and for domestic care. If masculinity is never objectively achieved but must be constantly reasserted, then physical exclusion from the arena where it might be proved levelled a damaging blow to the endeavour. In the early seventeenth century, Shepherd has questioned whether the man who lacked wages but lived on a charity pension 'retained much of a claim to patriarchal manhood' and this emasculation of the dependent man had a long history.[20] The need to supplicate for relief made the acquisition of feminine attributes in communication with others almost a requirement. A final turn of the screw in the early nineteenth century rendered any previous collective activity (such as trade-union activism, or evidence of political radicalism) prior to the need for welfare as threatening to the relieving authorities.

In 1991 it was argued that 'the wielding of authority over dependants in the home proved a foundation for men's public prominence' but for the poor man it was his only outlet.[21] Male dominance for the poor boiled down to responsibility for (and control over) immediate family; there was no other sphere in which it might operate. As a facet of this issue, one of the long-standing indicators of male worth was householder status,[22] so the jeopardy or break-up of the family home would be devastating, and this may always have seemed a risk after the widespread introduction of workhouses in the 1720s.[23] Additionally, for any man aware of Malthusian strictures, the rights of fatherhood would have appeared as under threat; resentment against Malthus's perceived arguments was widespread. Charles Shaw resentfully recalled 'We were a part of Malthus's "superfluous population".'[24] In short, by the early nineteenth century, the masculinity of poor men, always at risk of being undermined, became very shaky indeed. The development of Victorian masculinity, which had a strong domestic component, may have been of marginal assistance to the poor man, but the ideal of 'dutiful husbands and attentive fathers' sat more comfortably with the middle class who could choose to devote themselves to the family fireside, than it did with the impoverished unemployed and sick man who was effectively chained there.[25]

Having said this, ill-health was a vital way for adult men to justify their neediness and for this reason it features prominently in male pauper letters. However, the discussion thus far has aimed to point up the conflict inherent in men's reflections on their own illness. A pauper letter was a semi-public discussion of health and illness and for men was tantamount to an evaluation of their own claim to manhood. To admit illness or incapacity but still maintain a convincing claim was to walk a fine line indeed.

Male pauper letters

To paraphrase Linda Colley, pauper letters must be read both textually and contextually,[26] and thus the rest of this chapter will be devoted to a consideration of individuals whose writing illustrate both the material and rhetorical deployment of ill-health in male pauper letters. It will start with an example of the abject, halting letter which lacks fluency and is expressive of piteous need, the man who had little if any remaining claim to stereotypical masculinity, and will then move on to other examples that deploy more sophisticated phraseologies and were written either calmly or only with irritation. The final example deals with an author whose wrathful account, the chapter will argue, permits a rare example of psychological distress, illustrative of working-class masculinity under siege from the threat of mental disturbance, which he characterized as substantially caused by poverty.

Of course, interpreting the tone of pauper letters is fraught with difficulty. In particular subtleties of phrasing might now be lost. Thus it is entirely possible to read a resentful growl where a desperate whimper was intended, albeit that emphatic expression of anger may be less open to doubt. Furthermore, writers were not supplying a transparent account of their needs. Deprivation was doubtless a material reality but in all cases there is a tacit, largely unquantifiable gap between depictions by paupers and their lived household circumstances. Therefore what follows is a study of the deployment of accounts of ill-health, no matter how accurate or fictional, against (where possible) evidence of their impact (did they receive the relief they asked for, or were their predictions for their own futures justified?).

Sickness or injury could give rise to some of the most vivid accounts of material deprivation, and could be used to frame a case for abject helplessness. Such a state mimicked 'feminine' powerlessness. Walter Keeling's letters provide an illustration of this point. Keeling was a disabled ex-serviceman who wrote seven letters to his home parish of Colwich in Staffordshire from Hull, his preferred place of residence, between 1784 and 1798. At the time of his first letter he was aged approximately 45. He was explicit about his physical suffering, since he referred to lameness, an eye infection and a hernia, but he also talked in general terms about fevers or bad humours suffered by himself, his wife and son or the generally deplorable condition of the family. In November 1795, for example, he offered in mitigation of his claim for relief 'my Wife hase Been Verrey Badley this maney years Not able to help hir Self and me getting Old and Lame in my Leg and Side Where my Bowels was Lett out'. In the course of his correspondence he cited charges incurred for both doctor's visits and nursing. He did occasionally adopt the standard tactic of the pauper letter, the threat to return home and prove expensive, but not always and not in his case a characteristic of a threatening style, as his tone was apologetic and observational rather than sharp. In 1788 he was considering his family's return without him, emphasizing his own incapacity, when he predicted 'my Fameley will Come by Water the Next month if the wether Permits as I am not able to Come my Self'. Yet at the same time he feared that his temerity might not stand in his favour, since he prefixed this information with, 'Sir I hope you will not be angery with me for Wrighting to you'. Keeling's humility is tangible, and only escapes total self-abasement in his decision to write at all.

One alternative to this rhetoric of helplessness was to frame a request in a tone of a sensible appeal to reason. The contrast of men's letters with those written by their wives points up the very striking similarities which could pertain between male and female writers when the tone of letters is pegged at the level of the ostensibly objective request, but also the different role of illness for one-time breadwinners and their so-called 'dependents'. The correspondence of Philip and Frances James, along with the supporting letters from doctors and parish officers on their behalf, provides a good example. The Jameses wrote 14 letters between 1832 and 1837 (nine authored by Philip and five by Frances) from their home in Leicester to their parish of settlement in Uttoxeter, largely because Philip's 'liver complaint' prevented him from working. Their tone was not uniformly reasonable, and ranges from desperate to plaintive but they both often strived for a note of objectivity by effectively appealing to the reasoning of the Uttoxeter authorities. In June 1834, Philip contended 'Consider for a moment, I have not been able to do but a fortnights work since I left you which was Christmas time', so inviting or instructing the recipients to see the situation from his point of view. Five months later Frances argued on her husband's behalf 'As *you* have seen him and know the circumstances of the case *you* will feel certain that he is yet unable to work.' Furthermore, the Jameses sought and found external (by implication impartial) confirmation from apparently independent sources. Three different surgeons endorsed the letters to confirm that Philip was indeed suffering from a serious illness that rendered him incapable of work. Nonetheless, in the judgement of a local Leicester correspondent, Thomas Pickering (overseer of St Margaret's parish in Leicester), the couple could be assessed quite differently. Pickering wrote that 'the woman is considered deserving and industrious' but he was circumspect about Philip, whom he dealt with dismissively, saying 'the man is no great things'. In this way the Jameses provide the perfect example of a family where male illness strengthens a wife's public persona as someone who copes, while it degrades the status of the man himself.

Deferential language (in the manner of Keeling), or the adoption of apparent man-to-man or indeed woman-to-man objectivity (as with the Jameses), could provide conduits for effective persuasion; the alternative was anger. Anger of different stripes finds periodic expression in pauper letters but was problematic for writers given what it implied about the relationship between the writer and reader. Anger disrupted the expectations of parish officers and vestries. Anger in illness was doubly awkward. Illness was one of the grounds for otherwise able-bodied adults to claim legitimate relief, and therefore one of the types of application for relief inclined to rouse the particular suspicions of overseers who were anxious to weed out malingerers. Yet the wretchedly ill felt more than usually justified in their expression of anger when their glaring needs were not addressed. Thus, anger in strategic writing like the pauper letter might be regarded as a desperate resort.

A more dispassionate reading of anger, though, would characterize it as the occasional appearance of the 'hidden' transcript of the pauper. Here the usually silent discourse of the pauper's-eye view of relationships between parish authorities and their subordinates breaks through into the public domain. Lynn MacKay has argued convincingly that the emergence of the hidden transcript at the Old Bailey explains a spate of convict refusals of the royal pardon.[27] Anger in pauper letters is neither so public nor so tense, since paupers always retained a moral right to some form of relief, and convicts did not have a right to a pardon. The former risked greater irregularity in relief payments, or receiving relief in a less palatable form, while the latter literally put their lives at stake. Furthermore, a written repudiation of vestry wisdom may have lacked the immediate emotional impact of an angry outburst in person, in that the satisfaction and euphoria of breaking the silence (a recognized feature of releasing authentic opinions) may well have been attenuated by the physical separation and non-verbal communication of the participants.[28] At first sight, therefore, anger cannot be viewed as strategic. However, it could become so, particularly when combined with fluent, controlled forms of expression, though the relationship between strategy and material effect can only be measured where parish responses to individual letters are discernible.

The letters written by or for John Sayer are an object lesson in the maintenance of almost patrician dignity and reproof in the face of parish obstinacy. Sayer was seemingly between 40 and 50 years old when he wrote to the rural Staffordshire parish of Colwich in 1810 from his home in Oxford. His opening letter adopts a rather grand manner.

> Labouring on a Bed of Sickness & having no resource to fly unto for support ... but to the parish of Colwich ... I am reduced to this Necessity of applying to you for relief and respectfully request you will be so good as to remit me by return of post a sum sufficient to enable me to pay my rent for six weeks and to procure me some necessaries which my present unfortunate situation requires – Your own discretion will guide you as to what sum you may please to send, and you may be assured it will be discreetly applied to the relief of my necessities.

This emphasis on discretion is quite unusual, since this is not the quality which most pauper correspondents expected from either their overseers or from themselves. Less confident writers tended to ask for a specific sum or to quote a minimum figure. Of course, Sayer may not have written this letter. He certainly did not write all of his own correspondence, since the first of his letters was in one hand but the remainder were in another and with a different, somewhat less confident, style. Even so, Sayer's case retains a certain power based on content if not tone. Like the Jameses, Sayer too backed up his story with an outside authority, but he did not bother with mere surgeons. He referred the overseers of Colwich to no less a person than

Charles Wolseley esquire, a powerful local landowner destined to inherit his father's baronetcy and Sayer's former employer to boot. When his initial appeal failed and no money was forthcoming, Sayer's remonstrances to the parish officers included the threat of incurring Wolseley's anger, and a personal attack on the Colwich authorities: 'after writing to you a month back & not to Receive any answer Shows how unthinking you are and as Long as you Can Get What you want your selves you Care nothing about that one in Distress'.

The later months of 1810 brought Sayer material relief in the form of at least £3 sent to him enclosed in a letter from Colwich, so the combined force of Sayer's appeal and Wolsely's influence yielded a positive outcome in the short term. An unusual twist in Sayer's case was that, unlike many pauper writers, he was eventually compelled to return home. Even so, he was clearly a pauper with a rare degree of influence given the power of his former employer/friend. This showed itself ultimately in the pains taken on Sayer's behalf (and the expenses incurred) from the time of his return to Staffordshire until his death in July 1822, including the minute interest that Wolsley expressed in Sayer's affairs. How many landowners would have chased up their local parish officers to enquire icily why they had not bought a pauper a shirt, as Wolsley did in January 1813? In Sayer's case the threat to return home and prove expensive proved amply justified.

Depression in male pauper letters

What recourse was open to the man who lacked a powerful ally? Depression or low spirits could be pressed into rhetorical service by the pauper writer, albeit with less assurance of success. The tension between male expectation and the reality of experience at work and home has been assumed to be very damaging. Keith McClelland has argued that the tight association between manliness and work (for his purposes increasingly in the period 1850–80) meant that unemployment potentially heralded 'not only . . . economic but also . . . psychic depression'.[29] He acknowledged that little was known about how men coped with this, but assumed that loss of employment engendered feelings of shame, incompleteness and compromised dignity. Nonetheless he has identified telling shreds of evidence, citing the case of Robert Knight of the boilermaker's society, who commented that workers 'must make the best of the sunshine we now enjoy, for as certain as night will return, so surely will the clouds of depression again surround us with gloom, loss of work, and consequent suffering to ourselves and families'.[30] The meteorological metaphor permits Knight a poignant mode of expression that might otherwise have proved awkward to couch.

Oppenheim's study of depression in Victorian England highlights some of the difficulties, both with effective retro-diagnosis and with contemporary reactions to masculine experiences of melancholy, low spirits, or ultimately nervous breakdown. These symptoms in women chimed with their stereotypical depiction as emotional and intuitive, whereas depression in men, supposedly rational and purposeful, ran counter to many of the prevailing assumptions about the causes of mental distress: 'nervous exhaustion brought men perilously close to the feminine condition'.[31] She also argues that over the course of the nineteenth century, psychiatrists did not dispel this apprehension but instead interpreted male depression in ways that only shored up or exacerbated stereotypes of masculinity, regarding male hysteria, for example, as particularly linked to effeminacy. In other words, the prevailing context for masculine depression only got more difficult.

A further complication for the poor man was the suspicion of shamming or malingering attached to hysteria. Not all nervous disorders carried this additional burden; neurasthenia (labelled in 1869) was regarded as exclusively physiological in origin and therefore more respectable. Nonetheless, the able-bodied poor had always been dogged by the suspicion that unemployment entailed wilful withdrawal from labour. This apprehension waxed and waned along with discourses that emphasized the presence of the undeserving poor, but in the context of this chapter the early nineteenth century was a particularly acute moment for the able-bodied but low-spirited poor. Sentiments had been hardening towards the poor for some time and the Poor-Law-abolition movement of the 1810s, while unsuccessful in absolute terms, gave voice to the widespread belief that the poor were inviting dependency and idleness. Poor men may have been pushed into unemployment by trade depression, but contemporaries at this time often chose to blame them for their plight.

Over the course of the nineteenth century, doctors increasingly assumed that nervous exhaustion was peculiarly characteristic of commercial and professional middle-class men, and was associated with the need to earn a middle-class income and the fear of financial loss. They reasoned that members of the aristocracy held a relatively unassailable position, and that workers enjoyed no social standing, but the middle-class were continually striving to uphold their position and consequently drove themselves into overwork, insufficient rest and anxiety. This theory chimed with the doctors' preference for somatic explanations of mental illness and was apparently confirmed by the cohorts of men seeking help for nervous complaints outside of asylums. What contemporaries could not see or include in their analysis, what seems glaringly obvious to us now, was the pressure on all social groups to maintain their position in relation to the 'other', no matter how elevated or lowly. There was potential for minute gradations along the continuum of the working classes and impoverished and consequently for status-related stress.[32]

Autobiographies are one plausible route into the subject of working-class male depression. Francis Place is one of the few autobiographers to allude to their own mental distress (in his case, during a period of unemployment while blacklisted after a strike), and in retrospect the emotion that Place associated with this period was shame; he deeply regretted the way in which his own distress prompted him to vent what he regarded as his own bad temper on his wife, to the increase of their mutual misery.[33] Perhaps more typical than Place was William Aitken, whose own journalism issued a strong call to faith in both reason and the ultimate success of the campaign for the working-man's vote but whose mental state was deteriorating privately such that he committed suicide; the inquest into his death provided a brief but perhaps predictable story of ill-health, consequent unemployment and ensuing despair.[34]

Other narratives such as criminal petitions give general testimony to the mental health of their authors.[35] Pauper letters also speak sporadically, if in coded terms, about depression. They do not construct it as a coherent or self-contained part of a larger story, in the way that an autobiography might conceive a bout of depression as an episodic issue. Rather, pauper depression features as part of the ongoing struggle to impress letter recipients and readers with the sincere deprivations of poverty. It is part and parcel of the same continuum which seeks to describe material loss or inadequacy but few authors become so involved in the emotional implications of their account that they begin to unfold their psychological decline or suffering.

Samuel Parker, a woolcomber from Uttoxeter in Staffordshire, did attempt to describe his own depressed mental state in the course of his correspondence with his home parish. His letters cover a relatively short period, seven missives dated February 1833 to March 1834, but the length and detail of his writings (augmented with additional letters from local overseers, his wife and his vicar) are unusually rich in revealing a fear of despair that forms a coherent depiction of extreme poverty. What is particularly unusual in Samuel's case, however, is the combination of psychological insight with fluent angry expression; his words speak of dejection but his tone ranges from firm request via reproachful resentment into flashes of fury.

Samuel had been born in Uttoxeter some time before August 1799. It seems likely that his father, Thomas, was a tenant farmer, renting land from the Blount family just outside Uttoxeter, but that his family suffered declining fortunes. Samuel was apprenticed to a firm of woolstaplers in the town, served his full apprenticeship and went on to work for the same masters as a journeyman for a further year. He then travelled to Kidderminster in Worcestershire to seek work in carpet weaving some time before 1830, when he married local girl Nancy Powell. By 1832 he was living in his mother-in-law's house with his wife and two children and at the time of his first letter, his wife was expecting their third child. Awkwardly for Samuel, Kidderminster was effectually a 'one-industry town' and those who could not find work in carpet production were compelled to look elsewhere for employment.[36]

Samuel's letters, in addition to speaking at great length of his family's material misfortunes, made constant reference to the state of his mind and emotions. Throughout his letters, he maintained a running commentary on the state of his own spirits (either on what they were, what he hoped they might be, or what he feared they would become). The prospect of receiving sympathy from the Uttoxeter authorities was encouraging: the initial expectation that letters would be answered promptly encouraged him to keep his spirits up. Of course, an independent spirit was hurt by the necessity to ask for help; without a strong cause, they would not be so low spirited as to ask. His first letter refers to his initial application for poor relief some months earlier, and the fact that his lack of success 'caused my Mind to be very much put about'. His search for work entailed a lengthy tramp, giving him not only a hungry belly and sore feet but also an aching heart. The depths of his dejection were revealed in the possibility of his growing careless, apparently a reference to the idea that lack of external encouragement and opportunity might render him indifferent to his own fate and that of his family. In his first letter he predicted in abstract terms 'when the Husbands has brought there Family to the Parish leave them and grow careless care not for Imprisonment nor nothing else'.

He predicated his lack of motivation on the idea that acute lack of resources would compel him to return to Uttoxeter (the familiar plaint to return home, recast here in more melodramatic fashion). He conceived this as compulsion to break up his homestead; in other words he was explicitly tying his mental state to his ability to support his family home in the town of his choice and the avoidance of the workhouse ('the last habitation [he] ever could think of').[37] Any compulsion to return was therefore perceived as critically undermining the endeavour of independence. Also he was constructing a picture of his own mental health as dependent on the well-being of the rest of his nuclear family. In July 1833 he elaborated: 'knowing there sad Distress it as almost been to much for me and brought me to Desparation nearly drove me careless not careing for one thing nor the other'.

Parker also referred more than once to imprisonment, apparently alluding to the contemporary practice of punishing with temporary imprisonment those men who abandoned their families on the parish. However, far from succumbing to this fate he anticipated ways to use this policy to his best advantage. In one angry moment he pledged:

> . . . it was in my mind for us to be brought to the Parish and so I would leave them quite Incumbent upon the Parish and I to take no Notice of them till it might be if I resigned myself or was took too I should expect the Jail to be my Portion then would by my time to have it Exposed in the Publick Newspapers.

This extraordinary twist on the standard threat to return home may be unique; it is not a strategy featured in any of the 758 Essex pauper letters assembled by Sokoll.[38] On the whole though Parker was not inviting imprisonment, but rather stressing the flawed precepts of a society that would permit this to be the consequence of poverty. He drew explicit parallels between poverty, depression, what we would now recognize as loss of self-esteem and moral wrongdoing (if not actual illegality) when he wrote 'when a Person as lost the Spirit of Independence owing to Degradation through not being a little released out of poverty it brings on every thing that is bad till a person becomes a bad Member to Society'. What Parker was in effect doing was ascribing his anticipated 'carelessness' or fear of debility to the anxiety and overexertion which later Victorian doctors were so keen to reserve for the careworn middle classes. In Parker's case of course he was underworked, driven initially to an exhausting tramp in search of employment and then condemned to stressful idleness in Kidderminster itself. His loss of workplace identity, worry for his growing family and boredom made as potent a mixture as overwork could ever do. In his case, distress was given an extra twist by the fact that his regretful pleas for help appeared to make no impact at all. The timing of his letters (and those of his wife and vicar) make it clear that they had no effect whatsoever and no money was sent.

Samuel had a keen capacity for imagining the emotional responses of his readers (including their loss of patience; on one occasion he admitted 'I might be thought very rude'). Thus, 'It appears no feeling entreaty will do . . . not a Glymp's of the least Sympathy towards us'. He castigated the overseer's unfeeling silence, 'not having the Heart that could feel for another'. He implied that conscience would ultimately chastise the hard-hearted, who were fated to be 'Tormented in there minds for acting so Indiscreetly towards there fellow creatures' and be brought to 'a stool of Repentence'. At the core of his testimony, Samuel was arguing for an emotional dimension to parish welfare, the kind of insight that is generically absent from many parish documents (such as overseers accounts) and fugitive even in letters.[39] Financial relief represented mental alleviation. Hard cash was transmuted in these terms into emotional currency, in Samuel's words 'a little encouragement' which would be the means of soothing his anxiety since it would 'cause the mind to be set at rest'. In the absence of bankable sympathy, his mind remained 'vexatious and unruly'.

Samuel's letters do not, so far as we can ever know, contain a full list of the symptoms of his low spirits, and it is neither feasible nor desirable to try and identify his complaint as hypochondriasis or anything else. What he does do is point to a range of debilitating symptoms that explicitly tie material want to nervous disorder and distress. Having said this, although Samuel refers to his own 'shattered state' and blasted hopes, at no time is it obvious that he falls irredeemably into the despondency he predicts. In a sense, the continued flow of letters itself contradicts the idea of deep paralysing depression. It seems, though, that they had no decisive impact on their recipients; if the Kidderminster overseer is to be believed, none of Samuel's letters jogged the consciences of the Uttoxeter officers.

At the conclusion of his correspondence (when he secured work at Bridgnorth) Samuel fades from view. His industrial prospects were bleak and it is likely he suffered increasingly from the unemployment that dogged his thirties. Woolcombing and carpet weaving in Kidderminster experienced turbulent fortunes, with brief periods of boom punctuating longer spells of decline. One of the leading manufacturers folded in 1838 and Samuel's some-time employers were bankrupted in 1858.[40] Even so, his spirits apparently never received the fatal blow he anticipated in that he was never forced to remove permanently to Uttoxeter. He lived in Kidderminster until his death in 1875 aged 76.

Conclusion

The impact of gender on experiences of illness and on the responses of parishes ran very deep. Illness was particularly problematic for working men in the multiple ways it undermined their masculinity and claims to identity. The need for material survival and consequently for parish relief might effectively sweep away all personal considerations and subordinate them to the sometimes desperate pragmatism of need. Keeling's attempts at self-representation made no reference at all to his spirits and were confined to a strict delineation of practical wants. This approach was not unusual, but acute deprivation did not always result in uniform servility, or in a voluntary surrender of manhood. Fluent letters could frame elegant, dignified requests (as in the case of Sayer) whose initial lack of success prompted a rather commanding, indignant expression of reproach. A powerful friend could be a great asset, and while doctors and clergy were often ignored by parish officers, major landowners and ratepayers were not easily dismissed. They could give peculiar weight to pauper requests, though their presence in such a capacity is admittedly rare. Without external support of this kind, and facing a dreary but typical scene of poverty, writers could only fall back on emotion. For this reason men's letters sometimes gave vent to anger, a tone that may have been anti-strategic in terms of securing relief but may be unusually revealing for the modern reader, particularly where anger reveals its quiet sibling depression. Parker provides a rare example of the written protest that was possible where the frustrations of a slow, unforthcoming correspondence could be expressed by a fluent, literate and self-aware man. In other words he was able to say exactly how he thought poverty jeopardized his health by undermining his state of mind. He does not stint in his references to his feelings, particularly the slow crushing of his spirits, but conveys them with a passionate anger that shores up his identity rather than diffuses it. He defends the notion that anger comprised socially appropriate illness behaviour in his own case, and epitomizes the idea that an angry letter could constitute a masculine, if attenuated, assault on the parish.

Notes

1 Grell, O. P., Cunningham, A. and Jutte, R. (2002), *Health Care and Poor Relief in 18th and 19th Century Northern Europe*. Aldershot: Ashgate, chapter 1.

2 Fissell, M. (1991), *Patients, Power and the Poor in Eighteenth Century Bristol.* Cambridge: Cambridge University Press, pp. 99–100.

3 Lorber, J. (1997), *Gender and the Social Construction of Illness.* London: Thousand Oaks Sage, p. 1.

4 King, S. (2005), '"Stop This Overwhelming Torment of Destiny": Negotiating Financial Aid at Times of Sickness under the English Old Poor Law, 1800–40', *Bulletin of the History of Medicine*, 79, 228–60.

5 Tomkins, A. (2006), *The Experience of Urban Poverty 1723–82: Parish, Charity and Credit.* Manchester: Manchester University Press; Tomkins, A. (forthcoming, 2012), 'Poverty, kinship support, and the case of Ellen Parker, 1818–1828', in S. King (ed.), *The British Experience of Poverty.* Woodbridge: Boydell and Brewer.

6 All of the letters quoted here are given in full in King, S., Nutt, T. and Tomkins, A. (2006), *Narratives of the Poor in Eighteenth-Century Britain Volume 1. Voices of the Poor: Poor Law Depositions and Letters.* London: Pickering and Chatto, pp. 205–97.

7 Rose, S. O. (1992), *Limited Livelihoods. Gender and Class in Nineteenth-Century England.* Berkley: University of California Press, p. 138.

8 Seccombe, W. (1986), 'Patriarchy stabilized: the construction of the male breadwinner wage norm in nineteenth-century Britain', *Social History*, 11: 54; Rose, *Limited Livelihoods.* pp. 15 and 127–8.

9 Vincent, D. (1981), *Bread, Knowledge and Freedom: A Study of Nineteenth-Century Working Class Autobiography.* London: Europa, p. 54, argues that accounts of marriage in working-class autobiography seem to stress not romantic love but shared experience and interdependency, the mutual struggle through hardships characterized by the same hopes and fears, triumphs and disasters.

10 Shropshire Archives, P81/7/958.

11 Shepard, A. (2003), *Meanings of Manhood in Early Modern England.* Oxford: Oxford University Press, p. 221.

12 Ibid.

13 Ibid., p. 222

14 Colley, L. (1992), *Britons: Forging the Nation 1707–1837.* New Haven: Yale University Press, pp. 263–8. Colley cites primarily the Queen Caroline affair as a cause around which all women of all social standings could rally via public petitioning but I think the principle, that 'stressing female helplessness *and what was due to it* in this way could – up to a point – serve women's interests', is also applicable to the more local, personal circumstances of very poor women in their dealings with parishes.

15 Rose, *Limited Livelihoods*, p. 15.

16 Shoemaker, R. (2001), 'Male honour and the decline of public violence in eighteenth-century London', *Social History*, 26, 190–208

17 Davidoff, L. and Hall, C. (1987), *Family Fortunes: Men and Women of the English Middle-Class 1780–1850.* London: Hutchinson, pp. 110–12; Lorber, *Gender*, p. 4.

18 Rose, *Limited Livelihoods*, pp. 15, 23, 27.

19 Oppenheim, J. (1991), *Shattered Nerves: Doctors, Patients and Depression in Victorian England.* New York: University of Pennsylvania Press, p. 145. See Haynes, J. B. (1989), 'Working class perceptions: aspects of the experience of

working class life in Victorian Leicester', *Transactions of the Leicestershire Archaeological and Historical Society*, 63, 23–46, for an example of work looking at masculinity and trades unions.

20 Shepard, *Meanings of Manhood*, p. 214.

21 Roper, M. and Tosh, J. (1991), 'Introduction: historians and the politics of masculinity', in M. Roper and J. Tosh (eds), *Manful Assertions: Masculinities in Britain Since 1800*. London: Routledge, p. 13.

22 Tosh, J. (1999), *A Man's Place: Masculinity and the Middle-Class Home in Victorian England*. New Haven: Yale University Press, pp. 2–3. Pretensions to manhood had long been based partly on solvency. See Shepard, *Meanings of Manhood*, pp. 178, 189–91, for evidence taken from sixteenth century Cambridge University Commissary court cases.

23 Shepard, *Meanings of Manhood*, p. 206.

24 Shaw, C (1969), *When I Was a Child*. Wakefield: S.R. Publishers, p. 97.

25 Tosh, *A Man's Place*, p. 1.

26 Colley, L. (2002), *Captives: Britain, Empire and the World 1600–1850*. London: Jonathan Cape, p. 93.

27 MacKay, L. (2003), 'Refusing the Royal Pardon: London capital convicts and the reactions of the courts and press 1789', *London Journal*, 28, 23–4.

28 Scott, J. C. (1990), *Domination and the Arts of Resistance*. New Haven: Yale University Press, pp. 208–9.

29 McClelland, K. (1991), 'Masculinity and the representative artisan in Britain, 1850–80', in Roper and Tosh, *Manful Assertions*, p. 78.

30 McClelland, K. (1987), 'Time to work, time to live: some aspects of work and the re-formation of class in Britain, 1850–80', in P. Joyce (ed.), *The Historical Meanings of Work*. Cambridge: Cambridge University Press, p. 186.

31 Oppenheim, *Shattered Nerves*, p. 141.

32 Nonetheless, some late-twentieth-century historians have been tempted to echo the assumptions of Victorian commentators. Thus, Mangan, J. A. and Walvin, J. (1987), 'Introduction' in J. A. Mangan and J. Walvin (eds), *Manliness and Morality: Middle-Class Masculinity in Britain and America, 1800–1940*. Manchester: Manchester University Press, p. 4, assumed that working-class men and women gave little thought to masculinity and femininity.

33 Vincent, *Bread*, p. 54. However, Gagnier, R. (1991), *Subjectivities: A History of Self-Representation in Britain, 1832–1920*. Oxford:Oxford University Press, has characterized autobiographies as stylistically about restraint rather than disclosure.

34 Vincent, *Bread*, p. 200

35 Carter, O. (2001), 'Early nineteenth-century criminal petitions: an introduction for local historians', *Local Historian,* 31, 143.

36 Rose, *Limited Livelihoods,* p. 120.

37 Vincent, *Bread*, p. 53 refers to the workhouse as a place where the family was dismembered.

38 Sokoll, T. (2001), *Essex Pauper Letters 1731–1837*. Oxford: Oxford University Press.

39 Parker is unusual in this but not unique, since his sentiments are echoed by a pauper signing himself P. N. Stewart in a letter to Barnacre (Lancashire) from

Leek in Staffordshire, 3 April 1822; Stewart's references to his mental state are reminiscent of Parkers. He refers to 'feelings that I cannot express' and being 'very neare to distraction'. He too makes an appeal to the overseers as emotional individuals, 'husbands and fathers'; will they be 'worthy the character of men with human feelings'? Stewart goes further than Parker though in envisaging his own death in a ditch 'to stop this overwhelming torment of destiny'. I am indebted to Steve King for this reference.

40 Tomkinson, K. and Hall, G. (1975), *Kidderminster since 1800*. Kidderminster: Private Publication; Rose, *Limited Livelihoods*, chapter 5.

4

'I have once more taken the Leberty to say as you well know': The development of rhetoric in the letters of the English, Welsh and Scottish sick and poor 1780s–1830s

Steven King and Alison Stringer

Introduction

On 12 December 1784, Walter Keeling, an old man resident in the north-eastern town of Hull, but legally settled[1] in the town of Colwich in Staffordshire (encountered already in the chapter by Alannah Tomkins), wrote to the overseer of the poor of the latter parish. He wanted to

> Lett you know that we are in Hull and that wee are obliged to take a fornished Room which wee Pay 2 Shillings a wiek [week] for it which my wages will not aford and if you will be so kind as to Send me one ginney to Boy [buy] me a few goods I Shall Never Send no more While I live and

if not I Shall Bring my familey over Immediately Which I can Esey gett a hose [sic] Pass Sir: if you will be so kind as to Relive me this time I hope with gods help it will be the Last time kind Sir I hombley Thank you for all your goodness I am Sorrey to Troble you but I cant help it if I had but few goods I hope I Shall Do will as I have got a place of work where I hope to Stay While I Live.[2]

This letter is a classic of its genre, combining formulaic expression (it is the last time Keeling will trouble his home parish, something that almost all writers promise) with submissive posturing (he is sorry to trouble the parish and thankful for their favours to him) and threats (he will bring his family back to Colwich at considerable cost). It melds rhetoric, fact, aspiration and despair into a seemingly self-contained narrative, somewhat removed from the more formal petitions often found on the continent and in English speculative begging letters.[3] Such narratives, which provide proof of high levels of basic literacy in the population,[4] were generated by the complexity of the English (and Welsh[5]) laws of settlement and poor relief. Crudely, while labouring people were more or less free to migrate,[6] if they fell into poverty they could attempt to claim poor relief funded by communities only in their parish or township of settlement, defined by place of birth, marriage, the serving of an apprenticeship or payment of rates for a set period of time. As with Walter Keeling, falling into poverty could occur at a considerable distance from the parish of settlement, necessitating either that the pauper moved back 'home' or wrote back 'home' asking for relief in the host community. While the earliest commentators implied that pauper narratives were rare, subsequent historians such as Thomas Sokoll, Alannah Tomkins and myself have suggested that substantial caches exist.[7] Even for places where the originals have not survived, supplementary records (such as ratepayers minutes recording the reading aloud of such appeals and overseers' transcribed letter-books, which recorded both appeal and response) prove that many more letters were sent than have been preserved.

Such letters[8] become much more common in English and Welsh archives after 1800. This may reflect a number of issues: the fact that population and urbanization were both increasing rapidly, so that formal lines of communication replaced face-to-face interaction; that the scale and intensity of migration had increased;[9] or that the economic basis of the poor law and inter-parish relations changed after the ability to redeem banknotes for bullion coin at the Bank of England was suspended in the 1790s and coin-hoarding by merchants and others required new, paper-based, accounting and money payment systems.[10] However we explain the rising number of pauper letters, a related observation is that the Scottish poor law appears to have generated no analogous body of pauper appeals. Instituted later than its English counterpart, the Scottish poor law replaced a ramshackle system of charity-based payments and had a radically different philosophy and underlying entitlement structure, and a more institutionally and process-based operating system, than its English and Welsh counterpart.[11] Certainly in the nineteenth century, pauper petitions and examinations, not pauper letters, dominate the narrative landscape.[12] This said, and as is equally the case with Wales, large numbers of letters were written by paupers with Scottish origins[13] to English parishes where such paupers thought or claimed they may have gained an intermediate settlement to their Scottish roots.

Unsurprisingly, using letters such as that of Walter Keeling poses potentially intractable problems. The physical condition of many pauper letters is poor, and they range in orthographic quality from punctuated copper-plate hand to barely legible colloquial English. However they are written, there are also questions of provenance and accuracy. Did the person who signed the letter actually write it? What role was there for scribes or group dictation? Do such letters report fact or are they embellished? After all, these were appeals that local officials were under no obligation to respond to. While the law of the Poor Law placed an onus on communities to relieve the 'deserving' or 'impotent' poor, it said little about how this group were to be defined and treated, so that entitlement under the law was often a matter of local custom and circumstance. In the sense that pauper letters were the public articulation of a set of private circumstances, there may have been a real incentive to filter information. Even if we can establish provenance (for instance via continuity of handwriting over a letter series), how do we handle related questions of representativeness? That is, were the pauper letters that survive representative of all of those sent, and did the rhetoric, fact and artefact of poverty constructed in pauper letters reflect the same experiential circumstances as those who remained in their parish of settlement and fell into poverty there?

These are serious matters, reviewed in-depth in the introduction to this volume, but their potential impact can also be overblown. Local officials had numerous overlapping mechanisms for checking the veracity of claims made, and where these were employed paupers were invariably found to be broadly truthful. Similarly, there is little evidence from the internalities of letter collections that scribes or stylistic letter-books were used to construct narratives and shape their rhetoric. This does not mean that pauper narratives had no input from others; indeed, there is evidence from urban collections that neighbours consulted successful claimants in order to find out what was successful. However, such consultation does not make the resultant pauper narrative any less truthful or useful. And while orthography may be a problem, nascent schemes for the classification of letters according to structure or rhetorical type provide some checking mechanisms.[14] In similar fashion, vestry minutes provide a checking mechanism for the representativeness of pauper letters; those who remained in their parish of settlement still had to represent their oral case to local officials and there is no evidence that their framing of such cases differed much from that seen in pauper letters. In one respect, however, thorny problems remain, viz. the particularities of Welsh and Scottish paupers. For these letter writers, problems of literacy were compounded by issues around language, particularly those who came from Welsh-speaking communities. And, of course, whereas English pauper letters tended to be written from neighbourhoods and communities where Englishness pervaded, there is much evidence that Welsh and Scottish migrants had more isolated living arrangements.[15] They would have been unable to call upon certain rhetorical devices – for instance, suggestions that local officials consult respectable people in the host community to establish the veracity of claims – that the English took for granted. Such problems tended to push Welsh and Scottish pauper narratives towards the more simplistic, petition-like, end of the typological spectrum.

The rest of this chapter draws on a set of pauper letters (and associated official and supportive correspondence) collected as part of a wider Wellcome Trust project on sickness and poverty in the period 1750–1850. Numbering some 9,000 items in total, the narrative database covers the counties of Berkshire, Cumberland, Devon, Dorset, Lancashire, Leicestershire, Lincolnshire, Norfolk, North Yorkshire, Nottinghamshire, Northamptonshire, Oxfordshire, Somerset, Staffordshire, West Yorkshire, Westmorland, Wiltshire, Worcestershire and Warwickshire. While essentially rural counties predominate in the locational sample, the wide migration fields of people from these places means that the full spectrum of community typologies (rural, urban, industrial, service, town hinterland etc.) are well represented in terms of host communities. Indeed, there is even a bias towards letters from urban areas.[16] Deploying this narrative database, the chapter moves first to discussion of a typology of the rhetorical and strategic devices used by paupers to try and establish entitlement to out-parish relief in their *individual* letters. A subsequent, and much more substantial, section analyses how paupers developed their narratives of sickness over the course of *multiple* letters to their parish of settlement. Multiple letter writers abound in the underlying sample, some producing more than seventy narratives in their 'pauper career', and this section will focus on three such serial writers who seem to exemplify particular developmental trajectories. The analysis is driven by a deceptively simple question: how did the out-parish poor, when faced with the necessity of applying for relief over and over again, sustain the urgency, physical and emotional impact of their (predominantly health-related) afflictions? Due to the repetitive nature of their requests, these multiple correspondents must have employed some kind of developmental technique, embellishing themes which produced the required response and abandoning those which did not. In turn, they must have asked themselves, or seen their narratives informed by, a wider set of questions than those who wrote single narratives or who represented their case in person. How did such writers feel their plight was seen in the distant parish? Did the overseers and vestry remember them and their letters, and did the pauper expect such memory? To what extent did they feel trusted and how did they continually maintain their credibility? And ultimately, how did multiple writers respond to the rejection or simple disregard of their requests?

Rhetorical and strategic devices

Walter Keeling's letter suggests several of the devices used by paupers to try and establish entitlement in a poor law system in which law, custom and precedent combined to shape who was seen as deserving and how they were treated. As Alannah Tomkins has noted earlier in this volume, outright anger and confrontation of officials was relatively rare.[17] Rather, and as Steve Hindle has also argued,[18] servility, gratitude and respect were the basic building blocks of the standard pauper narrative. As an extension of this strategy, paupers would often (as with Keeling) apologize for approaching their parish or for offending the sensibilities of the 'gentlemen' ratepayers. How far the rhetoric of servility and deference was transposed into reality is more difficult to gauge; even the most malingering, irksome and aggressive paupers seem to have been given a hearing by local officials and ratepayer bodies and to have received relief notwithstanding constant admonitions by the same officials.[19]

At the level of individual letters, paupers also deployed, singly or in tandem, four other rhetorical and strategic vehicles. First, the dramatization of their situation. Thus, paupers almost always stressed that they approached their parish of settlement out of desperation and last resort, often having tried every other means short of crime to secure their welfare. To remain with the example of Walter Keeling (for continuity of argument rather than because he is exceptional or particularly well documented), in various letters he claimed that he was 'Sorry to Troble you but I cant help it', 'you can easily conceive to what a condition I am reduced . . . I hope out of your Humanity you will consider my case', 'my Trobles has been Verrey grate', and 'I am in Grate Want at Present and have had a grate Deal of Troble this Summer in Travling from Place to Place'. The latter claim is particularly interesting, at once evidence of his attempts to make do by moving from place to place in search of work but also confirmation that he had reached the end of his attempts to retain independence. Other paupers claimed that they had been driven to apply for relief because of high prices, unemployment, persistent sickness, a life of labour and uncontrollable circumstances such as their children becoming unemployed and returning home seeking support. For the sick poor at least, such claims were invariably accompanied by the dramatization of the symptoms, prognosis or impact of diseases or other afflictions. Walter Keeling, for instance, referred to the 'deplorable condition of my self and Family' and noted that that 'for the space of seven or eight weeks I and Family all laid sick of a Fever; being Oblidged to hire a Nurse as none of us could help another'. Incidents like this magnified the impact of other more ingrained problems such as encroaching blindness, 'I have Verrey Bad Youmer Fell in my Eyes as I have Been Sumtimes all most Blind for this 2 Months', and the impact of old age, 'I am in grate Distress as my Wife Has Been Verrey Bad In a fever for this Two monthes and me a old man Verrey much Trobled With a pain in my Side Verrey un able to Work'.

For the sick and ageing pauper in particular, dramatization of the situation seems to have been a common approach.[20]

A second set of rhetorical avenues centred on the character of the writers. We have already seen that illness and unemployment could compromise male identity and generate a narrative of depression in pauper letters. More widely, pauper letters frequently contained both positive and negative rendering of individual identities. On the negative side, paupers might sometimes point to their humiliation in the host community, their inability to go out because of their ragged appearance, their inability to perform the roles of parents, sons and daughters, their shame at pawning the very clothes from their backs and their fear for their reputations associated with the breaking of social codes over the repayment of debts to shopkeepers, friends and neighbours. On the positive side, most pauper letters referred to the aspiration that the writer would eventually be restored to independence. Walter Keeling expressed this sentiment on many occasions, often repeating the thrust of his 10 November 1795 letter that 'I have had Nothing from you this maney years I Shall Never Troble you no more'. Most of those who wrote multiple letters would also at some point give yardsticks of their honesty in depicting their circumstances. This might include invitations for the officials in their settlement parish to inspect the pauper and ascertain the situation for themselves, reference to their standing in the host community, the enclosure or appendage of testimony from others in their locality (doctors, landlords, vicars, etc.), and, occasionally, reference to widely reported incidents that helped to explain their appeal. In the latter case, paupers in the underlying sample refer variously to national reportage of cholera outbreaks of the sort traced by Beate Althammer later in this volume, unemployment in the industrial districts, riots, price inflation, closure of ports, steam engine boiler explosions and large-scale fires. It was also surprisingly common (if not always a successful tactic) to get others to write on behalf of the pauper. Walter Keeling noted disapprovingly on 27 January 1788 that 'Even our minister Which Will not Lie has sent you Porishons [sic] in two Letters but you Neve Would Send him anser and Now I am Porswaded by him and other Gentlemen to Send my Familey to you the Next month.'[21]

This letter from Keeling introduces a third set of rhetorical and strategic devices centring round a notion that we might define as 'forceful logic' or alternatively as 'threat'. Thus, it was common for paupers throughout the underlying sample to threaten to return home themselves or, even worse, to remain where they were but send their families to the settlement parish without the main breadwinner. Such logic was almost always accompanied by a notation that this action would result in considerable costs of travel, relief and (because of the sickness that might accompany the long-distance removal of the destitute) sickness relief. Walter Keeling's letter of 27 November 1786 is a classic of its type, asking for relief 'otherwise I shall be oblidge to make application to the Parish, which may prove fatal to me and Family, and very expensive to you, as no Doubt is, but they would be for removing me and Family at your expence which must prove very considerable'.[22] It is interesting against this backdrop that neither Keeling nor many other paupers in the underlying sample asserted any right to poor relief. What was more common was to imply rights by talking about and asserting the moral duty of either parish or official. We have already seen Keeling asking the parish overseer to act with humanity, and more widely serial letter writers in particular seem prone to talk about the needs of the parish to protect dignity, meet its godly obligations and act to support the weak, feeble and sick in particular. However they tried to heap imagined obligations onto officials, it is also clear that some paupers, especially where repeated letters were ignored, became more hostile. Such hostility might confine itself to strong admonition for not replying to letters or giving less than was asked for. Occasionally, however, it spilled into threats, threats that the pauper would call in the magistrates, that the actions of the officials in the settlement parish would be made widely known in the host parish, and that a failure to act would push desperate families and individuals into criminal or immoral actions. Sick paupers were particularly prone to adopt this strategy in the face of a refusal to help.

A less aggressive, and fourth, rhetorical device was to freight appeals in pauper letters with claims to particularly strong connections with, and thus deservingness in, the settlement parish. Most crudely, this might take the form of noting that the writer had recently and persistently been home to the settlement parish. Other variants included reporting intelligence from the settlement parish brought by relatives or contact (thus giving the illusion of a connectedness), stressing that merchants or carriers from the settlement regularly saw the pauper in the host parish, or asking the overseer and other officials to pass on news to relatives and friends back home. Such sentiments were usually encased in a linguistic register referring to 'my' parish, place or home. A surprising number of paupers also reported their family history as part of their appeals, at once emphasizing the depth of their connection with a place and substituting for the pauper not appealing in person. Such reportage might encompass references to employment history, parental and grand-parental names, brothers, sisters and even friends and sponsors in the locality. One letter even reminded the overseer that the writer had built his fathers house when he was resident in his parish of settlement! The most sophisticated rhetoric of this type was that which claimed personal connection with currently or previously serving officials, effectively personalizing a relationship in which the decision of who to relieve and with what forms of welfare was at the discretion of the individual. Sick paupers were particularly likely to adopt this tactic. Walter Keeling pursued this strategy when he wrote on 29 July 1787 to Mr Turner (presumably a previous overseer) because 'I Dont know overseer of the poor Hoping that you Will be so Kind to give thees few Lings [sic] to him'.[23]

There is more work to be done on the spectrum of rhetorical strategies employed in pauper narratives, both for Britain and the Continent.[24] In particular, we can observe that the strategies employed by those paupers with Welsh settlement parishes, or Scottish paupers writing as part of the English system in order to try and establish an English entitlement, were consistently among the simplest in the entire sample. Welsh paupers were much more likely to focus on servility, gratitude and the costs associated with their coming home than their English counterparts, perhaps reflecting the fact that their narratives were disproportionately likely to be met with a strict interpretation of the Old Poor Law: that the pauper must return to Wales in order to garner relief, unless they were willing to accept a 'token' level of relief in their host parish. The Welsh version of the Old Poor Law was almost certainly considerably harsher than its English counterpart.[25] Scottish paupers, of course, had no rights to relief in English parishes unless they could establish an intervening settlement, and the letters of Scottish paupers were invariably more circumspect than those of their Welsh and English counterparts. In particular, threats were likely to trigger deeper investigation into the family circumstances of Scottish paupers, and the precarious position of Scottish migrants in the English welfare system probably explains why most pauper letters from this group focused single-mindedly on the legal definition of settlement counterposed with the appeal that officials act with humanity. Scottish paupers were also consistently among the most dramatic in their description of disease, the consequences of poverty and the depth of their suffering. In short, such paupers shaped their narratives to reflect their marginal position among the marginal. These observations must await further development in future work.

Development of rhetoric in letter series

This rhetorical and strategic range is important. The key question, however, is how paupers employed and interlinked discrete strategies in order to make, maintain, or re-establish a case over a series of letters. To explore this matter, we can turn to three paupers who wrote multiple letters to very different settlement parishes. The first writer, William King, represents an older (60 years of age in 1834), more educated and articulate pauper. The second, Thomas Earl, a Scot writing from Southampton but settled in the Wiltshire parish of Bradford-on-Avon, was less comfortable with writing. Although described by his local overseer as 'getting old', he had young children at home and his eldest boys had only just been placed as apprentices. Neither of these men was at the time of writing a 'pensioner', receiving a previously agreed payment from their home parish. Rather, they applied for and were granted discretionary casual (albeit relatively regular) relief. Our third writer, Elizabeth Brand, provides a letter series very different in content, tone and execution to the previous two. She was writing on behalf of her sick and aged mother, who received a regular stipend from the parish of

Thrapston (Northamptonshire). Although Elizabeth Brand was not strictly a pauper, her letters address the issues of 'rights' to welfare and the nature of poor law administration when faced by the issue of sickness. We turn first, then, to William King.

Thomas Sokoll's edition of Essex pauper letters contains 14 narratives written by William King[26] of Bethnal Green (London) over a period of six years to the overseer of his home parish of Braintree, between 20 November 1828 and 2 October 1834.[27] He had a fairly regular pattern of correspondence, penning two letters a year, one in the early-to-mid-winter and one at the beginning of the summer. Did King expect the overseers to remember his earlier letters – that he suffered from asthma, and that his wife had been sick and under the care of a doctor – or did he reiterate afresh every time? Did he feel the need to describe new complaints, in order to avoid repeating himself, or was the family's ongoing suffering from various chronic diseases used in a cumulative way? And can we ascertain how successful the requests were? In short, was there a development of King's rhetorical strategy over the course of his fourteen requests for assistance?

First, let us consider how prominent the issue of sickness itself was in King's letters.[28] Of the 14, ten were directly concerned with the health of either King himself or members of his family. Complaints ranged from the specific – 'asthma' (20 November 1828 and 4 March 1834), rheumatism (also 4 March 1834) and an outbreak of what was probably cholera, 'the affliction wich has Carryed off so Meny of our fellow Creatures of Late' (11 May 1833) – to unnamed but still identifiable problems – 'bad in my breath' (30 April 1829) and 'very hevey inward complaints' (12 March 1830). King also complained about being 'very ill' (20 November 1828 and 16 December 1831), of 'much illness' (17 July 1833) and 'past and present afflictions' (4 March 1834). Towards the end of the series he was increasingly concerned with the afflictions of old age: 'failings of nature' (31 July 1834) and 'Great weakness and Sinking' (September 1834). The issue of sickness also took various roles in the letters. Sometimes ill-health was the central reason for King's application, either due to his inability to work ('I So Unable to do what Might do to Make Us a Little Better off', 17 July 1833) or the actual financial cost of formal medical care: 'My wife is Very ill I Yust Now Brought Medecine from Shordith for her from the Doctors' (20 November 1828).[29] On most occasions, however, ill-health was used as a device to illustrate the desperation of the family's situation, along with their pawning clothes in order to buy food, their ramshackle accommodation and the shame of owing money to neighbours.

Against this backdrop, the narratives from King were by no means rhetorically static. His first letter combined many of the rhetorical vehicles mentioned above, calling attention to his desperate plight ('I am in Very Low Circumstances'), his need for understanding and humanity on the part of the official, his fortitude and self-reliance ('I yust Bore Up Under My Gret affliction of Mind'; 'it tis My Hope Not to Send again till I am More than forced to do it'), his plight as a consequence of circumstances beyond his control ('My work such I Do is Now Very Slack'), and his altered and compromised identity ('We Keep our trabble from the World all we Can . . . [we] have Been obliged to Part with our Poor Cloase such as they are to get Meal'). At the rhetorical core of the letter, however, was King's emphasis on his reluctance to even *trouble* the parish. He had avoided doing so for as long as possible and wished to avoid doing so in the future, a theme he returned to in one form or another in this letter no fewer than eight times: '[I] have Refrained to trabble them till this time'; 'I Yust bore Up Under My Gret affliction of Mind Partly owing to My Being obliged to trabble My Parrish'; 'I Greatly fear twill be My Sore trial be on Soume greater Dependence to My Parrish'; 'We have Made the Most trying Shifts till Now'; 'Let the Gentlemen Consider how Little I have trabbled them'; 'tis My hope Not to Send again till I am More than forced to do it'; '[My Girl] I hope will be no Expense to My Parrish'; 'I Long for the time to take a House and Pay so Much for it a Twelve Month as May Make me a Parrisoner in London'. In other words, it had cost him considerably in terms of self-respect to be forced to apply for relief. From his intention to attend the vestry personally (but physically prevented by his asthma and 'other complaints') to his desire to legally settle in London (and therefore no longer be the responsibility of Braintree), King distanced himself from any suggestion of idleness and reliance on charity. He was, in effect, seeking to evidence his honour and compromised identity in the face of intolerable sickness.

King's technique of repeating, restating and reiterating his essential self-reliance and fundamental distaste at being an object of charity obviously succeeded, for in his second letter (written five months later on 30 April 1829[30]) he noted 'when you Sirs Sent Us the Last Pound'. In this second letter, however, he changed rhetorical direction, making only two references to this desire to be no trouble. In place of this rhetoric he substituted a theme which came to dominate his later letters: that if the vestry could really understand his plight they would, in an act of dramatic empathy, be moved to relieve him immediately; highlighting in other words the moral duty of the parish to act. In this second letter, King also referred to the first, stating that in his initial correspondence he had not entered into the unpleasant details of his 'Very Trying Circumstances' because he felt 'allmost ashamed to Lower the feelings of the Kind Gentlemen' with a litany of woes. He went on to describe how during the hard winter his local parish officers had given the family bread 'though we Do Not Blong to Bethnal Green', in effect calling attention to the failure of duty of his settlement parish.[31] This placing of his 'wrechedness' in the public domain, so fought against in the last letter ('We keep our trabble from the World all we can'), is not unusual. Many paupers invoked the dismay of their friends and neighbours as a demonstration of the severity of their distress and a way of informing overseers that they had 'witnesses'. King took the rhetoric one step further by claiming to be the subject of a newspaper article: his 'wrechedness apeared in the News and in a Small track Likewise wich I Now Can Produce if Needs be'. In turn, this theme of public proof – confirming the veracity of the reported distress and, indirectly, William's spotless character – recurred in every subsequent letter. On 25 February 1830,[32] King wrote that he and his wife had suffered greatly over the winter, but his principal cause of misery was shame: of money owed, of being unable to look after his daughter and of relying on friendship ('wich hangs on a Very Brittle thread'[33]). His dignity and self-respect were compromised by his poverty. This psychological rather than physical oppression (a theme we have also seen in the chapter by Alannah Tomkins), combined with the fact that he had consistently avoided 'trabbling' the parish over the previous 40 years of 'Painfull distress' despite being advised by others to do so, constituted a strong moral case for the parish to do its duty. As a final flourish, he threatened (again supported by 'two or three friends') to return to Braintree for good.

William King did not hear from the parish, and wrote again just over two weeks later, on 12 March 1829.[34] His language in this narrative was more urgent – he definitely 'Cannot Do without Soume Help'. He restated and added to the list of indignities to which his family had been subject, compromising their identity: above all his wife's ring – spiritual symbol of the eternity of their marriage – had to be pawned in order to get food, offering only corporeal and temporary relief. King himself suffered from 'Very Hevey inward Complaints' (note the plural) and offered quite simply that 'Nature failt [failed]'. Suggesting that the vestry could not possibly have seen his earlier letter as it would certainly have moved them to send assistance, King felt he must 'leave My case in thear Consideration. I trust they will Never forget Poor King Next Monday'. This is a particularly important letter, representing King's first move towards the tones of rebuke which peppered his later correspondence.

On 16 December 1831,[35] King wrote thanking the vestry for twenty shillings but lamented that it was not a larger sum. Dramatic themes of chronic ill-health ('I am But Very ill and my wife the same'), miserable accommodation ('Poor Cold Mean Place') and loss of dignity ('our few Cloaths a Mostly all out or My wife Might apear More tidey') apparent in every letter were dealt with in a much more succinct fashion than previously. There were none of the statements of proof and witnesses, none of the reluctance to trouble the vestry and rather less sentiment. This letter addressed the practicalities of poverty to a greater extent than the psychological pressures foregrounded in earlier narratives. If they did not receive some relief 'we Must Suffer More Loss and other Painfull feelings', but this was by way of an ultimatum, rather than setting out current misery as a trigger to provoke generosity.

From this point, King's letters took on a fairly consistent pattern: opening with thanks for previous relief, and then setting out reasons why it was never quite enough, how his standing in the community was compromised by debts to tradesmen and neighbours and his deserving nature. Increasingly, King used the technique of stating certainty that, if witnessed first hand, his plight would move the vestry to greater generosity: 'if Sir you Realy Knew our wants and feeling you and Most of the other Gentlemen would Be anxious to assist Us'[36] or 'it would Be Very Painful to you to witness our Distress'.[37] Similarly, as King's confidence grew in the light of successful appeals, he rebuked the vestry for not sending the money on time. In order to collect his allowance, King had to meet Mr Haywood the carter in Whitechapel, a distance of one and a half miles from his home in Bethnal Green. To make this journey only to be disappointed was 'Both Dangerous and Painfull',[38] and the accusatory tone was in stark contrast to that of supplication in earlier letters. On 17 July 1833 he wrote: 'Send it by Mr Hayward at once at the opointed time as tis So hard and Unpleasent to him and all Partys to Go So far. I make Not Doubt but the Gentlemen will Grant Me thus favour Not Being willing to ad Repeatd Disopointment to one who is all most drivn to dispair'[39] Thus, while William King's detailing of his own and his wife's ill-health actually changed little over the course of six years,[40] the rhetorical scaffolding that tied sickness with deservingness moved from repetitive unwillingness to be a burden on his parish, despite very real physical, financial and spiritual oppression, to (not very) veiled implications of neglect. On 4 March 1834, King wrote:

> I Most Heartly thank you all Sirs for the Last 20 Shillings But am Sorry I had to Be So Very Trabblesome to Mr Hd By having to Go So Meny times to white chapple, Did you Know Sir what Either I or My wife Suffer By it you would No doubt Pervent it.[41]

It is not, one suspects, Mr Haywood the carter who was put out. King noted his age and infirmity in these later letters, rather than repeated descriptions of his various complaints. The asthma and rheumatism remained, but it was the generalized 'failings of Nature'[42] and the 'Great weakness and Sinking'[43] of sixty hard years which he felt would provoke the most sympathetic (and generous) response.[44] This was a complex rhetorical development, informed by an expectation that his letters would be remembered and his deservingness accumulated layer-by-layer.

A very different letter writer was Thomas Earl, a sometime Scot and sweetmeat seller living in Southampton but settled in the Wiltshire parish of Bradford-on-Avon. He wrote eight letters back to his home parish between 14 December 1832 and 4 March 1835.[45] All but one referred to sickness, often as the central reason for his application. Where King bemoaned a general lack of health, using it as an adjunct to his general misery, Earl placed his various injuries and illnesses right at the centre of his argument: 'Dear Sir I am once more throw poverty and affliction abliged to Send to you for support'.[46] On 24 February 1833[47] Earl wrote that he was unable to ply his trade due to a bad back and a chest (or possibly kidney) problem. It was a struggle even for him to start the letter: 'with Great Pain of Body I take pen in hand'. Thus the recipient was in no doubt from the very start that the situation was desperate. It emerged in this first letter that these problems stemmed from being unable to afford good clothing

> Now I cant Get out of dors to Get aney thing for them having travelled So Long without Shoes that will keep out water and badley clothed I have Got a Chill in my Lines and Saterday last I was pading up my feet fell a Side and Cricked my back So that I am not able to Rise out of the Chair without help.[48]

At first glance, Earl's letters would appear rather less sophisticated than those of King. Yet, they contain a subtle subtext that has at least something in common with the Essex pauper. Earl had been in his physical state for a long time, and showed commendable stoicism about it: he had 'travelled so Long without shoes that will keep out water', and as a result of having to make do without shoes he had injured himself. His letter ended by repeating his opening gambit: 'I should have Roat to him [James Chapman, through whom Earl receives his relief] but am not abel to sit up.' Such a turn of phrase both dramatized the situation and also gave it a pointedness: Earl was in such pain that he could only write one letter, reinforcing the importance of this single narrative. The parish responded with £1.

Earl's next letter was written nearly three months later (20 May 1833).[49] Like William King he demonstrated considerable confidence that his plight would have been remembered: 'I have Once more taken the Leberty to Say as you well know We have had a Great deal of affliction.' And like King he also praised actions of the officials in his host community before asking for any help from his settlement parish: 'I should say thank the Lord for the kind assistance the Gentelmen gave at this place they Gave in Giving us a Letter to the Despencery by which means My wife is in a great measure restored to health.' The implication is clear – if his plight was taken seriously by Southampton's vestry, then Bradford-on-Avon should have few additional qualms in paying his rent. Lest those qualms should loom large, Earl reminded the parish that if they would not help, his entire family of seven must return to Bradford, thereby highlighting the economy of a little expenditure now (2s 6d a week) to avoid larger bills in the future. Characteristically, he ended with a flourish: 'the last time I sent to you my wife was not abel to be moved but she Can now and must without help is Given'. His wife's recovery, therefore, could be traced to the favourable actions of Southampton and stood in contradistinction to the attitude of Bradford, which might necessitate a long journey home.[50] Again, Bradford responded with cash, a sovereign.

Despite promising not to bother the parish again, Earl suffered another accident in November 1833 and wrote for relief.[51] Again, he demonstrated his abilities as a rhetoricist. It was 'Misforten' – circumstances beyond his control – which prompted the request and it was 'Much a Gainst [my] inclenation to trouble' the vestry, implying a commendable discomfort with financial dependence. He 'Canot Get half a nof in the Summer to live as we ought' so he had struggled on in poverty, not bothering the parish since May, and he had sought to support his family himself until the very clothes he stood up in ('I have traveled untel I have Neither Shoos nor shorts') had fallen apart. However, the last straw was that

> On Saterday last I went to help to make Ready for to bury Mr Dryer and Carrying Som Lumps of wood I fell Down a Cross 5 Bricks and hurt my Right Side So that we cant tel where the Ribs is broke or not but I am Quite disabled to travel but I must try my frends to get me in to the Despencery if they will be So kind therefore Gentelmen if you do not Send a Speedy Releaf you will have us all brought home to you as soon as I am abel to be moved.

His last injury was sustained while padding up his feet because he was too poor to afford shoes. This one happened while he was assisting with the funeral of his brother-in-law. Earl gave a detailed account of the accident, what he was carrying, how many bricks tripped him up, but a fairly sketchy account of the injury itself. Tellingly, there was no surgeon's note with this letter; the supporting testimonies were from two laymen, who 'believe this statement to be correct'. Again he threatened to return home, but softened it with a reminder of his enfeebled state: 'as soon as I am abel to be moved'. Earlier in the year, Earl had bargained with the Bradford overseer that if they agreed to May's request, he would not need any more relief that year. It would not be over-reading this later letter to suggest that Earl had to find extra ways to enhance the legitimacy of his new application. Thus, while he listed quite legitimate problems (lack of trade, no prospect of trade, the search for trade hampered by lack of clothing), it was a 'misforten', an injury sustained while doing his civic and familial duty, which has driven Earl to break his promise. In normal circumstances a physical injury such as broken ribs may have been sufficient to qualify a father of five for help, but in the light of his previous pledge to survive unaided the appeal required extensive background detail. This is a strong example of the development of rhetoric by a serial letter-writer. Earl had to remember and refer to his own previous correspondence, assume that the vestry would also remember it and modify his current claim in the light of his earlier one.[52]

Illness took a central role in the following letter too. In that of 8 October 1834,[53] Earl reported that the whole family had suffered from a severe 'bowell complaint': Thomas had been 'Very ill this Last week', and 'Thorsday Last my wife was taken in the night in the Same Complaint' so severely they feared for her life, and two of the children were 'Very bad'. Earl repeated his earlier rhetorical technique of being very specific about the details of the misfortune; rather than simply stating that the entire family had suffered he listed each individually, giving timings and severity, and importantly describing details of treatment undertaken. Martha Earl, in danger of her life, took some Daffey's Elixir and recovered a little. For a family in poverty this was significant – proprietary medicines were not cheap – but such a reference also served a rhetorical purpose, highlighting recourse to self-dosing before consulting the (even more expensive) doctor. The letter continued with more descriptions of the failure of the Earl's garden (an attempt to shift for themselves), and with another threat to come home, balanced by the promise of work in the future if they were allowed enough relief to tide them over until the railway was started. Earl also applied pressure by stating how good the local overseer have been, writing to Bradford on Earl's behalf and even trying to see the Bradford overseers (without success) when passing through.

By 19 January 1835[54] Earl has progressed from paying for proprietary medicines to the engagement of not one but two doctors. While the previous precision as to the nature of illnesses was missing from his letter of this date, timings were again very specific:

> My wife has been ill and Under The Doctor's hands this last three months and is now Very ill and our daughter was taken very bad on friday after Chrismas day and is under a nother doctors hand but she is a Little beter and I have been very bad in the bowl Complaint but am now beter.

Earl's letter was considerably briefer than his usual narrative style. The family health problems took centre stage, with Thomas simply stating that there was no work to be had and his family was in 'a starving state'. There was no explanation as to why the daughter was treated by a different doctor, or intimation of what Martha's prognosis might be. Nor was there a request for money to pay the two physicians. Earlier letters often mentioned specific sums of money or bills which needed paying, allied with descriptions of why Earl was unable to meet them himself. This letter simply stated the gravity of his family's situation, and assumed this to be sufficient evidence of their need.

The final extant letter was written in March 1835.[55] Over the last two years Martha Earl had progressed from being not 'abel to get out of Dors'[56] to being ' a great measure restored to health',[57] then 'never well',[58] 'very ill',[59] so ill they 'thought she Ould have died',[60] 'under the Doctor's hands . . . and is now Very ill',[61] through to 'bedridden . . . [and] at the point of Death'.[62] She had been attended at least three times by doctors, including at the dispensary, and yet the only time Thomas Earl's application was supported by a doctor's note (20 May 1833), Dr Fowler only referred to 'an illness which produced great debility'.[63] In this final letter Earl seemed to struggle, for the first time, to convey the gravity of his situation. He repeated the fact that his wife was at death's door, his two youngest children were not expected to last the week, that he went out to sell his 'sweetmeats' but that it brought in little money, and that if Bradford would not help him then he would be brought 'home'. Despite Martha's continuing illness, Earl was unable to get the doctor to give him a note, as 'if it was known that we had aney thing from our parish They Could not be allowed the privilege of a Letter from the Despensary'. There was movement here away from the apparently carefully constructed earlier letters, where Earl made his case strategically, conscious of previous promises and references, giving details of ill-health in a judicious and effective way. Here, for the first time, the language and construction resonated desperation. The postscript was particularly telling, asking the overseer to contact Martha's sister to let her know that his wife is seriously ill, and that she had better come and see her.

Where Earl's letters had built upon each other up to this point, forming a series which progressed in a coherent fashion, being both self-referential and developmental, this final letter broke the pattern. Previously Earl's own illnesses and injuries prevented him working, or his wife's maladies illustrated his compounded problems. In this last letter, Earl effectively echoed William King: it was the psychological impact, the oppression, of poverty and illness and of being unable to look after his family, which formed the emotional lever of this narrative. His wife's chronic illness, so much a feature of earlier correspondence, was no longer an adjunct, but the central theme. Martha was at death's door, and 'what Little her Stomake will take I Cant Get for her'. This is the last surviving letter from Thomas Earl, and it reads as such. There is a finality to it which implies he had exhausted his literary ingenuity. He summed up: 'Gentlemen I have nothing more to say but beg for a Speedy ancer what to do.'

The Brand family represent a very different narrative and poverty-type. Over a series of six letters written between June 1827 and October 1829[64] first William and then Elizabeth Brand of east London pursued the parish of Thrapston (Northamptonshire) for relief 'due' to Sarah Pole, Mrs Brand's mother. These letters are particularly interesting as they were written not by the claimant herself but by the carers of a Thrapston pauper. Thus they carry no language of supplication (other than the formal niceties of 'your humble servant' and 'I beg the favour') and, in the first instance, no reference to deservingness, threats to return home or illustrative detail as to the socially demeaning affects of poverty and illness. Instead the Brands wrote with the language of right. They looked after Sarah Pole, using money issued to her by the parish to which she belonged. It was *her* money, her due, which they were requesting. However, in order to add moral and practical urgency to the request for the cash, both Brand and his wife developed in these letters a narrative about the physical frailty of Mrs Pole, and the expense this *added* to looking after her. Although they did ask for extra cash due to her illness, it was not the main issue; they only used that illness as a point to add leverage to their demand for money owed.

In the first letter[65] (undated, but it appears in the letter book between letters of 30 November and 15 December 1826), William Brand set out his position in unemotional and businesslike terms: 'I am under the necessity of writing to you respecting my wife's mother who receives a weekly allowance from your parish I should be obliged by a remittance by Mr Jno. Mays'. It is clear that Brand was treating this as a financial arrangement rather than a nurturing one. The money was due to his mother-in-law, and it was from 'your' parish, the implication very obviously that the responsibility for her keep lay with Thrapston. Brand then gave instructions as to how he would like to receive this money; the word 'remittance' is notable as this is usually employed by overseers. It is a term of bureaucracy rather entreaty, aligning Brand with the parish authorities rather than the pauper in question. He conveyed the need for the (owed) money not by asking for sympathy for Sarah Pole's afflicted – and therefore deserving – state, but by noting that this illness was costing large amounts of money in drugs ('her continued illness often requires the whole sum per week for medicine'), money which it was not the duty of the Brands to spend. The only note of personal appeal in this first letter ('my business being very dead I find it impossible to keep her and my family too') distanced Brand from responsibility for his mother-in-law. He was *not* a pauper and she was most definitely an adjunct part of the household. The letter ended with the confident statement 'Shall therefore expect to here from you soon as possible', Brand being secure in the knowledge that this was not a request for alms, but to all intents and purposes a bill.

The second letter concerning Sarah Pole, in August 1827[66] came from the daughter, whose approach was rather less detached. Mrs Brand wrote concerning money *outstanding*: 'Having requested the favour of Mr Mays for this 3 weeks past to ask you to be so kind as to send my mother's money but have been disappointed.' The tone here was less one of business and more one of feeling wronged. She had frequently spoken to the carrier, Mr Mays, concerning her mother, and asked him to convey both letters and verbal messages about Sarah Pole's 'afflicted state'. Later in this second letter Elizabeth Brand modified her statement that the money was her mother's, asking the overseer to 'send me something'. The letter concluded by subtly chastising the overseers. Claiming to have reiterated her mother's illness to Mays, she put the words of criticism into his mouth, saying that '[he] think it not behaving with that generosity he expected from the gentlemen of Thrapston'. Elizabeth used Mays – presumably a trusted agent of the overseers as he conveyed money and messages between Thrapston and London – to support her case. She was merely 'disappointed' not to have received money in the light of repeated descriptions of her mother's affliction, whereas upon hearing the story Mr Mays felt that the overseers of Thrapston had behaved parsimoniously. This was a rhetorically skilled letter.

Six months later,[67] Elizabeth Brand was again chasing the Thrapston overseers for money 'due for the use of my mother', reverting to the purely financial approach adopted by her husband in the first narrative. She set out money paid, money due (£6) and the method by which she wished to receive it. She made it clear that this was not a begging letter; she was merely arranging to be paid for a bill. However, this straightforward, businesslike, tone began to dissipate with her next letter. On the 23 February she wrote:

> I went to meet Mr Mayes in Smithfield and feel myself much disappointed as my mother is a poor invalid and supporting of her is the means of keeping me very much behind hand hope you will consider it in the right light and remit me a trifle more in addition to what is my due there is £6:0:0 this day 23rd Feb 1828 for the use of my mother I hope if any of the gentlemen have himself in London they would be kind enough to call and see my aged mother and then they will find I have send the truth she is a poor object of charity I will be sure to meet the Wagoner on Saturday next I have a long way to come I hope I shall not be disappointed.[68]

The fact of her mother's frailty came much earlier in this letter; not as additional evidence in the demand for money owed, but as the reason for it. There was criticism implicit in the description of her mother as a 'poor invalid' and the fact that the 'supporting of her' was preventing the Brands from moving forward; Thrapston's laxness not only neglected their 'poor object of charity', but also had an adverse affect upon the lives of those who looked after her in their stead, making them out of pocket and inconvenienced ('I have a long way to come'). In the previous letter, Elizabeth adopted the semi-official language of her husband's first, casting the Brands in the role of partners with the parish in the duty of caring for an elderly parishioner. In this later letter, and in the face of being apparently disregarded by the overseers, Elizabeth's tone moved towards one of accusation. She had been denied her 'due', and suspected that Thrapston doubted the veracity of her claim to extra money on account of her mother's illness, inviting any of the 'gentlemen' to come to London and confirm that she did 'send the truth'. While up to this point Elizabeth Brand did not overtly refer to her, or rather her mother's, *right* to financial aid from the parish (other than calling it her 'due'), there was an undertone of expectation. Elizabeth hoped that the overseers would consider her claims 'in the right light'.

The final letters in the Brand series were written in August and September,[69] again taking the form of a 'bill' and a follow up. At the end of August Elizabeth wrote with an itemized account of money owed, stating times (29 November 1828 to 3 September 1829) and amount (£8). Accepting that it might not be possible to send the money immediately, Elizabeth requested an indication of when she would receive it: 'you would oblige me by writing a line when you can send it, as it is very ill convenient to wait week after week on Mr Maze and not get it'.[70] As with the first letter, there was no supplication, no description of why her mother needed the money (it was 'due') and no promises of undying gratitude. The letter was almost word-for-word in the pattern of those written between overseers themselves when arranging 'remittances' between parishes. If anything, this letter was slightly *less* courteous, it being clear that the Brands considered themselves to be acting beyond the call of duty in their support of Sarah Pole. Indeed,

Elizabeth repeated her criticism of the parish, stating the trouble which she was put to even waiting to receive her mother's money. One month later the Thrapston overseers had still not sent the cash, and in a style apparently unique in letters about relief, Elizabeth expressed her indignation:

> We are astonished that you have not sent up the money due to my Mother Sarah Pole as it is now getting a great deal over the time, I shall expect you will send the money without fail on Saturday next.
> Your humble servant etc
> E Brand[71]

It is quite clear that Elizabeth felt that this money was *owed* to her mother, not a gift or charity. 'Disappointed' had changed to 'astonished' – an expression of surprise and frustrated expectation rather than dashed hope – and her hitherto implied criticism of the workings of Thrapston bureaucracy became more overt. She now expected (contrary to all former experience) she would be sent the money 'without fail' the following Saturday.

Although this last letter did not mention her mother's sickness, it is a clear demonstration of the assumption of a right to relief. In previous correspondence Elizabeth Brand has employed all manner of tactics to extract what was clearly a long-standing allowance from her mother's home parish, with limited success. She had not once, however, resorted to the cajoling, supplicant tone of the vast majority of other sick and distressed applicants. When she referred to her mother's affliction it was to provoke shame in the overseers, not pity. She accused them of neglecting their duty to an aged parishioner. Rather than using her mother's frailty as a lever of pathos (such as 'take pity on my poor sick mother') she was much more forceful in her rhetoric (along the lines of 'how dare you ignore my poor sick mother?').

Conclusion

The importance of effective written language to paupers living away from their settled parishes cannot be overestimated. When faced with abject destitution the only potential source of relief was a group of distant officials who were unable to witness their misery at first hand. Thus the letters of such paupers had to perform a range of functions, not only convincing overseers of the applicant's legitimacy, deservingness and veracity, but also developing a linguistic register which added emotional weight to their application. Indeed, at a time when ill-health was the prevalent state and the recipients of such letters were just as likely to be suffering from a debilitating range of conditions as the senders, a considerable rhetorical ability was vital. It is clear from the examples set out above that simple statements of incapacity were not considered adequate qualification for relief – the psychological and social impact of ill-health flesh out the narratives in the vast majority of applications. Loss of dignity, compromising of social connections and simple 'distress' loom large, even when – as seen through King and Earl – the writer or his family were under the attention of the doctor and therefore incontrovertibly ill. Along with loss of earnings, added expenditure and the inherent misery of sickness, the poor felt the need to justify applications with extensive circumstantial evidence. Whether it was William King's 'Gret affliction of Mind' at the prospect of being dependent, Thomas Earl's punishing struggle to purchase nourishing food for his ailing wife ('what Little her Stomake will take I Cant Get for her'), or Elizabeth Brand's being kept 'very much behind hand' by Thrapston's laxity in paying her 'poor invalid' mother's pension, circumstantial evidence could be very important.

In short, the out-parish poor were by no means without tools in the negotiation of relief. Where those who applied in person could demonstrate the physical evidence of their afflictions, letter writers had financial and social leverage at their disposal. Threats to return home with extensive and expensive families, and contrasting the humanity of local – yet legally unobliged – authorities with the behaviour of their home parish, are common strategies throughout the sample. Elizabeth Brand's invocation of a third party's poor opinion of an administration's behaviour is more unusual, but by no means unique. More importantly, it is clear from our serial letter writers that rhetorical strategies developed over a number of letters. The out-parish poor expected their plight to be remembered from one letter to the next, and they consistently sought to generalize the specific reason for writing into a wider case for ongoing or supplemental relief. Indeed, many of the letter series are rhetorically sophisticated. What is also significant is that the out-parish poor expected that, if they approached the issue in the right way, their letters to be successful. While the language of rights is rarely seen in pauper letters, except perhaps where parishes were perceived to be reneging on their commitments, the underlying expectation of a favourable hearing, empathy, humanity and care for a fellow parishioner is resolutely clear in these pauper narratives. While the poor in general may have been losing their legitimacy in the eyes of ratepayers in early nineteenth-century England, we must be wary of suggesting the same for the sick poor.

Notes

1 On the British settlement laws, see Snell, K. D. M (2006), *Parish and Belonging: Community Identity and Welfare in England and Wales 1700–1950*. Cambridge: Cambridge University Press.

2 For Walter Keeling and references to the letters used here, see King, S., Nutt, T. and Tomkins, A. (2006), *Narratives of the Poor in Eighteenth-Century Britain, Volume 1: Voices of the Poor: Poor Law Depositions and Letters*. London: Pickering and Chatto, pp. 219–23.

3 On petitions and comparative material, see Fontaine, L. and Schlumbohm, J. (eds) (2000), *Household Strategies for Survival 1600–2000*. Cambridge: Cambridge

University Press; and van Voss, L-H. (ed.) (2001), *Petitions in Social History*. Cambridge: Cambridge University Press.

4 See contributions to Raven, J., Small, H. and Tadmor, N. (eds) (1996), *The Practice and Representation of Reading in England*. Cambridge: Cambridge University Press.

5 England and Wales were subject to the same welfare laws from 1601 onwards.

6 Pooley, C. and Turnbull, J. (1998), *Migration and Mobility in Britain Since the Eighteenth Century*. London: UCL Press.

7 Hitchcock, T. King, P. and Sharpe, P. (eds) (1997), *Chronicling Poverty: The Voices and Strategies of the English Poor 1640–1840*. Basingstoke: Macmillan; Fontaine and Schlumbohm, *Household Strategies*; King, Nutt and Tomkins, *Narratives of the Poor*; Sokoll, T. (2001), *Essex Pauper Letters 1731–1837*. Oxford: Oxford University Press.

8 Not to be confused with settlement certificates. By 1800 the ability of English and Welsh parishes to issue settlement certificates – pieces of paper acknowledging that a migrant and their family 'belonged' to the parish issuing the certificate and that the parish would pay relief if the person slipped into poverty – had been in place for more than a century.

9 Williamson, J. G. (1990), *Coping with City Growth During the British Industrial Revolution*. Cambridge: Cambridge University Press.

10 Hutter, M. (2007) '"Visual Credit": The Britannia Vignette on the notes of the Bank of England', in Cox, F. and Schmidt-Hansa, H. (eds), *Money and Culture*. Frankfurt: Peter Lang, pp. 15–36.

11 On the Scottish welfare system and poor law, see Mitchison, R. (2001), *The Old Poor Law in Scotland: The Experience of Poverty, 1574–1845*. Edinburgh: Edinburgh University Press.

12 See Gestrich, A. and Stewart, J. (2007), 'Unemployment and poor relief in the West of Scotland, 1870–1900', in King, S. and Stewart, J. (eds), *Welfare Peripheries*. Frankfurt: Peter Lang, pp. 125–48.

13 Because the pauper acknowledged Scottish roots or because their names were Scottish.

14 Sokoll, T. (2006), 'Writing for relief: rhetoric in English pauper letters 1800–34', in Gestrich, A., King, S. and Raphael, L. (eds), *Being Poor in Modern Europe*. Frankfurt: Peter Lang, pp. 91–112.

15 See Pooley and Turnbull, *Migration and Mobility*.

16 King, S. (2008), 'Friendship, kinship and belonging in the letters of urban paupers 1800–40', *Historical Social Research*, 33, 249–77.

17 See chapter 3.

18 Hindle, S. (2004), *On the Parish? The Micro-Politics of Poor Relief in Rural England 1550–1750*. Oxford: Oxford University Press.

19 King, S. (2007), 'Regional patterns in the experiences and treatment of the sick poor, 1800–40: rights, obligations and duties in the rhetoric of paupers', *Family and Community History*, 10, 28–49.

20 For references to the individual letters, see King, Nutt and Tomkins, *Narratives of the Poor*, pp. 219–23.

21 Ibid.

22 Ibid.

23 Ibid.

24 A major project on pauper narratives in Germany is currently being coordinated by Professor Andreas Gestrich at the German Historical Institute, London.

25 King, S. and Stewart, J (2001), 'The history of the poor law in Wales: Under-researched, full of potential', *Archives*, 36, 134–48.

26 He was possibly a cobbler. In a letter of 12 March 1830, he mentions that he 'might Mend ore Make a few Slop womans Shoes'. See Sokoll, *Essex Pauper Letters*, p. 122.

27 Ibid., pp. 111, 116–17,118–19, 120–2, 124–5, 131–4, 139–40, 143, 147–50.

28 There is not the space here to discuss how contemporaries might have conceived of and labelled sickness.

29 This description comes as a postscript rather than in direct conjunction with the illness described in the letter. There are implicit warnings here: 'skilfull' probably meant to imply that the doctor would be expensive, but the fact that he had done King's wife good might be interpreted as value for money. See Sokoll, *Essex Pauper Letters*, pp. 111–12.

30 Sokoll, *Essex Pauper Letters*, p. 116.

31 Ibid.

32 Ibid., 120. It is unclear if King survived nine months without aid or if and intervening letter has been lost.

33 Ibid., p. 121.

34 Ibid.

35 Ibid., p. 131.

36 Ibid., p. 133, 18 October 1832.

37 Ibid., p. 139, 11 May 1833.

38 Ibid.

39 Ibid., p. 143.

40 The exception was when the whole family suffered an infectious illness in 1833. See Sokoll, *Essex Pauper Letters*, p. 139.

41 Ibid., p. 147.

42 Ibid., p. 148, 31 July 1834.

43 Ibid., p. 149, September 1834.

44 Ibid., p. 121.

45 Hurley, B (2004), *Bradford on Avon Applications for Relief From Out of Town Strays*. Devizes: Wiltshire Family History Society.

46 Ibid., p. 17.

47 Ibid., p. 15.

48 Ibid.

49 Ibid.

50 The implication is reinforced by a note from Martha's doctor, R. Fowler, saying that she had been very ill and was only just on the road to recovery.

51 Hurley, *Bradford on Avon*, p. 16.

52 Earl was successful, being awarded his usual relief of 20 shillings.

53 Hurley, *Bradford on Avon*, p. 17.

54 Ibid., p. 18.

55 Ibid., p. 19.

56 Ibid., p. 15, 24 February 1833.

57 Ibid., p. 15, 20 May 1833.

58 Ibid., p. 16, 22 March 1834.

59 Ibid., p. 17, May 1834, in a letter written to his sister.

60 Ibid., p. 17, 8 October 1834.

61 Ibid., p. 18, 19 January 1835.

62 Ibid., p. 19, 4 March 1835.

63 Ibid., p. 16.

64 Northamptonshire Record Office 325P/194, 'Thrapston Letter Book'.

65 Ibid., letter 44.

66 Ibid., letter 81.

67 Ibid., letter 109.

68 Ibid., letter 110.

69 Ibid., letter 119. Dating on letters is awry here suggesting some error in the binding.

70 Ibid., letter 144.

71 Ibid., letter 147.

5

Poverty and epidemics: Perceptions of the poor at times of Cholera in Germany and Spain, 1830s–1860s

Beate Althammer

Introduction

'Asiatic' cholera caused shockwaves when it first appeared on the European borders in the early 1830s. Originally this epidemic disease had only been known on the Indian subcontinent, and although it had begun to spread over large parts of Asia and the Near East in the early nineteenth century, European worries had not yet arisen. Europe, a fortress of progress and civilization, so many had believed, would not be affected by the nasty and dirty sickness from the swamps of Bengal. But when cholera broke out in Russian Poland and crossed to the eastern provinces of Prussia in 1831, public concern was enormous, even in regions much further to the west. Rumours were disseminated, public prayers held. Hundreds of books, pamphlets and newspaper articles were published on this new threat that frightened and at the same time fascinated the collective imagination. Cholera seemed to be not just another normal malady, but rather an approaching disaster, something like a new form of plague. It developed very fast and violently. The symptoms were drastic and revolting. Half of those falling sick died, often within hours. Authorities developed frantic countermeasures but were seemingly unable to stop the disease. For the medical profession it was a severe setback: none of the many propagated preventive and therapeutic remedies really helped, and – until after the bacteriological turn of the 1880s – no agreement could be achieved about causation or transmission.

Historians have written extensively on cholera, but at least in German historiography – which has turned to the subject later than its British or French counterparts – the focus remains limited. Several studies have described the first outbreak in eastern Prussia in the summer of 1831, state policy to contain it and reactions of the population during the initial turbulent month of cholera-hysteria.[1] Other studies have been devoted to the famous Hamburg epidemic of 1892, the last in Germany, during which perceptions and reactions were already strongly influenced by the new bacteriological paradigm.[2] But very little attention has been paid to the period inbetween.[3] Reflecting this lacunae, the picture of German, and especially Prussian, policies to control epidemic disease has been distorted. Drawing on Ackerknecht's theory that there was an affinity between conservative regimes and contagionist disease control on the one hand, Liberal convictions and anti-contagionist explanations of epidemic disease on the other,[4] Prussia is commonly presented as a classic example of poor public-health planning. Right up until the most recent contribution to German cholera history, the study of Olaf Briese,[5] Prussia has been described as an authoritarian state that clung to contagionism and consequently to repressive, bureaucratic and militaristic strategies of disease control, with devastating collateral effects for the poorer parts of the population.

There is some truth in such assertions. Prussia, like most other European states, at first adopted a contagionist position. It was then generally believed that cholera was a contagious disease caused by a substance transmitted from person-to-person or through objects. Correspondingly, in the summer of 1831 the Prussian government mobilized the same measures of containment as had been used effectively against plague in early modern Europe. Military cordons were set up along the eastern frontier and could only be passed after long quarantines. When this first line of defence failed whole cities and regions were quarantined; the sick were forcibly isolated in hospitals and the dead hastily buried in separate graveyards. By the 1880s the Prussian state was a strong supporter of the rise of bacteriological explanations of disease, which gave new legitimacy to controlling and isolating measures at times of epidemics. This new approach was equally infused with militaristic rhetoric: like the old contagion, the bacterium was an external material foe that had to be warded off, combated and exterminated.[6] Yet, contagionism did not lead to bacteriology in any linear fashion. The middle decades of the nineteenth century were dominated by anti-contagionist theory in Germany as well as in other parts of Europe. Even in late 1831, while the first cholera pandemic was still in progress, the Prussian government revoked most of the compulsory measures which had proved unsuccessful in stopping the disease but were causing serious harm to the economy. By the time cholera reached the western provinces in summer 1832, military cordons were already history and during the following pandemics of the 1840s, 1850s and 1860s there were no restrictions to mobility, little by way of quarantine measures and no separate graveyards. Although Prussian laws always maintained a moderate contagionist stance, practice completely adapted to the anti-contagionist convictions propagated by most of the medical profession in the mid-nineteenth century.[7] These anti-contagionist theories were heterogeneous, ranging from belief in cosmic or telluric phenomena corrupting the atmosphere to the assumption that local pollution from swamps, sewers, latrines and all kinds of filth triggered epidemics. Their common ground was the ancient notion of miasmas and their common conclusion was that isolation and quarantine were useless because no person-to-person transmission had to be feared.

Debates between contagionists and anti-contagionists are an established theme in medical history. But what consequences did swings in contemporary scientific theory and state policy have for public perceptions of and reactions to cholera in the middle decades of the nineteenth century? One reason why the pandemics of the 1840s, 1850s and 1860s have been studied much less than the first (1831) and last (1892) is perhaps that they generated fewer written sources. Official and public attention seems to have fallen off, anxieties cooled. But how is this to be explained? The most evident reason is that cholera turned out to be less murderous than initially feared. It was no second plague and rarely killed more than 3 per cent of the population of any locality; most regions lost many fewer inhabitants or were not touched at all. Nonetheless, cholera remained dangerous and in Prussia the objective risk did not diminish. On the contrary, the number of victims rose with each new epidemic wave and the last state-wide cholera pandemic of 1866–7 was the worst of all. Still it generated surprisingly little comment when compared to 1831. It has been argued by some historians that the population simply 'got used' to cholera. Others have suggested that helplessness in the face of the disease led to fatalism and silence, or that after the initial cholera-panic a more rational attitude was adopted. A widespread, though often only indirectly implied, assumption is that the abolition of drastic contagionist containment measures enabled a more relaxed attitude. These, in part contradictory, explanations indicate that in fact very little is really known about the mid-nineteenth century epidemics.

This chapter addresses social reactions to cholera, and especially the narrative patterns developed to analyse the disease, using a comparative approach. Initially it will focus on the most western province of Prussia, the Rhine Province, and especially on its two largest cities, Cologne and Aachen, with 90,000 and 50,000 inhabitants respectively in the mid-nineteenth century. The first pandemic reached the region in the summer of 1832 and mainly affected Aachen, generating a mortality rate of about 7:1000, while the rest of the province was largely spared. The following pandemic waves caused more casualties. In 1849 Cologne witnessed 1,450 deaths, more than 16:1000 of the population.[8] Aachen lost a moderate 4.3:1000, but the directly adjoining suburb of Burtscheid suffered a mortality rate of 27:1000 and in 1866 another 18:1000. Neighbouring industrial towns like Elberfeld, Barmen and Essen also experienced mortality rates of up to 20:1000. Despite the fact that the threat from cholera was, objectively measured, increasing, public concern faded. Never again was there so much discussion and rumour about cholera as in 1831, when the disease had not yet reached the province. It will be argued that this attitude was connected to prevailing perceptions of cholera as a disease of the poor, a perception that also shaped the measures of medical and material relief organized.

In a second section, reactions to cholera in the Rhine Province will be contrasted with those in Barcelona, in the north-eastern Spanish region of Catalonia. Its socio-economic structures were not so very different: like the Prussian Rhine Province, Catalonia was among the early industrializing regions of continental Europe, and Barcelona was an important industrial and commercial city, with about 170,000 inhabitants in mid-century. There was a similar polarization between rich and poor to Aachen or Cologne, and the local bourgeoisie was just as influenced by capitalist convictions. Yet, reactions to cholera were completely different. Anxieties ratcheted up rather than down, and mid-nineteenth-century epidemics caused extraordinary panic and mass flights from the city. This contrasting pattern of behaviour, it will be argued, cannot be explained by a divergent scientific knowledge or containment policy, for the anti-contagionist paradigm was accepted in Spain as clearly as it was in Germany. Nor does the fact of higher mortality rates (see Table 5.1) in Barcelona in and of itself offer an adequate explanation.[9] Rather, the chapter will argue, different social relations and perceptions of the poor strongly influenced reactions to cholera. We will in short be dealing with narratives about the poor and their place in local society. While the focus is slightly different to other chapters in the volume, narratives about the poor are, as the editors argue in their introduction, crucial to an understanding both of the genealogy of language in pauper narratives and the agency of the poor themselves.

Table 5.1 Cholera mortality in Cologne, Aachen and Barcelona (absolute numbers and per 1000 of population)

Cologne			Aachen			Barcelona		
Year	Deaths	‰	Year	Deaths	‰	Year	Deaths	‰
1832	1	0.0	1832/3	269	6.9	1834	3,521	30
1849	1,450	16.1	1849	216	4.3	–	–	–
1854/5	15	0.1	1855	115	2.1	1854	4,800	27
1866/7	858	6.9	1866	152	2.3	1865	2,200	11

Aachen and Cologne

When news arrived in the summer of 1831 that the military cordon on the eastern border of Prussia had failed and that cholera was spreading, the disease – although still far away – became the talk of the day among the population of the Rhine Province. The regional authorities were seriously worried, sure that the industrial cities in the Prussian west were extremely vulnerable to cholera because of their large pauperized working classes whose living conditions had been undermined by high food prices and unemployment in the preceding years. The medical officer of Aachen predicted that the epidemic 'would rage terribly among our 13,000 poor' and that more victims were to be expected than in the towns of eastern Prussia, where there were 'no factories and by far fewer needy and impoverished people'. If factories closed down during a cholera outbreak, he warned, the number of destitute, 'who, as experience has shown, must be very predisposed to absorb the contagium', would rise even further.[10]

The provincial authorities pressed local administrations to prepare early for the pending catastrophe. Already in the summer of 1831 sanitary boards had been constituted in the larger cities. These boards planned hospital facilities and the then still prescribed isolation and quarantine measures, but also discussed how the living conditions of the poor could be ameliorated in order to strengthen their resistance. The city representatives on these boards were unenthusiastic from the start because everything had to be paid for out of local funds, but for some weeks in the autumn of 1831 they were nonetheless willing to seriously consider far-reaching plans. Thus, the sanitary board of Aachen talked about distributing cheap food and warm clothing, subsidizing rents and even building barracks to supply additional housing for poor families.

As winter came, however, all such ambitious and expensive plans lapsed, never to be revived. The Aachen sanitary board justified the burial of its crisis plans with the argument that cholera was not developing as dramatically as initially feared: the 'character' of the disease seemed to be weakening as it travelled west, and it might not reach the Rhine Province at all. Besides, the general economic outlook was more favourable: factories were resuming production and food prices were falling so that no large-scale support of the poor would be necessary even if cholera should emerge in the city.[11] The municipal authorities did not deny that misery among the lower classes remained but, as the Aachen poor relief administration argued, trying to change this was pointless because of 'the way of life of the local poor' who would only misuse donations: if they were given warm clothing they would pawn it, and if soup kitchens were established they would sell the food, feed it to pigs or even throw it away since it was not to their liking.[12]

Clearly, the local authorities were trying to absolve themselves from action by downplaying the danger and heaping the blame for poverty on the unreasonableness of the poor. Their superiors in the district government initially warned against ceasing preparations but eventually consented. Even when cholera was coming dangerously close in early summer 1832, now from the west, from France and Belgium, countermeasures were only resumed on a very limited, strictly medical, level. There was no more talk about improving the material conditions of the poor to strengthen their resistance, about the danger of factory closures or the necessity of supporting thousands of unemployed. Both authorities and the general public behaved more calmly than in the previous autumn: there were no alarmist rumours, no special prayers held,[13] and when cholera actually broke out in Aachen at the start of September 1832 everyone seemed determined to hang on to the normalities of life.

In fact, cholera passed Aachen without causing any notable disturbances in public life. There was no disruption in business, schooling, theatre performances or other social events. The same is true for the later epidemics of 1849, 1855 and 1866. Especially in 1849 there was a marked tendency in Aachen to deny the very existence of a local outbreak: the city authorities remained silent and the newspapers joined this endeavour by not reporting local cholera deaths. Even in retrospect the town council asserted that only a few scattered cases had occurred in Aachen.[14] In Cologne it was not so easy to ignore cholera completely that same summer, since the number of deaths rose dramatically from the end of July: at the peak of the epidemic there were more than 50 burials per day, as against a trend of six or seven in 'normal' periods. Nonetheless, authorities and newspapers played down the epidemic as much as possible. The leading local paper, the *Kölnische Zeitung*, did not comment on the ongoing epidemic for weeks; when it finally broke its silence in mid-August, it was only to complain that the non-local press was unscrupulously exaggerating the state of illness in Cologne. In truth, it asserted, the epidemic was developing very mildly: 'It can therefore only make the local resident smile when he hears that some people even let themselves be deterred from visiting Cologne by these distorted reports, while in the same Cologne fear of the illness has almost disappeared.'[15]

The determination not to let cholera disturb normality was successful in Cologne as well as in Aachen.[16] Apart from some advertisements in local papers for 'remedies against cholera', almost the only outward sign that something unusual and troubling was occurring was an intensified practice of piety by parts of the population. A parish brotherhood, for example, organized a procession to ward off cholera in mid-July 1849. This did not, however, please the local authorities: they asked the archbishop to stop such religious demonstrations, since they would harm the health of participants and make a depressing impression on the public.[17] Another parish called for contributions to a church-building project as a work of repentance in order to stop Divine punishment.[18] And in the last phase of the 1849 epidemic, the parish of Saint Severin, which had suffered badly, celebrated its patron saint's feast much more extensively and solemnly than usual.[19] These certainly were signs that parts of the population were morally shaken by cholera and that at least some priests and stout Catholics were willing to acknowledge this fact, using it at the same time to promote piety. Nonetheless, the impact of the disease on civic life remained muted.

One important factor that helped the middle and upper classes to downplay cholera was the conviction that it mainly affected poor people. Countless official reports, medical tracts and newspaper articles steadily repeated this argument, thereby implying that the upper strata of society were quite safe. Not material poverty alone, but a slovenly, disorderly and intemperate lifestyle was depicted as the prime reason for infection. An Aachen newspaper, for example, had reported in the autumn of 1831 that the first cholera victims in the east Prussian city of Königsberg were 'very poor people devoted to drink' who tended to a repulsive greediness and had devoured 'stinky fish'.[20] After cholera had actually reached Aachen in summer 1832, the local physician, Joseph Hartung, assured his middle-class patients that the well-to-do were affected only 'by way of exception'; he was convinced that the poor were almost exclusively affected because of their abundant consumption of indigestible food.[21] In July 1849, when cholera was threatening Cologne, local newspapers asserted that everywhere so far 'poor, badly nourished individuals addicted to alcohol, crowded together in unventilated streets and flats', were the prime victims, while from among the rich 'almost only those are snatched who wilfully provoked the illness'.[22] One stated that 'cholera is, with irrelevant exceptions, an illness of the proletariat'.[23] Many similar narrative claims from the 1850s and 1860s could be cited. Newspaper commentators were not necessarily pitiless towards the poor: some explicitly stated that social conditions were to be blamed. But this did not change the general impression that only the lower classes were easy prey for cholera.

This impression was soon adapted likewise by leftist authors, who presented themselves as defenders of the poor. At the beginning of the 1849 epidemic Cologne's *Westdeutsche Zeitung* still defiantly asked, referring to the passive attitude of the local authorities, 'does the town council maybe believe cholera would make a difference between its members and the proletarian?'.[24] However, a few days later it had changed its mind and asserted that 'the old observation holds good that almost exclusively the proletariat is afflicted by the epidemic'.[25] It concluded, although in the rhetoric of class struggle: 'Remember, proletarian! It is a proletarian sickness, and what do the moneybags care about the poor!'[26]

The officers of the provincial administration were not always comfortable with this characterization of cholera as a sickness affecting solely the lower classes. Indeed initially in 1831 they even tried to suppress such newspaper articles[27] because they feared the poor might be upset and the rich would lose all interest in preventative measures. Later, however, the same provincial officers adopted similar arguments pointing not only to material distress, but also to the bad habits of the poor. During the epidemic of 1832 the district government of Aachen asserted that not lack of work and wages, 'but disorderliness, laziness, ignorance and uselessness owing to lack of skill' were the main reasons for the widespread poverty which was promoting cholera.[28] The district government of Cologne reported during the epidemic of 1849 that many poor people were succumbing because they were 'ignoring all advice and continuing a most irregular way of life'. Material or medical help were not lacking, it was just that 'it was not possible to regulate these crude people and to bring them to properly use the support so friendly offered to them'.[29]

As highlighted above, cholera had been closely associated with poverty from the start but these narratives mark a notable shift in emphasis. In 1831, when cholera had not yet reached the Rhine Province but was perceived as a general threat, the ruling classes had been willing to do something against material distress to ward off the epidemic. They were willing to do so not only out of humanitarian feelings for the poor, but because they feared for their own safety: cholera might spread from the poor to the wealthy and provoke economic disturbances and consequently social unrest. When such fears faded, the narrative of cholera as a sweeping catastrophe became inconvenient in the eyes of opinion leaders. Not cholera but this narrative seemed to be endangering business and social stability. From 1832 onwards, the urban ruling classes did everything possible to ignore or at least to play down the disease. To do this successfully, however, they first of all had to dominate their own individual fears of infection. These fears had not simply vanished, but they could be contained by steadily repeating in public narratives that only the others, the poor, the foolish and disorderly, were endangered. The more depraved cholera victims were depicted, the safer honourable citizens could feel. At the same time they could excuse themselves from expensive preventive and relief measures, which would only cause a stir without helping against the habits oft the poor.

Scientific theory sustained these contentions and thus helped the upper classes to suppress their fears. Contagionists and anti-contagionists agreed that the individual constitution was a crucial factor in explaining why only some inhabitants of an affected locality fell ill at times of epidemic. Insufficient food, defective clothing, overcrowding and filth, but also all kinds of extremes and excesses, were considered as important predisposing causes that weakened the body, making it susceptible to contagions or miasmas. This theory of predisposing causes was rooted in ancient humoralism and had taken a new life in the eighteenth century, fitting well with enlightened notions of individual responsibility and control over ones own fate.[30] It became a dogma during the cholera decades of the mid-nineteenth century as authorities and physicians all over Europe recommended a regular, clean, well-balanced and moderate way of life as the surest way to conserve health.

The middle and upper classes gladly adopted the theory of predisposing causes since its dietary rules mirrored bourgeois virtues and values, helped them to feel safe and to differentiate themselves from the poor who could or would not live as recommended by science. The dietetic interpretation of disease, however, also pressed the bourgeoisie to stay demonstratively calm in the face of cholera. Its rules prescribed to keep not only the bodily constitution, but also the mind, in a balanced state: extreme sentiments, especially the negative ones of anxiety and fear, were esteemed as very harmful. Therefore it was vital to maintain a semblance of normality and to avoid everything that would disturb the mind.

The complicated question of whether the wealthier parts of the population really were comparatively safe from cholera is not addressed here. However, the autosuggestion of the middle and upper classes that they were immunized by their solid lifestyle has influenced the statistical data available. As the district government of Cologne noted during the epidemic of 1849, there were probably many more victims than registered by the police due to the reluctance of respectable citizens to admit deaths from cholera in their own families and neighbourhoods: 'Since cholera attacks preferably the poor, the so called proletarians, and kills them almost exclusively, it is called a beggars disease and it is considered a disgrace to lose ones relatives from it.'[31] In turn, this suppression of deaths in wealthier families strengthened the image of cholera as a disease of the poor.

Although the urban upper classes did all they could to ignore cholera, downplay its danger and put the blame for illness on the lifestyle of the poor, they still had to offer some medical and material assistance to the victims. They were obliged to by the state, and it was also in their own interest to prevent scandalous scenes. Activities were coordinated by local sanitary boards (established under a Prussian law of 1835 as permanent institutions but only really convened during epidemics), comprising local officials, notables and doctors. During the first cholera epidemic of 1832, special sub-commissions were also appointed in each parish to control cleanliness, inspect the houses of the poor and supply aid to the sick. Later these tasks were left to the regular institutions of poor relief, which could act more discretely.

The poor relief system of the Prussian cities was based primarily on outdoor relief. It was executed by parish commissions and honorary overseers who supervised the paupers in their homes. During the first half of the nineteenth century the level of pauperism in Aachen and Cologne was high; usually about 10–15 per cent of the population received desperately inadequate outdoor relief. In cholera years there was no marked rise in relief spending. Thus, during the Cologne epidemic of 1849 some parish commissions pleaded for extraordinary resources to secure the endangered poor, many of whom were living in absolute distress without bedding or clothes.[32] Their applications were, however, rejected by the sanitary board with the (by then) common argument that this would be too costly and moreover useless, since 'such support would soon be mostly wasted again'.[33] Only in the worst affected parishes were some extra blankets, mattresses and soup distributed to the sick. This official aid was supplemented by private charitable donations, but they do not seem to have been very important.

The authorities were similarly reluctant to engage additional doctors. The treatment of poor cholera patients in their homes was left mostly to the regular parish doctors who worked for the poor relief administration alongside private practice. When the number of sick rose as drastically as in Cologne during the epidemic of 1849 – there were about 2,800 cholera cases in the course of four months – these doctors were quickly overwhelmed. Some of them pleaded for additional staff and one doctor wrote angrily: 'It is an old experience which cannot be ignored by any administration that exceptional events require exceptional means; and that cholera is such an event surely does not have to be discussed.'[34] This was exactly the interpretation of cholera that the city authorities were trying to deny and consequently very few extra doctors were engaged. The same austerity was maintained with respect to other categories of staff such as porters for the sick and dead, though this at times provoked public annoyance. A letter to a local newspaper in August 1849 complained about tired porters who simply set down the patient they were supposed to bring to the hospital and went for a beer, 'while the poor victim lay on the street screaming with painful cramps, so that in the neighbouring houses shutters and doors had to be closed in order not to hear the misery'.[35] The poor relief administration confirmed that such incidents were frequent and caused commotion on the streets, so that the employment of more porters seemed inevitable after all.[36]

During all epidemics the majority of the sick stayed at home. Nursing was left to families, assisted at times by sisters from religious orders. Only those who had no relatives, lived in all too miserable conditions or expressly wished so, were brought to hospitals. Force was not used. Usually special hospitals were set up, but in 1849 the sanitary boards of Aachen and Cologne refrained from such efforts: cholera patients were admitted to the open wards of general hospitals. Anti-contagionist convictions, economy, and the desire not to rouse alarm or to upset potential neighbours of special hospitals, supported this decision. To refrain from all extraordinary activity could even be defended as the most circumspect attitude, since according to the theory of predisposing causes rousing alarm might trigger sickness. Looking back on the first pandemic of 1831, the Prussian statistical office argued in 1849 that the drastic measures initially taken to contain cholera had 'filled all minds with horror and made persons with a weak constitution all the more susceptible to it'.[37] Based on the same argument, the Aachen town councillor and physician Heinrich Hahn successfully pleaded against opening a special cholera hospital in 1849, since this step might actually provoke a severe epidemic outbreak.[38]

Local authorities also argued that the poor disliked hospitals and especially cholera hospitals. There was indeed considerable mistrust on the part of the lower classes, most notably during the first pandemic of the early 1830s. Europe-wide rumours circulated about dreadful things happening in cholera hospitals and doctors were suspected of conducting experiments on the poor or even deliberately killing them. In many places such fears led to resistance and revolts.[39] The Rhine Province had no cholera riots, but rumours spread here too. The physician Joseph Hartung reported from Aachen in 1832:

> About the cholera hospital of this place the wildest rumours were spread, and it was striking to me that some of them were the same as I had found circulating among the people of Berlin and Vienna, especially that one man had not taken the medicine given to him in the hospital for inner treatment, but poured it into his boot secretly, and behold! the boot completely corroded to powder, proof enough that the sick were being poisoned on purpose . . . No wonder therefore that most from the poor classes concealed their sickness as long as possible and refused medical help and especially resisted with all their might, as long as they could utter their will, transfer to the hospital.[40]

Later, fear subsided though it still flickered sporadically, as in Cologne in 1849.[41] The mistrust on the part of the poor was not completely irrational. While nobody appears to have been purposely killed the therapies applied against cholera were, when judged by present-day medical knowledge, useless and often harmful.[42] Methods based on traditional humoralism, above all bloodletting, purges and emetics, were still generally used. They were complemented by irritating drugs which were supposed to stimulate the nervous system, and by sedatives to calm it down. Stimulation was also intended by external methods such as hot and cold baths, rubbings, or burning the skin with acids. Most doctors did not allow cholera patients to drink much: the rapid dehydration of the body was not recognized as the most fatal symptom of cholera.

In sum, very little was done to help the sick and poor at times of cholera. This was in part due to the state of the medical art but mainly reflected the attitude of the upper and ruling classes, whose main concern was to play down the danger, keep businesses running and to save money. Indeed, doing as little as possible was the main characteristic of urban cholera policy in the Rhine Province. Moreover, the same can be said with respect to long-term reforms. Some historians have asserted that cholera was an impulse for the modernization of urban sanitary provision. With reference to the Rhine Province – and indeed most parts of continental Europe – this seems questionable, or at least the impulse took effect only with great delay. In Germany a sanitary movement did not begin to organize until after the last cholera pandemic of 1866–7; urban sanitary reforms on a broad front were initiated only from the 1870s onward, several decades after the great cholera shock of 1831.[43] Aachen and Cologne were no pioneers in this respect. During the middle decades of the nineteenth century, sanitary conditions were quite deplorable in both cities. This was remarked, for example, by an English traveller, Thomas Banfield, who visited Cologne in 1846: he wondered about the 'strange neglect' of public hygiene in this wealthy commercial town and

pointed to the danger of epidemics.[44] Local notables, however, saw no need
to act. In the summer of 1866, as cholera was threatening again, one town
councillor of Aachen, a pharmacist, warned his colleagues that the old and
rotten sewers, which were leaking and polluting the ground water, could
cause serious harm. Yet, the majority of the council, led by the influential
Dr Hahn, rejected such alarmism. In Hahn's opinion, Aachen was 'thank
God a very healthy city'.[45] This contention ignored the fact that the overall
mortality rate, which had fallen back in the first half of the century, was rising
markedly again in the 1860s and lay well above the Prussian average.

The only sign of a new hygienic awareness was that during the cholera
pandemic of 1866–7, which was to be the last affecting the Rhine Province,
disinfectants were spread abundantly. This at least was a change compared to
1849, when nothing at all had been done in Aachen and only a single man had
been employed in Cologne to disinfect the dwellings of cholera victims. The
attempts at disinfection were motivated in the first place by miasma theory
and more specifically by the groundwater theory developed by the Bavarian
hygienist Max von Pettenkofer. They were supposed to neutralize the sick-
making perspirations of excreta, whereas the assumption that cholera was
transmitted by drinking water played no major part.[46] And although a shift
towards hygienic preoccupations was beginning to take effect in 1866–7,
this did not fundamentally change the dominating narrative pattern that
had been established in 1832: cholera was not described as a collective
catastrophe, but as a normal disease that mainly seized the lower classes
due to their living conditions and habits. It did not require any spectacular
response, interruption of public life, nor extraordinary relief measures for
the poor. On the contrary, the best thing to do was to do nothing unusual.

Barcelona

The pattern of reactions to cholera described for Aachen and Cologne
emerged in many European regions. Yet there were also completely differing
reactions, entwined with a different narrative of cholera. The city of
Barcelona is a good example. Cholera arrived here for the first time two years
later than in the Rhine Province. From northern Germany it had jumped to
England, from where it was transported to Portugal and then across Spain
from west to east. As in Prussia, the Spanish government initially reacted
with military cordons and quarantines but abolished such policies when it
became apparent that they had failed. The inhabitants of the as yet unaffected
region of Catalonia watched the progress of cholera intensely, like those of
the Rhine Province had done in 1831. Whereas worries had subsided in the
Rhine Province at the end of 1831, the contrary was true in Barcelona. Here
anxiety increased from day to day in the summer of 1834.

One important reason for this rising sense of panic was that alarming
news not only about the progress of the disease, but also about serious

collateral incidents, was arriving from Madrid. In the Spanish capital, the outbreak of cholera was accompanied by bloody riots. Reacting to a rumour that friars had caused the illness on purpose by poisoning wells, a mob sacked several monasteries and nearly 80 monks were killed.[47] Barcelona newspaper readers were thus getting the impression that both a dangerous epidemic and a breakdown of public order was approaching. From the end of July 1834 daily prayers to ward off cholera were held in more than a dozen churches and letters to the local newspapers attacked the city authorities for insufficient preparation. While several decrees regarding preventative measures – with similar aims to those discussed in Aachen in the autumn of 1831 – had been published, little was happening in practice. One letter writer complained that if cholera could not be stopped, at least dispositions should be made immediately so that the population could face it well nourished and clothed and provided with medical help. He predicted that hopeless chaos would arise if action was taken only when 'the enemy is already among us'.[48] The most drastic sign of rising fear was, however, that from mid-August many families who could afford it began to leave the city for the countryside. The stream of emigrants increased sharply when cholera actually reached Barcelona in mid-September: 'The people left by thousands every day', one eyewitness noted.[49]

This form of reaction was not limited to the first cholera epidemic of 1834. The second one, reaching Barcelona in late July 1854, was accompanied by an even greater mass flight:

> In the last days of July and the first of August the population left the city, and the railway stations of the east and north line were crowded with people of every age, class and sex, fighting for the seats in order to be among the first to escape. Only those who were among them can describe the reigning confusion . . . The city was depopulated within a few days.[50]

Contemporaries estimated that about 100,000 people, or two-thirds of the inhabitants, departed. When cholera broke out for a third time in Barcelona in 1865, reactions were not quite as frantic, but again a substantial part of the population left. The consequences were always the same: factories and shops closed down; the poor who had no means to leave the city were left without work and income; food prices soared; and an administrative chaos developed, for many civil servants, doctors and even priests absented themselves as well. Economic and social life came to a·standstill.

It is true that casualties were higher in Barcelona than in Aachen or Cologne. Yet, this cannot explain the mass flights from the city since they always took place at the very beginning of the epidemics when nobody could know how mortality rates would develop. Nor can they be explained by a differing scientific knowledge or containment policy. In Barcelona 1834, as in Aachen 1832, there were still some last remnants of contagionist measures, but the sick were not isolated, and departure from neither of the cities was prohibited. By 1854, anti-contagionist convictions had won the day in Spain as much as in Prussia. The theory of predisposing causes was also widely known. In countless official proclamations and medical tracts the Spanish public was informed that a moderate, cleanly way of life and a calm state of mind were the best protection against cholera. Yet, the middle and upper classes of Barcelona were clearly not convinced that bourgeois virtues immunized their bodies. They rather believed that everyone, irrespective of class, dietary lifestyle and constitution, was endangered by the miasmas hovering over the city. They closed down their enterprises and escaped to the supposedly healthy air of the hilly hinterland.

The lower classes were left to the improvised emergency measures of those officials, doctors and voluntary helpers who remained in the city despite their fear. To organize help for the poor was more difficult than in the cities of the Rhine Province. On the one hand the numbers of needy and sick were much larger. On the other, there existed no established system of outdoor poor relief to serve as an infrastructural basis, while the institutions of indoor relief had no spare capacity. Considering these problems and the chaotic circumstances, the emergency measures organized during the epidemics were quite impressive.[51] Special hospitals were opened, doctors engaged to treat the poor in their homes and money subsidies distributed to afflicted families. As in the Rhine Province, cholera patients were not forced into the hospitals, which were viewed with some mistrust in Barcelona too and could not have accommodated all of the sick in any case. For the homeless, beggars and vagrants it was a different picture, at least in 1834; such people were rounded up and interned in an establishment outside the city walls. They were perceived as a danger 'infesting' the streets, as an order of the Interior Minister had formulated it, but they were at the same time considered as highly endangered and therefore sheltered in a supposedly safer place during the epidemic.[52] For the same reason, inmates of the cities poorhouses, especially children and lunatics, were transferred to establishments in the countryside.[53] Finally, something had to be done about the large number of unemployed: for them, soup kitchens and public works were organized.

The city of Barcelona spent enormous sums on these measures to support the sick and poor during epidemics, much more than Aachen or Cologne. In Cologne (1849), the extra expenditures caused by cholera totalled 10,578 Taler, a sum that did not seriously stress the communal budget. In Barcelona (1854), however, the city government had to raise a loan of one million reales (or, converted into the Prussian currency, 70,400 Taler) just to finance the most urgent emergency measures.[54] Voluntary contributions were much more substantial as well. The subscriptions launched in Barcelona to finance relief in 1834, for instance, yielded approximately 200,000 reales (14,100 Taler) whereas the subscription organized in Cologne (1849) yielded only 1,315 Taler. The differing sums were partly due to the way these subscriptions were launched. In Cologne there was no official call to help the poor; the subscription was the initiative of a private charity organization which published a cautiously formulated appeal asserting (conforming to local conventions) that Cologne was luckily so far only 'mildly' affected.[55] When one of the poor relief administrators, to whom the collected money was passed on, published a note of thanks stating how badly his parish was suffering, he was criticized as 'tactless' by an anonymous advert.[56] The authorities and bourgeoisie of the Rhine Province did not wish any heartrending publicity, even though this would surely have stimulated donations. In Barcelona, however, the authorities took the lead with emotional appeals, symbolically acknowledging how hard the situation was for the poor. In August 1834, for instance, the city government invited 'all friends of humanity and public order' to contribute: 'If Divine providence has intended a time of bitterness for us, may it at least pass in this great city without giving the simple part of the population needy of protection reason for complaining about the pitiless negligence of the wealthy and protective part.'[57]

Of course this was merely rhetoric, and despite all efforts the support mobilized was completely insufficient. In sum, the lower classes suffered much more in Barcelona than in Aachen or Cologne, not only from the disease itself, but also from unemployment and hunger. Their sufferings were, on the other hand, not played down. In many official declarations the epidemics were addressed as times of havoc and distress. They were viewed as catastrophes, as exceptional events which required exceptional means. This does not mean that the ruling classes of Barcelona would not have preferred to hush up and ignore cholera. If it had been feasible, they would surely have liked to react similarly to those of the Rhine Province, for the sake of business, social order, the city's budget and public health. They likewise believed that anxious feelings would only worsen the situation and therefore intended to keep up normality as far as possible. In 1834, for example, the local authorities made the theatre continue performances so that the remaining inhabitants would find some distraction.[58] In 1865 they forbade the ringing of church bells for cholera victims and instructed the hearses to avoid central streets.[59] Nonetheless, all such attempts to veil cholera collapsed in view of mass emigration. Since ignoring cholera was utterly out of the question, the authorities turned their attention to demonstratively supporting the lower classes in order to keep them from making serious trouble. Paternalistic gestures were needed to stabilize the situation.

The morals and lifestyle of the poor were rarely addressed to explain their sufferings. Whereas the theory of predisposing causes became the most important explanatory factor in the Rhine Province, it remained marginal in Catalonia. Cholera was not depicted as an illness provoked by the internal constitution of the individual body, but as an external foe that had invaded the city, threatening everyone alike. This absence of moralizing reproaches was at least partly dictated by the behaviour of the rich. Emphasizing the dietary sins of the poor would not have been very convincing since the upper classes obviously did not trust in dietary rules for their own safety. And if someone tried to link illness to the habits of the poor, this quickly provoked the counter-reproach of hypocrisy. A good example is a poem which a benevolent citizen sent to the local newspaper during the epidemic of 1834. In friendly words the author admonished the lower classes to eat and drink moderately and to abstain from all excesses in order to safeguard themselves from the disease. Promptly 'a day labourer' answered, also in poetic form, repudiating such advice and stressing that not the poor but the rich were continuing their usual gluttony despite cholera: they just retreated from the city to their country houses and believed that 'for them the illness was as far away as if it were in Oran.'[60]

Explicit criticism of the rich, and especially of factory owners who deserted their workers, becomes more frequent in written sources only from the late 1860s, when a radical workers press developed.[61] Nonetheless, even in earlier decades the lower classes were quite capable of demonstrating their disapproval, and this was a further reason why authorities and newspapers abstained from any remarks which might have offended them. In situations as critical as during epidemics nobody wanted to upset the lower classes of Barcelona, whose inclination towards collective action was notorious. While no major disturbances actually occurred the ruling classes were well aware that any spark could have trigged off similar incidents as that in Madrid in 1834. This fear was magnified by the fact that cholera repeatedly coincided with revolutionary upheavals, as already in 1834 when the civil war between Liberals and Carlists was shaking Spain. Most acutely this coincidence influenced the experience of cholera in 1854: in the weeks immediately preceding its appearance in Barcelona, there had been a *pronunciamiento*, an overthrow of government in Spain, which was accompanied in the Catalan capital by militant demonstrations, machine breaking and workers' strikes.[62] Public order was already profoundly destabilized before the first cholera cases occurred helping to explain why the ensuing mass flight from the city was even more spectacular than 1834 or 1865.

In the eyes of those officials and notables who stayed in the city, the most important task was to contain chaos. They would not risk further annoying the working classes, but rather needed their cooperation. This in turn strengthened the self-confidence of the workers, who could present themselves as the more reasonable and reliable part of the population, in contrast to the egoistic and panicky rich. During the epidemic of 1854, for instance, the local workers associations published a statement, calling the factory owners to calm themselves, come back to the city and open their factories. 'They can be sure that the workers don't want anything else but to work, in order to maintain their families, and to enjoy the civic freedom which has been happily conquered through our glorious *pronunciamiento* and is always defended by our popular authorities, who are never deaf towards our just requests.'[63] With this statement the workers acknowledged on the one hand that they badly needed the return of their employers, but at the same time they were talking about the conquests of revolution and the protection of the authorities, who were in fact making all kinds of concessions to the workers in order to restabilize society. They even relied on workers to patrol the city as security guards.[64] The extraordinary crisis occasioned by the intersection of revolution and cholera virtually forced the local authorities to accept the workers as respectable partners.

Thus, while the experience of epidemics strained the relationship between rich and poor, joint efforts to cope with them could on the other hand forge new bonds of loyalty. The workers' associations demonstrated to the local authorities that they were able to help keep order, while some officials – such as Governor Pascual Madoz, who energetically led the emergency measures during the epidemic of 1854 – earned great respect from all classes. A few factory owners who did not follow the general impulse to flee also gained prestige in the eyes of their employees. This is illustrated by a letter from the workers of a large cotton mill to the owners, thanking them for the help offered during 'the disastrous, bloody time of cholera, which has engraved a sad and indelible reminiscence of the year 1865 into memory'. When the disease broke out and 'many victims fell from its terrible blows', they wrote, 'everything around us was mourning, lament, hopelessness! . . . What would become of your many workers in the midst of so much devastation, so much havoc?' But then, 'as if by magic', the factory owners organized medical and material help. 'In a horrible time, when often a brother flees from a brother, a friend from a friend and a husband from a wife, you have offered us relief; you have saved our lives; you have treated us like loving fathers.'[65]

Epidemics roused extremely strong sentiments in Barcelona, sentiments of fear, panic, mourning and sometimes hate on the one hand, of solidarity, respect and gratitude on the other. At the end of such a stirring experience, a solemn ritual was needed before returning back to normality: all epidemics were closed by an official ceremony that started with a grand procession in which local authorities, town councillors, professional corporations and military troops took part, followed by a mass with Te Deum in the cathedral. Official proclamations announcing the ceremony recalled the sufferings during the terrible time that had at last passed, and helpers were publicly honoured for their brave efforts.[66] The authorities of Aachen and Cologne, in contrast, never considered making such a public fuss. At the most, as in Cologne 1849, a small memorial tablet was discreetly presented with thanks to the Sisters of Mercy who had cared for the cholera-sick in the hospital.[67] The retrospective commemoration of epidemics was also much more pronounced in Barcelona than in the Rhine Province. Here not only the customary medical reports were published, but also popular illustrated pamphlets which related the past catastrophe, the heroic deeds of some individuals and the final rescue from greatest danger (see Figure 5.1). This said, general sanitary conditions in Barcelona remained even more precarious than in Aachen or Cologne, one reason why cholera was to return again in 1885.

FUERTE DISPUTA ENTRE LAS MUGERES Y EL COLERA EN SU DESPEDIDA.

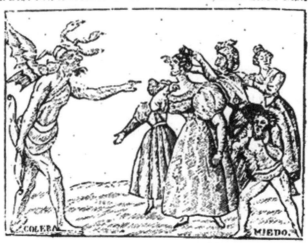

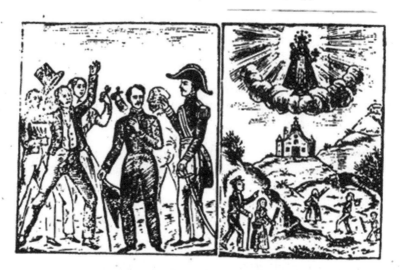

RELACION VERIDICA
de los estragos ocasionados por el Cólera en la ciudad de Barcelona en los meses de Agosto y Setiembre, de 1854, y número de las víctimas ocasionadas por tan terrible mal.

FIGURE 5.1 Illustrations from popular pamphlets relating the havoc caused by cholera in the city of Barcelona in 1854.
Source: Benet, J. and Martí, C. (1976), *Barcelona a mitjan segle XIX. El moviment obrer durant el Bienni Progressista (1854–6)*. Volume 1, pp. 427 and 445.

Conclusion

When Asiatic cholera began spreading across Europe in the early 1830s, perceptions of this new disease were relatively homogeneous throughout the continent. Once it arrived, however, local outbreaks were treated in completely different ways by the societies of different countries or regions. The largest cities of the Prussian Rhine Province and the capital of Spanish Catalonia were presented in this chapter as two contrasting forms of reaction, which were in turn entwined with different narrative patterns. In Aachen and Cologne the dominant narrative of cholera described it as a normal illness that affected almost exclusively the poor, was promoted by an inadequate lifestyle and could be warded off by obeying dietary rules based on the ancient theory of predisposing causes. Epidemics did not require any extraordinary countermeasures. On the contrary, it was best to do little. In Barcelona a much more dramatic narrative of cholera developed. Epidemics were experienced as times of havoc and disaster, triggering off panic, chaos and an interruption of societal life. The disease was depicted as an indiscriminate killer which could only be escaped by flight. The poor were seen as affected most in Barcelona, too. This was, however, usually not attributed to their habits, but to the breakdown of the economy. Their sufferings were publicly acknowledged, and extraordinary measures of relief were deemed necessary.

These contrasting narratives cannot be explained by one single factor but by a confluence of circumstances, not all of which have been analysed in this chapter. One important factor, for instance, was the memory of earlier epidemics. Spain had experienced intense yellow fever epidemics in the early nineteenth century, with much higher mortality rates than cholera ever achieved. In the Rhine Province, there were no such terrifying memories of epidemic disease. Another factor was the notorious political instability of Spain in the nineteenth century, which undermined trust in the capabilities of the authorities. Fear that epidemics might be accompanied by a breakdown of public order was magnified, as mentioned above, by the repeated coincidence with revolutionary upheavals. Through their flight, of course, the middle and upper classes contributed to further destabilizing society.

The urban bourgeoisie of the Rhine Province was much more confident that order would not be disturbed. Prussia was a more stable state and its administration much more efficient. The chronological proximity of epidemics and revolutions was relatively common in throughout Europe,[68] including Aachen and Cologne where the revolutions of 1830 and 1848 had occasioned some turmoil. By the time cholera arrived in 1832 and 1849 respectively, however, social unrest had already been crushed. There were no lower-class associations that could impress the bourgeoisie, as was the case in Barcelona. The most important spokesman of the short-lived workers movement of Cologne in 1848, the physician Andreas Gottschalk, himself became a victim of the 1849 epidemic; his burial was attended by a large crowd, but this was no demonstration of strength. The poor of Cologne and Aachen were really in no position to forcefully articulate demands or influence the dominant narrative of cholera.

Thus, a third factor explaining different reactions to cholera, and the one which has been stressed most in this chapter, are the relations between rich and poor. The urban middle and upper classes of the Rhine Province could stay calm in the face of cholera because they felt sure of themselves and their position in society. They were able to convince themselves of their superiority and that the social distance separating them from the poor would not be crossed by the disease. When they depicted cholera victims as poor, foolish and depraved, they were not confronted with loud protests. By pointing to the faults of the victims they could not only strengthen their own feeling of immunity, but also excuse themselves from expensive relief measures, play down the sanitary problems and continue business as usual. The bourgeoisie of the Rhine Province managed to suppress its own fears of infection and at the same time to avert any disruption of the economy, from which the poor in fact would have suffered most.

The upper classes of Barcelona were not so self-assured. Tormented by the memory of yellow fever, rattled by frequent political upheavals, aware of the defects of public administration and scared of a working class always ready to protest, they felt incapable of maintaining the calm state of mind that was, according to contemporary science, so important in the time of cholera. By following the impulse to flee, however, they lost the authority to moralize the poor. The only narrative of cholera compatible with their behaviour was that of an extremely dangerous external foe which threatened rich and poor alike. Through this pattern of interpretation, epidemics became traumatic experiences for the inhabitants of Barcelona and left deep marks in the collective memory.

Notes

1 Dettke, B. (1995), *Die asiatische Hydra. Die Cholera von 1830/31 in Berlin und den preußischen Provinzen Posen, Preußen und Schlesien.* Berlin: de Gruyter; Ross, R. (1991), 'The Prussian Adminstrative Response to the First Cholera Epidemic in Prussia in 1831', Unpublished PhD, Boston College. On Great Britain, see Morris, R. (1976), *Cholera 1832, the Social Response to an Epidemic.* London: Croom Helm; Durey, M. (1979), *The Return of the Plague: British Society and the Cholera 1831–2.* Dublin: Gill & MacMillan; Gill, G., Burrell, S. and Brown, J. (2001), 'Fear and frustration – the Liverpool cholera riots of 1832', *The Lancet,* 358. On France, see Sussman, G. (1971), 'From yellow fever to cholera: a study of French government policy, medical professionalism and popular movements in the epidemic crises of the Restoration and the July Monarchy', Unpublished

PhD, Yale University; Kudlick, C. (1996), *Cholera in Post-Revolutionary Paris. A Cultural History*. Berkeley: University of California Press.

2 Evans, R. (1987), *Death in Hamburg: Society and Politics in the Cholera Years, 1830–1910*. Oxford: Oxford University Press. On the last epidemics in Italy, see Snowden, F. (1995), *Naples in the Time of Cholera, 1884–1911*. Cambridge: Cambridge University Press.

3 For smaller studies, see Jahn, E. (1994), *Die Cholera in Medizin und Pharmazie im Zeitalter des Hygienikers Max von Pettenkofer*. Stuttgart: Steiner; Mühlauer, E. (1996), *Welch ein unheimlicher Gast: Die Cholera-Epidemie 1854 in München*. Münster: Waxmann. On Italy, see Stolberg, M. (1995), *Die Cholera im Großherzogtum Toskana. Ängste, Deutungen und Reaktionen im Angesicht einer tödlichen Seuche*. Landsberg: Ecomed.

4 Ackerknecht, E. (1948), 'Anticontagionism between 1821 and 1867', *Bulletin of the History of Medicine*, 22, 1–22. See also Baldwin, P. (1999), *Cantagion and the State in Europe, 1830–1930*. Cambridge: Cambridge University Press.

5 Briese, O. (2003), *Angst in den Zeiten der Cholera: Über kulturelle Ursprünge des Bakteriums*. Berlin: Akademie-Verlag; Briese, O. (1997), 'Defensive, offensive, Straßenkampf. Die rolle von medizin und militär am Beispiel der Cholera in Preußen', *Medizin, Gesellschaft und Geschichte*, 16.

6 On the rise of bacteriology in Germany, see Gradmann, C. (2005), *Krankheit im Labor: Robert Koch und die medizinische Bakteriologie*. Göttingen: Wallstein; Sarasin, P. et al. (eds) (2007), *Bakteriologie und Moderne. Studien zur Biopolitik des Unsichtbaren 1870–1920*. Frankfurt: Suhrkamp.

7 This certainly is true for the western parts of Prussia, as is evidenced by the correspondence of the regional authority (*Oberpräsidium*) of the Rhine Province. See Landeshauptarchiv Koblenz (hereafter LHAK), 403, Nos 6877, 6961–2.

8 This figure is taken from the final report by the Cologne district government, 5 December 1849 (LHAK, 403, No. 6961, pp. 233–4). In London, the worst cholera epidemic caused a mortality rate of 6.6:1000; in Berlin it never rose above 8.7:1000. The Hamburg epidemic of 1892 killed 13.4:1000.

9 In Spain there was another pandemic in 1885. For a detailed account of the mid-nineteenth-century epidemics as well as further bibliographical and archival references, see Althammer, B. (2002), *Herrschaft, Fürsorge, Protest. Eliten und Unterschichten in den Textilgewerbestädten Aachen und Barcelona 1830–70*. Bonn: Dietz, pp. 467–598.

10 Hauptstaatsarchiv Düsseldorf (hereafter HSTAD), RA, No. 1125, ff. 49–50: 11 September 1831.

11 HSTAD, RA, No. 1125, ff. 198–9 and 205–7: reports from the sanitary board to the district government, 6 December 1831 and 13 January 1832.

12 HSTAD, RA, No. 1125, ff. 61–6: report from the poor relief administration, 27 December 1831.

13 The Prussian king had called for special prayers to be held in September 1831. The diocese of Cologne, to which Aachen belonged, had responded but official prayers ceased at the end of the year and were not revived. LHAK, 403, No. 2318.

14 Town council session, 15 February 1850, cited by Schröter, H. (1983), 'Die Cholera in Aachen 1849', Diss. med., Aachen, pp. 76–7.

15 *Kölnische Zeitung*, 15 August 1849.

16 The annual report of the local Chamber of Commerce only mentioned in passing the affliction of workers and no negative effects on business at all. Handelskammer Köln (1850), *Jahres-Bericht für das Jahr 1849*. Köln. The continuation of social events is documented by adverts in the local press.

17 Announcement in *Kölnische Zeitung*, 17 July 1849; protocol of sanitary board and letter (draft) to archbishop, 18 July 1849, in Historisches Archiv der Stadt Köln (hereafter HASTK), 400, V-2Da-32, ff. 33 and 35.

18 Appeal titled 'Die St. Mauritiuskirche und die Cholera', *Kölnische Zeitung*, 19 August 1849. A similar call was launched by a Catholic association of Aachen on the eve of the 1866 epidemic, although without expressly mentioning cholera: *Echo der Gegenwart*, 14 July 1866.

19 Report from the parish board, *Kölnische Zeitung*, 31 October 1849.

20 *Cholera-Zeitung*, 4 October 1831. This special cholera newspaper was edited by the medical officer of Aachen, Zitterland, from October 1831 in order to combat false rumours, inform and calm the population; its publication was stopped in early 1832, before cholera actually arrived in Aachen.

21 Hartung, J. (1833), *Die Cholera-Epidemie in Aachen*. Aachen: Privately published, pp. 67 and 80.

22 *Rheinische Volkshalle*, 12 July 1849, and *Kölnischer Anzeiger*, 20 September 1849, both cited from Dautzenberg, M. (2002), 'Die choleraepidemie in Köln 1849', Diss. med. Köln, pp. 85–8.

23 *Kölnische Zeitung*, 21 September 1849.

24 *Westdeutsche Zeitung*, No. 44, 15 July 1849.

25 Ibid., No. 59, 2 August 1849.

26 Ibid., No. 87, 2 September 1849.

27 LHAK, 403, No. 2301, pp. 23–5: report from the censorship officer in Aachen, 10 December 1831.

28 LHAK, 403, No. 2349, pp. 109–11: report from district government Aachen, 11 October 1832.

29 LHAK, 403, No. 6961, pp. 200–1: report from district government Cologne, 21 September 1849.

30 See, for example, Coleman, W. (1974), 'Health and hygiene in the *Encyclopédie*: a Medical doctrine for the bourgeoisie', *Journal of the History of Medicine and Allied Sciences*, 29, 211–44; Hamlin, C. (1992), 'Predisposing causes and public health in early nineteenth-century medical thought', *Social History of Medicine*, 5, 43–70.

31 LHAK, 403, No. 6961, pp. 199–200: report to the Prussian state government in Berlin, 21 September 1849.

32 HASTK, 650, No. 423, ff. 33–54: applications by several poor relief commissioners dating from early August 1849 for extraordinary support.

33 HASTK, 400, V-2Da-32, fo. 85: protocol sanitary board, 6 August 1849.

34 HASTK, 650, No. 423, ff. 85–7: petition from parish doctor Cassel, 10 September 1849.

35 Cutting from *Allgemeiner Anzeiger*, 26 August 1849, in HASTK, 400, V-2Da-32, behind fo. 104.

36 HASTK, 650, No. 423, fo. 55: report dated 21 August 1849.

37 'Uebersicht der im Preußischen Staate im Laufe des Jahres 1848 an der Cholera Gestorbenen, verglichen mit der Anzahl der an derselben Seuche in den Jahren

1831, 1832 und 1837 Gestorbenen', *Mittheilungen des statistischen Bureau's in Berlin*, 2 (1849), 293–327: 300.

38 Town council session, 31 July and 1 August 1849, cited by Schröter, 'Die cholera', 61–2.

39 See, for example, Sussman, G. (1973), 'Carriers of cholera and poison rumors in France in 1832', *Societas*, 3, 57–84; Morris, *Cholera 1832*, pp. 95–128; Kudlick, *Cholera*, pp. 183–92; Gill, Burrell and Brown, 'Fear and frustration'.

40 Hartung, *Die Cholera-Epidemie*, pp. 23–4.

41 Heimann, F. (1850), *Die Cholera-Epidemie in Köln im Jahre 1849*. Köln: Privately published, pp. 19–20.

42 Therapy is described in detail in contemporary medical reports as those by Hartung and Heimann. See also Goltz, D. (1998), '"Das ist eine fatale Geschichte für unsern medizinischen Verstand". Pathogenese und therapie der cholera um 1830', *Medizinhistorisches Journal*, 33.

43 For the rise of the German sanitary movement, see Hardy, A. I. (2005), *Ärzte, Ingenieure und städtische Gesundheit: Medizinische Theorien in der Hygienebewegung des 19. Jahrhunderts*. Frankfurt: Campus.

44 Banfield, T. (1848), *Industry of the Rhine, Series II: Manufactures*. London: Theobald, pp. 218–19.

45 Town council session, 20 February 1866 (published in *Echo der Gegenwart*, 25 March 1866).

46 Research that pointed to transmission by water was not unknown to German scientists, and the general public had heard about it, too. The *Kölnische Zeitung*, for example, had reported on 4 October 1849 about the findings of Dr William Budd in Bristol, which indicated that water polluted by excrements of the sick was the main transmitter and that it should therefore be boiled or distilled before drinking. This theory had no major practical effects until after 1866.

47 First news of the riots came to Barcelona by official pronouncements published in the *Diario de Barcelona*, 24 July 1834 and following days. The events in Madrid are described in detail by García Rovira, A. M. (1989), *Liberalisme i forces populars en la crisi de l'Antic Règim a Espanya, 1832–5*. Barcelona-Bellaterra: Universitat Autònoma de Barcelona, pp. 148–209.

48 *Diario de Barcelona*, 5 August 1834.

49 Ollé Romeu, J. M. (ed) (1981), *Successos de Barcelona (1822–35)*. Barcelona: Curial, p. 147: diary entry for 17 September 1834.

50 Pusalgas, I. M. (1855), *Cólera en 1854. Historia descriptiva y médica del cólera-morbo-epidémico que invadió la ciudad de Barcelona y algunos pueblos de su provincia*. Barcelona: Privately published, p. 37.

51 They can be reconstructed from the bulletins published in the *Diario de Barcelona* and from Arxiu Administratiu de Barcelona (hereafter AAB), Gob. A, Nos 3053, 3127, 3970, 3971, 3972.

52 *Diario de Barcelona*, 8 July 1834, 23 September 1834; *Articles sobre el Principat de Catalunya al 'Diccionario geográfico – estadístico – histórico de España y sus posesiones de Ultramar' de Pascual Madoz*. Barcelona: Curial, 1985, Vol. 1, p. 205.

53 Nonetheless, paupers were decimated by cholera. During the epidemic of 1854, 442 from among 2,200 inmates of the Casa de Caridad and at least 56 from the 291 lunatics in the Hospital de Santa Cruz died.

54 HASTK, 650, No. 423, fo. 112: final account dated 14 June 1850; AAB, Gob. A, No. 2693: letters from the mayor and deputy mayor of Barcelona dated 9 and 14 September 1854.

55 Advert from the charity Meisterschaft in *Kölnische Zeitung*, 2 September 1849. The final account was published in *Kölnische Zeitung*, 11 November 1849.

56 *Kölnische Zeitung*, 22 and 23 September 1849.

57 *Diario de Barcelona*, 10 August 1834.

58 The theatre announced that it would comply with this order, though adding somewhat sarcastically that actors might run short. *Diario de Barcelona*, 21 October 1834.

59 AAB, Gob. A, No. 3970–1, fo. 10–11: letters from the mayor, 12 August 1865.

60 *Diario de Barcelona*, 1 and 6 November 1834.

61 Especially during the yellow fever epidemic of 1870, which provoked the same pattern of reactions as cholera, the workers' paper *La Federación* criticized the rich sharply.

62 For the political context see Benet, J. and Martí, C. (1976), *Barcelona a mitjan segle XIX. El moviment obrer durant el Bienni Progressista (1854–6)*. Volume 1. Barcelona: Curial.

63 *Diario de Barcelona*, 10 August 1854.

64 Ibid., 8 August 1854.

65 Letter dated 12 November 1865, printed in *La España Industrial S.A. Barcelona en su 82. aniversario 1847–1929*. Barcelona, 1929, pp. 92–3.

66 See, for example, *Diaro de Barcelona*, 11 and 12 November 1834.

67 HASTK, 400, V-2Da-32: protocol sanitary board, 29 October 1849.

68 See Evans, R. (1988), 'Epidemics and revolutions: cholera in nineteenth-century Europe', *Past and Present*, 120, 332–56.

6

Living with insanity: Narratives of poverty, pauperism and sickness in asylum records 1840–76

Cathy Smith*

Introduction

The fearful extent to which insanity prevails among the poor is a subject of great and melancholy interest to all . . . Among the causes which tend to increase insanity, may be reckoned extreme distress and poverty; the use of ardent spirits; and exposure to cold.[1]

Those who are practically acquainted with insanity know the great amount of complicated distress and anxiety that falls upon such unhappy persons, when any member of their families is attacked with mental derangement. Industrious and regular habits are often interrupted . . . propriety of conduct is disregarded, the character is injured, employment is lost, every comfort is gradually sacrificed, and complete destitution is sometimes incurred in a vain attempt to overcome or conceal so serious a calamity.[2]

Indeed, it may be said with truth that, except what are termed the opulent classes, any protracted attack of insanity, from the heavy expenses which its treatment entails, and the fatal interruption which it causes to everything like active industry, seldom fails to reduce its immediate victims and generally also their families, to poverty and ultimately to pauperism.[3]

As these extracts from the *Derby Mercury*, *The Morning Chronicle* and *The Pall Mall Gazette* illustrate it is not hard to find contemporary recognition of the intimate relationship that insanity and poverty shared. In acknowledging that insanity both 'prevailed among the poor' and reduced its sufferers to poverty, these newspapers simply gave public voice to conclusions reached in nineteenth-century medical psychology and among those most acquainted with the growing lunatic population of Victorian England. Poverty and material deprivation were widely considered as both catalyst to and a consequence of periods of mental ill-health. Indeed, when Sir William Ellis published his *Treatises on Insanity* in 1838, only 'hereditary tendencies' ranked higher than poverty in his league table of causes of insanity.[4] For those who favoured physical explanations, aetiologies of madness readily attributed a diseased brain to social experiences such as anxiety and poverty, something explored elsewhere in this volume by Alannah Tomkins. As late as 1878, Daniel Tuke could do little more than reiterate the findings of his predecessors: 'Wherever there is most pauperism, there, as a general rule, will be the largest amount of insanity; not merely because insanity pauperises, but because malnutrition and the manifold miseries attendant upon want favour the development of mental disease.'[5]

It was difficult for contemporaries to conclude anything else. The nineteenth century witnessed a growing number of county asylums, especially after the lunacy legislation of 1845, only to see the demand for their services outstripped by a growing pauper lunatic population. The Reports of the Commissioners in Lunacy recorded an increase in the pauper lunatic population from 16,000 in 1849 to 72,000 in 1889.[6] Most asylums had to house far greater numbers than had been the original intention and many were rapidly forced to undergo programmes of expansion, including the Northampton General Lunatic Asylum (hereafter NGLA) and the Denbigh Asylum.[7]

Yet, while the link between poverty and insanity was and is inescapable, it has perhaps come to overdominate our assessment of how poorer families coped with insanity. The work of family historians tells us that labouring and working-class families were heavily reliant on the combined earnings of family members to survive. Financial contributions had to be made by men, women and children,[8] and women, according to Valenze, were key in holding together an economy of makeshifts.[9] Moreover, the poor had to be and often were 'the most dynamic of local groups in creating work opportunities'.[10] Given the emphasis on household survival strategies for the poor and the fact that contemporaries and historians can be prone to seeing them simply in economic terms, it is hardly surprising that families with limited material resources were felt to suffer the most from having an insane family member.

From this perspective, the increasing numbers of pauper patients admitted to county lunatic asylums is easy to explain. Poorer families were less able economically and thus less willing temperamentally to cope with their mentally ill relatives.[11] People who could not contribute to, and acted as a drain upon, the family and household economy were relinquished to the care of the authorities and often left to live out their lives within the walls of the asylum. As Scull argues, 'the availability of the institution [asylum] decreased the tolerance of all sections of society', but as he goes on to say, 'it was among the poor that this change was most marked'.[12] He used the words of Dr Nesbitt, medical superintendent of the NGLA between 1845 and 1860, to substantiate his claim:

> Persons in humble life soon become wearied of the presence of insane relatives, and regardless of their age, desire relief. Persons above this class more readily tolerate infirmity and can command time and occasion. Hence the asylum to the "poor and needy" is the only refuge. To a man of many friends it is the last resort.[13]

Thus, the availability of the asylum 'provided motive, opportunity and justification for families to disclaim responsibility' for their burdensome relatives.[14] For Anderson, too, families on low income in Preston were less willing to support their dependent kin.[15] Even among wealthier families, according to Suzuki, property rather than sentiment, was key to how a family dealt with insanity.[16]

Yet recent work on the families of pauper lunatics has revealed a more complex picture. Families and communities policed their insane, more often than not initiated the process of committal and determined the time of discharge. Lunatics were not readily surrendered to the asylum but often cared for at home or in the community for long periods of time.[17] Relatives, neighbours and paid keepers were all important in the extramural care of the insane. When asylums were used, it was often strategically, and the poor remained, as Bartlett has argued, uncertain about the asylum as an institution.[18] The role and voice of the poor was thus not lost in a period of increasing state intervention in the care of the mentally ill. More recently, too, the bureaucratic records generated by the asylums have been used to capture the emotional experience shared between the insane and those close to them.[19] Letters have shown how families engaged with the medical profession and supervised the care their relatives received.[20] As Roy Porter reminded us in 1985, it takes at least two people and frequently more to make a medical encounter; the full implications of this are beginning to come to the fore.[21]

At the same time we cannot ignore the fact that increasing numbers of paupers, working and lower-middle-class families chose at some stage to use their local county or private asylums. Not all of those admitted were single or without close family, not all of them were violent and in many instances families of fairly limited means paid for their relatives' admission. Sometimes this may have been because of economic circumstances in the way that Scull suggests, but as this chapter will argue it was also closely related to the family life-cycle and issues of household practicalities. Equally, the rate at which individuals were institutionalized might be interpreted not as a breakdown in emotional ties but perhaps as an investment in the health and future of a family member. As I have argued elsewhere, asylums did work in the short term for some patients and discharge rates were more significant than once presumed. Expectations of a 'cure' were not unrealistic.[22] Moreover, the willingness of families of limited means to secure private admission for their relatives, as costly as this could prove, suggests an emotional attachment to the insane. This, together with the financial support often received from relations, friends and even employers, illustrates a wider recognition for and sympathy towards the plight of those coping with mental ill-health. Nancy Tomes has argued that families took emotional decisions in relation to the fate of a family lunatic.[23] I would argue this could even be the case when that decision involved committal to an asylum.

The aim of this chapter is to explore how the lower, middle, working and poorer classes of Victorian Northampton dealt with mentally ill relatives. How was insanity experienced and managed at home? Why did families use the asylum? What impact did insanity have on a family and for how long? The focus will be on the narratives that are told as families engaged with their local asylum and poor law authorities. A combination of asylum records will be used with census material to explore the social and economic backgrounds of the insane and their relatives. Of particular interest in this chapter are the letters that were written to the NGLA finance committee soliciting charitable support to subsidize the weekly cost that asylum admission entailed. These letters were written by husbands for insane wives, wives for insane husbands and parents for insane children. Not infrequently a local person of standing would write on behalf of a family. More often than not this would be a local vicar or minister, but others included Northampton's mayor and local employers. Mostly, these letters were written for those of lower middle-class or working-class status; families not poor enough, at least initially, to need poor relief but whose financial resources were insufficient to afford private rates of admission.[24]

From the 1860s, verbatim copies of the letters written to the NGLA were recorded in the minutes of the asylum's Finance Committee along with the decisions made in respect of them. The letters detail family circumstances, financial standing and personal qualities to help elicit charitable support. Rarely did these letters take on the demanding tone that can sometimes be found among pauper letters in respect of poor relief and which are explored elsewhere in this volume.[25] This is not surprising given that the letters written to the NGLA were for charitable support, which was not a right. Interestingly, most of them did not talk emotionally about the asylum patient but instead focused on the family's situation and the difficulties experienced as a result of mental illness. Unlike the letters examined by Louise Wannell, they were not addressed to the medical superintendent and rarely talked about the treatment of an individual other than in terms of the patient's social status.[26] The aim of these letters was very specific – to secure a reduction in the weekly cost of admission. Obviously, the structure and content of the letters, even their authors, may have been strategically chosen on the basis of what was perceived to make a worthy charitable case, but seldom was charitable support given without substantiating evidence on family circumstances.

The detail in which these letters are recorded may owe something to the fact that the NGLA, after opening in 1838, registered as a charitable hospital from 1845 to 1876. Thereafter it became St Andrew's Hospital for wealthy and middle-class patients. Like many asylums built before the 1845 lunacy legislation, the NGLA was built by public subscription, but unlike most other subscription hospitals it never became a county asylum. It certainly performed this role in that most of the patients between 1838 and 1876 were paupers and supported by poor rates, but for local political reasons the asylum governing body exploited a loophole in the 1845 legislation allowing the asylum to register as a charitable institution.[27] Part of the argument behind this was that charitable status allowed the asylum managers to stay true to the original intention of those who funded the NGLA. This was to cater for '50 pauper patients and 20 class patients . . . The class patients for whom we wish to provide for are persons in indigent circumstances but above the need of parochial assistance.'[28] A concern for this social group was regularly voiced in the nineteenth century as those who suffered most from the debilitating effects of insanity.[29] The issue of charitable support was regularly discussed by the NGLA Committee of Management and in 1859 concern was raised that

> . . . we have not been acting up to the intentions of the benevolent individuals through whose liberality Northampton Asylum was built. In accordance, as they believe the wishes of those men, bringing the advantages of this asylum within the reach of what may be called the lower middle-class of our population – tradesmen and farmers in narrow circumstances and others whose means raise them just above the level of the Union Workhouse.[30]

Much like the Scottish asylums and many other English and Welsh county asylums, the charitable initiative was to be supported from additional funds raised by those who could afford to pay private rates of admission.[31] In order to benefit from this cross-subsidization, those considered for charity had to outline the circumstances of their immediate family, relatives and sometimes friends. Given that we rarely have insight into the lives of working families, the detail in these letters has proved invaluable for exploring the impact and consequences of living with insanity. They provide a different, but no less compelling and important, focus to the English pauper letters explored elsewhere in this volume.

Family circumstances and the 'insane' at home

The opening of a local asylum certainly gave the poor and those of limited means another option for the care of their insane. With the legal emphasis on public safety, those of unsound mind and considered dangerous or suicidal were quickly committed.[32] Yet for those who were neither violent nor suicidal, the care options were more varied. Table 6.1 uses the Quarter Sessions Lunacy Returns to assess the pattern of 'lunatic' care for Northampton between 1845 and 1874. These Returns represent one-day censuses of the lunatic population taken in December each year. This means that anyone who entered an asylum after December in one year and left before the following December would not necessarily appear in the returns unless they received another form of care such as in the workhouse or received parish relief living at home or in lodgings. Given the growing recognition that asylums discharged a significant number of patients in under a year, this must seriously underestimate the role the asylum played in the short-term care.[33] Equally, if families were not claiming poor relief

Table 6.1 Provision for persons of 'unsound mind' 1845–74 (%)

	Asylum	Licensed House	Workhouse	Lodgings	Family and Friends
1845	36	3	24	5	32
1850	40	2	31	2	25
1855	48	1	25	2	24
1860	55	0	23	3	19
1865	57	0	21	2	21
1870	54	0	22	3	21
1874	60	0	23	2	15

Source: NRO: QSLR for Northamptonshire.

Note: The 1874 returns were used because the 1875 returns have not survived. It should be noted that the 1874 Returns do not include the Northampton Union.

for their insane relatives they too would not feature on these returns. What the Quarter Sessions Returns do cover is the care of the long-term insane, and in this respect Table 6.1 shows that a growing percentage of the long-term insane were placed in the asylum. By contrast, the percentage of those placed in workhouses or lodgings remained relatively static and we see a decline in the relative number cared for by family and friends, particularly from 1845 to 1850 and again in 1874.

It is hard to draw too much from these figures especially in terms of trying to evaluate the relationship between poorer families and their insane relatives. Despite the growth in asylum use, the majority of the mentally ill looked after at home were classified as long-term congenital 'idiots' or 'imbeciles', with most considered to have been insane since birth or in infancy. This pattern of care in Northamptonshire is mirrored elsewhere. In north Wales, for example, Michael has shown the role 'relatives, neighbours and paid carers' had in looking after the lunatic and idiot poor.[34] The assumption often made then and now is that these individuals were rarely troublesome and relatively easy to look after, thus we could assume family ties were not tested in the way that they could be. Moreover, medical superintendents were reluctant to receive such cases into their asylums because they felt the congenital nature of the mental affliction meant a cure was unlikely and asylum admission would therefore have little effect. Relatively little work has focused on congenital 'idiots' besides Wright's work on idiot children and Houston's on the mentally incapacitated in Scotland.[35] However, the NGLA narratives illustrate that the behaviours, abilities and demands of the congenitally insane varied enormously. Some, like Benjamin A., could earn a basic living. When he lived at home, as he usually did, he could contribute to the household economy. In 1850, on one of his frequent short-term asylum admissions, Benjamin was described as 'a very useful and industrious person able to do a fairs day's work' when well.[36] When ill he became unmanageable and his family resorted to the asylum. This shows two things: first, the behaviour patterns of the insane might not be changeless, and second, that, as Houston has argued, there was no rigid dichotomy between institutional and community care.[37]

While Benjamin's 'idiocy' was not totally debilitating, for others the case was different. Thomas N. was admitted to the NGLA in July 1846 at the age of 23. His case notes describe him as a 'drivelling idiot, unconscious to the calls of nature', a condition he had been in since birth.[38] The 1841 census records Thomas N. living at home with his parents and three siblings.[39] His father and one younger brother were working as agricultural labourers. The 1845 Quarter Sessions Returns record Thomas being looked after by his mother for 1s 10d a week.[40] For such a small sum of poor relief, Thomas required considerable care and it is unlikely that anything other than familial responsibility and emotional ties kept Thomas at home. He did enter the asylum once but was removed by friends within six weeks of his admission and taken back to his father's house. It was recorded that no improvement had taken place in his condition and having removed Thomas from the asylum, his family had to take responsibility for the cost of his care.[41] Thus there is evidence to suggest that those on low incomes felt both care and responsibility for their insane, even over the long term and even though this may have been detrimental to their household economies.

Key to the fate of individuals like Benjamin and Thomas was parental support. Table 6.2 shows parents, mothers and fathers formed the majority of those recorded as carers. Census data and asylum records reveal many of these parents took on this responsibility until late in life and sometimes until their death unless the individual they were caring for died first. For example, Hannah G. was an idiot residing with her parents and younger brother at Culworth in 1841.[42] She was still residing at home with her family in 1851.[43] By this stage her father was 61 and her mother 56, while Hannah had reached the age of 31. In 1861 Hannah's parents were living alone and a Hannah G. of Brackley was recorded in the death register indexes for October to December in 1859.[44]

The death of parents inevitably had a major impact on the care of an 'idiot' or 'imbecile' child. When this happened, siblings might take on the responsibility and sometimes the congenitally insane were placed in lodgings. More often than not the loss of long-term parental care resulted in institutionalization. Richard A. was recorded as living with his parents in 1853 and then with his sister from 1860.[45] Alfred T. was a 'congenital idiot' who lived at home with his parents from 1845 to 1853. In 1855 he was being looked after by a Sarah Marlow and in 1858 he was admitted to the NGLA.[46] Likewise, William D. was registered with his parents in 1845 and 1850, then with a relative Lydia D. in 1855, but by 1860 he was in the workhouse.[47] When Mary K. was admitted to the NGLA in 1862, her case notes describe her as a 'congenital idiot' who had always lived at home with her mother, her father being dead for some years. When her mother died she was taken to the Union workhouse but as they were unable to manage her she was brought to the asylum.[48] Ann M., believed to be idiotic from the age of 11, was admitted to the asylum in March 1863.[49] She had been in the asylum once before but after a two-year stay her mother believed she could manage her at home. However, her mother died in 1861 resulting in Ann having to go to the Union workhouse until admitted to the asylum in 1863.[50] She remained in the asylum for the rest of her life. It is clear from such records that these 'idiot' and imbecile adults became very disturbed with the loss of their parents and the change in their domestic circumstances. Their admission to the asylum was often as a result of violent and unmanageable behaviour, this perhaps reflecting their sense of dislocation and loss.

Domestic care was not simply limited to those suffering from what were perceived to be congenital mental conditions. While husbands and wives feature little as carers in Table 6.2, there is much more evidence from asylum

Table 6.2 Carers listed in quarter sessions lunacy returns

	1845	1850	1855	1860	1865	1870	1874	Av. %
Parents	14	14	14	17	13	17	11	14
Mother	9	4	24	20	21	19	26	18
Father	3	1	10	13	26	15	24	13
Wife	1	0	1	3	5	6	3	3
Husband	1	0	1	0	1	4	3	1
Sister	10	4	3	9	6	6	14	7
Brother	5	2	9	8	7	4	3	5
Daughter	3	0	2	3	5	2	5	3
Son	0	0	1	1	1	4	0	1
Grandmother	0	0	0	0	0	1	1	0.3
Grandfather	0	0	0	0	0	1	0	0.4
Stepmother	0	0	0	0	0	1	0	0.4
Stepfather	0	0	0	0	0	1	0	0.4
Cousin	0	0	0	0	1	1	0	0.3
Relatives	5	0	5	0	0	6	0	2.0
Friends	22	37	5	13	4	6	1	13
Brother-in-law	0	0	0	1	1	0	0	0.3
Mother-in-law	0	0	1	1	3	0	0	0.7
Uncle	0	0	2	1	1	0	0	0.6
Aunt	2	0	0	0	0	0	0	0.3
Niece	0	0	1	0	0	0	0	0.4
Self	0	0	3	3	3	3	5	2
Not Stated	26	37	17	6	3	2	5	14
Total	101	99	99	99	101	99	101	

Source: As for Table 6.1

admission registers and case notes that they bore the brunt of mental illness in the short term. As Peter Bartlett and David Wright argue, 'situations of 'care' in the community existed long before a crisis precipitated institutional confinement with 'admission orders revealing that the "attack" of insanity had often been underway for months, if not years, before confinement took place'.[51] In Northampton, Jane J. was admitted to the asylum in 1863 with 'raving mania' that had lasted for ten months.[52] Her admission had been triggered by a change in personality 'from being a good wife; kind mother and amiable and agreeable companion, clean and tidy' to becoming 'cross, irritable and dirty, indifferent alike to the duties of her social position and decencies of life'.[53] This must have been particularly difficult to cope with, given that Jane and her husband Henry had four children at home. In 1861 the census shows their ages ranged between nine years and two months old.[54] The census also showed that this family had a sick nurse living with them, possibly supporting Nancy Tomes's claim that admission only came after families had 'exhausted every other form of extramural treatment they could afford' with their decision precipitated by 'escalating tension and desperation that culminated in a crisis'.[55] Certainly, there is evidence to suggest that the asylum was not the first resort. When George B. was admitted on 16 January 1865, his admission notes recorded that when he had felt unable to work he had put himself under medical treatment at the dispensary. This had enabled him to resume work until a fortnight prior to his admission when he had been 'overcome by undesirable sensations feeling that "everything went wrong"' with him, and he attempted to destroy himself and his children.[56] When James R. was suddenly seized by a stroke on the brain, he 'gave up his business directly and went to a friend in the country', but while there took Laudanum for suicide purposes and thus was admitted to the asylum.[57] While behavioural crisis could curtail care at home in other instances the cause of the insanity could prolong domestic treatment. For example, Hilary Marland's research on puerperal mania shows that the ambivalence contemporary medical professionals shared over this illness meant many who suffered were treated at home with only the worst cases being admitted to the asylum.[58]

The foregoing discussion clearly shows that domestic care was very important for the long-term congenital insane. Equally, there is evidence to suggest that the families of those suddenly stricken with mental ill-health would provide care for some time and explore extramural options before a crisis forced institutionalization. However, contrary to the findings of Nancy Tomes, the NGLA admission records suggest that more often than not a sudden development of suspected insanity was swiftly followed by asylum admission. Figure 6.1 illustrates the duration of illness before asylum admission as given by family and friends and recorded in the admission registers and case notes. This evidence shows that most patients were admitted within two months of their symptoms being manifest and a majority were admitted within four months. The pattern is similar for both

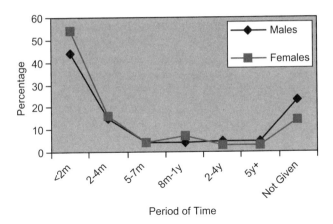

FIGURE 6.1 Speed of admission for pauper patients.
Source: S.A.H.A., Admission Registers R1, R2 and R3 1846–75

men and women, and resembles that found by Bartlett where 79 per cent of men and 77 per cent of women were admitted from domestic care to the asylum within three months.[59] Where admissions occurred much later, after five or more years, these were invariably congenital idiots or imbeciles who later in life had experienced a change in domestic circumstances as discussed above. A number of factors could explain this finding. Scull may be right in arguing the onset of mental illness pushed the emotional and financial resources of some poorer families and this forced them to initiate the process of committal at an early stage of the illness, but as Figure 6.2 shows, the speed of pauper admissions varied little from that of private admissions.

Figures 6.1 and 6.2 suggest that the speed of admission followed a very similar pattern for both male and female pauper patients and male private patients. Private female patients tended to be admitted later in the development of their mental illness. In Leicestershire while the majority were confined within three months of the symptoms of their illness developing, the figure was lower for private admissions (61 per cent private and 72 per cent pauper).[60] A further distinction that arises is in the treatment of elderly female patients. Table 6.3 shows a significant correlation in the marital status of private and pauper patients apart from the category of widowed females, suggesting that pauper families found it particularly hard to look after their elderly female population.

Domestic care remained central to the experience of the pauper congenital insane and it was usually the death or incapacity of carers, usually parents, which instigated a change in care arrangements and often institutionalization. Equally, perhaps contrary to what might be expected, those who could afford

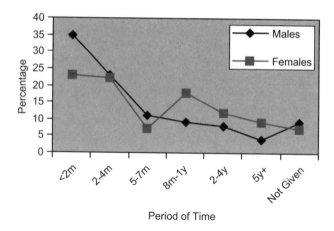

FIGURE 6.2 Speed of admission for private patients.
Source: As for Figure 6.1.

Table 6.3 Marital status of private and pauper patients (%)

	Private Patients		Pauper Patients	
	Male	**Female**	**Male**	**Female**
Single	46	46	38	32
Married	43	43	49	47
Widowed	10	11	10	21
Not Given	0	0	2	0.4

private admission more frequently admitted single adults, while a slightly higher proportion of married adults were admitted as paupers. This is rather different to the findings for nineteenth-century Ireland where unmarried paupers were most likely to face asylum admission.[61] Clearly, there is a local and regional dynamic to patterns of asylum use as John Walton's work has demonstrated.[62] But also, as Jonathan Andrews and Anne Digby have argued, further research needs to be undertaken on the different categories of private and pauper patient to draw firmer conclusions about the experience of mental ill-health according to socio-economic status.[63]

Were we to suppose that the pressures of an increasingly industrial and capitalist Victorian world pushed working and poorer families into giving up the support of their mentally ill relatives, the few examples here would question such a conclusion. Northamptonshire was not Lancashire but it is clear that poor and labouring local families continued to care for their congenital insane despite their varying needs and the limited poor relief they obtained. In this respect, household economics was not the basis on which care decisions were made. The question now is why we see a different pattern of care for those with a recent diagnosis of 'insanity' for whom the decision to commit came much earlier in their illness.

Institutionalization of the insane

According to Andrew Scull, the rate of certified 'madness' among the Victorian population rose from 12.66 per 10,000 in 1844 to 29.6 per 10,000 by 1890. The rate of asylum admission per 10,000 rose from 3.92 in 1855 to 5.51 in 1890.[64] While a change in domestic circumstances explains the admission of the congenital or chronic insane, this was rarely the case for those recently certified. Instead, for Nancy Tomes, it was a crisis – emotional, economic or both – that usually precipitated admission, 'some event or situation that could neither be ignored nor tolerated' finally tipping the balance 'in favour of the asylum'.[65] Similarly, admissions to the Devon Asylum show that decisions to certify were often taken at a point when the resources of individuals, kin and friends had diminished.[66] Dwindling economic resources might be one factor but admission records generally focus more on behaviour crises or a sudden deterioration in symptoms. Outbreaks of violence, attempted suicide, lewd behaviour, public embarrassment, sudden changes in temperament, deep depression or anything that brought the mental well-being of the family member to a head and/or was perceived to be too disruptive to family life could initiate asylum admission. For example, Fred M. (aged ten) was one of the youngest patients to be admitted to the NGLA, in February1865.[67] The 1861 census records Fred aged six living with his parents and three younger siblings. Fred's admission notes reveal how difficult it must have been for this young family. He was described 'as of filthy habits' and of being 'dangerously passionate – throwing knives and weapons at anyone who displeases him'.[68] It was also recorded that he bit and 'ill-used' the other children. It may well be that with three other young children Fred's mother and father reached a point where they could no longer cope and they had to think about their other children. The admission notes state he had 'been in this state of mind since birth' and so his parents had cared for Fred for ten years. David Wright's research on Earlswood, where Fred was eventually transferred to, shows that institutionalization was more likely to occur when it was the oldest child that became mentally ill.[69] The lack of elder siblings possibly caused a crisis in caring arrangements but perhaps equally the interests of Fred had to be balanced with those of his younger siblings. Thus, at times families had to think strategically about how they used the asylum.

The decision to admit Fred may also have been triggered by the particular point in his family's life-cycle which made his behaviour and the care he clearly required even harder to accommodate. Work carried out on poorer families has demonstrated that there were times in the family life-cycle when impoverishment was most likely to occur. Key stress points included the birth of a child or having a young family, perhaps starting out in business and certainly old age when income earning potential was reduced or limited.[70] Wall and Henderson have shown how poor families manipulated welfare provision to overcome short-term financial crises and Wright has suggested that the 'strategic confinement' of children took place at Earlswood Asylum for similar reasons.[71]

Given the clear links between mental ill-health and poverty it is no surprise to see that individuals were more vulnerable to mental ill-health and/or more likely to be admitted to the asylum at certain stages in the family life-cycle – a fact that was recognized early on in the contemporary literature. William Farr noted in 1837 how insanity often prevailed among adults when their responsibilities were greatest, that is when their children were young.[72] In 1844 the Commissioners in Lunacy had drawn attention to the fact that insanity most frequently attacked those aged between 25 and 40, the group with the largest family responsibilities.[73] Sixty per cent of those admitted to the St Andrew's Asylum, Norfolk, in 1814 were aged between 30 and 49.[74] This was similar to the picture for other asylums. Lancashire admissions between 1848 and 1850 were most common among men and women aged 30–40 years of age.[75] In 1864 the largest number of males admitted to Colney Hatch were between the ages of 30 and 35 and for women between 35 and 40.[76] Table 6.4 shows that most men and women admitted to the NGLA were in their 20s, 30s and 40s, with the average age consistently falling in the 40s for both men and women throughout the nineteenth century.

While the behaviour of the insane individual is the factor most focused on in the admission records, there is a real sense that at certain times this was more bearable than at others. The case notes of patients, and letters written to the NGLA, reveal more of the impact insanity could have on young families. Mary Ann N. was admitted to the asylum on 19 October 1863 with mania caused by parturition.[77] Her mania came at a bad time for her husband John. In a letter written on his behalf by the curate of Daventry, he was described as a 'young man' and 'tailor by trade' but whose customers 'are chiefly in the lower ranks of life and his trade cannot be very lucrative'.[78] With Mary Ann suffering from parturition we can assume they had recently had a baby and as the curate explained John 'was obliged to contribute to the support of his parents with whom he lives and further that he has incurred great expense on his wife's account before her removal to the asylum'.[79] At a time when John had a young baby, was living with his parents and trying to work, Mary Ann's 'occasional violence', extreme restlessness and excitability must have been too much to cope with. On her admission to the asylum it was noted that she needed the constant attention of a nurse to prevent her tearing her clothes and because she would only eat if fed.[80]

Table 6.4 Age distribution of NGLA pauper admissions 1846–75

Age Range	Male		Female	
	No.	%	No.	%
1–9	0	0	2	1
10–19	14	7	20	8
20–29	39	19	43	18
30–39	44	21	41	17
40–49	35	17	46	19
50–59	29	14	33	14
60–69	35	17	32	13
70 +	11	5	25	10
No Given	2	1	1	0.4
Total	209	101	243	100.4

Even for those above pauper status, the difficulties of managing mental illness with a young family were clearly demonstrated. Thomas T.'s letter to the NGLA Finance Committee reveals the problems he faced with the onset of his wife's insanity:

Gentlemen,
I am a butcher in a small way of business at 86 Bridge Street, Northampton. My wife is an inmate of the asylum at a charge to me of 1 guinea a week. I have a family of five children to keep and am put to the additional expense through the loss of my wife's assistance. It is impossible for me to continue paying the above charge. If I attempted it, it would ruin me and deprive me of the possibility of providing for the rest of my family or keeping on my business. I am willing to pay for my wife's maintenance all I can afford. I believe I should be able to pay 10 shillings a week at the most. I beg therefore to appeal to your kindness and consideration and to request that my wife be placed in such class of patients that that sum would be sufficient. My wife has already been 18 weeks at the asylum and there is no hope of her recovery. She was insane and in an asylum eight years since but recovered at that time. Should you not be able to assist me I should be compelled to apply to the parish which I am most unwilling to do and the result of which would be that I must reduce myself to a state of absolute pauperism and inability to keep myself before they would grant me assistance. This I humbly represent would be extremely hard.

I am now willing and have the opportunity to get a living but if crushed by expenses too great for my circumstances, my business must be discontinued and my whole family must become paupers.[81]
Thomas T., 14 January 1867

Catherine T. was admitted as a private patient in September 1866 suffering from mania, which was attributed to milk fever.[82] The 1861 Census records Thomas and Catherine living at 86 Bull Street Northampton with one daughter aged four. By the time Catherine was admitted in 1866 she has had a further four children.[83] At this stage Catherine was 30 years old and Thomas 33.[84] As the letter clearly indicates Thomas was struggling to run his butcher's business alongside looking after his children and wife. The records suggest that he had some support from Catherine's parents but this was not sufficient to prevent her committal. Catherine's admission notes record her as talking incoherently, 'beating herself, the bed and anything in her way' and that she had struck her mother the day prior to her admission.[85] The emotional stress of dealing with Catherine's illness with a young family was further compounded by the fact that Thomas no longer had her assistance in the home or the business.

Catherine was originally admitted at 21s a week, a sum that was clearly causing Thomas financial problems. By the time he wrote to the Finance Committee, Thomas has spent £12 12s on Catherine's care and unlike her previous admission she did not seem to be on the path to recovery. On the 17 January 1867 the Mayor of Northampton wrote in support of Thomas:

Gentlemen,
I have known Mr T. for several years and know him to be a very honest, hard-working man: from nature and the extent of his business I feel quite sure his statement is correct and that he would be unable to pay a larger sum than 10s a week.
P. Phipps, Mayor of Northampton.[86]

Thomas's character, station in life and plight meant he fulfilled all the criteria for benevolent consideration and charitable aid. The supporting letter from the mayor can only have added further weight to his cause and thus the Finance Committee decided to accept 10s a week, less than half the standard rate. Any charge that Thomas was exaggerating the consequences of Catherine's illness to the fate of his family and his business can be dismissed on the basis that he wrote again to the asylum in June 1867:

Gentlemen,
I feel it my duty to let you know the position in which I am now placed through misfortune. I cannot meet the demand I have received from the asylum to defray the expense my wife incurs. I have been obliged to give up my business. I have five little children to keep – I feel it to be an

impossibility for me to pay, so now I must beg to leave the case in your hands.[87]
Thomas T. 19 June 1867

Catherine was readmitted as a pauper patient and remained in the asylum for three years and five months. Her stay in the asylum prior to her becoming a pauper patient had cost Thomas £25 2s and in the space of eight months this had reduced the family to pauperism. Nor was the story of Thomas and Catherine unique. Richard T. wrote to the asylum in 1871 explaining that as a result of his wife's admission 'she has not been able to manage her household affairs, which has also been a considerable loss to me'. He went on to say that he had to pay for someone 'to take charge of the house and his two children having no relative who can undertake this'.[88] The Finance Committee reduced the charge to Richard T. from 21s to 5s, but like Catherine his wife also ended up in the pauper wards.

A more detailed idea of how such costs affected those on medium and low incomes can be found in other letters. In 1864 the Finance Committee received a letter regarding Mrs Sarah S., a patient admitted to the asylum suffering from melancholia.[89] A month after her admission Charles Gibbon, rector of Lutton, wrote to the asylum:

23 March 1864
Sir,
Mr Fitzwilliam forwarded to me your letter on the 29th respecting William S.'s wife
Mr S. has also come to see me with your letter of the first instance and he proposes to pay 12s a week for his wife's maintenance in the asylum. This in my opinion, is quite as much as he can be reasonably expected to pay. He is a blacksmith by trade and has been for many years a journeyman blacksmith in the village. His wages (I believe) are only £20 a year with his board. He also rents about 10 acres of land and keeps two cows. They have both been very industrious and have saved a little money or else he could not be able to pay even this amount for his wife. He is altogether a very worthy man and richly deserves any favor [sic] which the Committee may be able to show him under this heavy affliction.[90]
Charles I. Gibbon, Rector of Lutton

Sarah, like Catherine T., was originally admitted for 21s a week. The rate was reduced to 12s a week once the committee had heard of her husband's situation. She was discharged recovered on the 25 May 1864 and her stay at the asylum had cost £5 8s, representing 27 per cent of William's yearly salary. Perhaps not surprisingly, and certainly not unusually, Sarah's melancholia was linked to concerns about money. She was described as suffering from 'sorrow, fear and regret', saying 'she has no money and is in debt to everyone'.[91] The cost of her care may have been the reason why she was discharged on her husband's authority and there is no record of her ever being readmitted to the NGLA.

Even for those whose income exceeded Mr. S's the financial burden of an insane family member was difficult to bear. When the wife of a clerk to the Grand Union Canal was admitted in 1861, the local reverend wrote to the asylum asking for a reduction in the weekly cost.[92] Mrs C.'s husband earned £70 a year. His wife was initially admitted at 21s a week, which was reduced to 14s a week. If she had stayed in the asylum for a year, the cost, even at the lower rate, would have been in excess of 50 per cent of her husband's salary. Such detailed financial records of households are rare, but the proportion of annual income spent on asylum care at the NGLA was similar to the one case found by Wright for the Earlswood Asylum.[93]

While families with young children clearly struggled when faced with the cost of care for the mentally ill, it is equally the case that those at the other end of their life-cycle also found it difficult. Usually, as noted earlier in the chapter, the long-term chronic insane were cared for at home by their parents, but sometimes insanity developed later in life. At such times it appears, as David Wright found, that the NGLA was used strategically to help with the immediate crisis but also in these instances possibly for cure. Septimus W. was admitted to the asylum on 8 September 1866 suffering from mania caused by 'pecuniary difficulties'.[94] His mother Anne, a 65-year-old widow, wrote to the asylum on the 17 September 1866. Her letter stated she was 'without means' and with her two daughters entirely dependent on two further sons who were clerks in London.[95] Her daughters also kept a small school. The charge for Septimus was £80 a year. Two members of the church, a consulting surgeon and the Headmaster of the Merchant Taylor's School countersigned the letter. Even with such weighty support the case was deferred and ultimately turned down because in October 1866 Mrs. W. wrote again to express her disappointment at the committee's decision. This time she noted that friends have come forward 'to the best of their power with a Donation to the hospital'.[96] The committee responded by asking if the sum was reduced to 25s a week what sort of sum would Mrs W. and her friends be able to raise and what sureties could they provide. In December 1866 Septimus's case notes reveal that his friends were not able to pay for his maintenance and he was therefore taken to his mother's house in Brixton that morning.[97]

In 1871 the asylum received the following letter:

Lawrence Street
Northampton
Sir,
I have been advised by a friend to apply to the Committee of Directors of the Northampton General Lunatic Asylum through you to ask them to reduce the weekly charge for my son William G., as my income is very

small only £67 11s per year and I earnestly entreat you to do so at the lowest possible sum that your regulations will permit you, as the present charge would soon bring me to beggary. I formerly was a Hawker of tea, but am now unable being seventy-five years old, to do anything to increase my means.
William Barmwell G., 25 October 1871
P.S. Mr Whitworth of George Row who is, I think, one of your Directors has known me for many years.[98]

The secretary of the Finance Committee checked William's father's yearly income out of which he had paid the first instalment for his son's admission (£9 15s) from savings dedicated to doctors' bills or 'other extra expenses'.[99] While the minutes reveal William had three other brothers, they were not in a position to help. The Finance Committee 'resolved unanimously' to reduce the weekly charge to 5s, and William stayed in the asylum for four months before being discharged recovered at a total cost of £11 15s, or 17 per cent of his father's annual income. William was readmitted to the asylum ten months later, entering as a pauper lunatic, presumably having exhausted his father's funds. William stayed until his death just over two years later at the age of 37.[100]

As the extract from *The Pall Mall Gazette* outlined at the start of this chapter suggests, for anyone other than the 'opulent classes' the trade in lunacy was costly. Yet admissions to private asylums as well as private admissions to county and charitable institutions continued to rise in this period. Even those with incomes as low as £20 a year, like our blacksmith Mr S., were willing to pay significant if reduced weekly maintenance charges. This suggests that far from emotional bonds being severed because of the pressure that mental illness caused, families were willing to use whatever resources they had to ensure the best possible treatment for their relatives. Perhaps the optimistic prognostications of cure regularly voiced by alienists and reformers encouraged the use of the asylum despite the financial implications or, as Wright argues, it was possible that the asylum was used in the short term on a trial basis. The hope of cure clearly motivated the wife of Mr Thomas F. When he was admitted to the NGLA on 10 September 1864 his wife had borrowed part of the £13 13s required for his first quarter's stay. When it came to the next quarter's payment his wife was clearly struggling. She made a personal appearance before the Finance Committee stating that she was 'most anxious' to maintain her husband as a private patient 'while there was prospect of recovery'.[101] The NGLA Finance Committee suggested they would accept 12s a week and that she should consult her friends to raise the required sum. It would appear that Mrs Thomas F. raised the next quarter's money but then found herself in difficulty. The committee recorded in August 1865 that if Mr Thomas F. was not removed from the asylum he would be sent to his wife. Three weeks later it was recorded that he had been discharged 'not improved'.[102] Thomas's wife had clearly tried as hard as she could to obtain for her husband what she felt was the best treatment in hope of a cure for his mania.

Conclusion

Living with insanity, as these narratives reveal, could be time-consuming, difficult and costly. We cannot safely assume that congenital 'idiots' and 'imbeciles' remained at home because they were relatively easy to look after. Yet for these individuals the home remained the primary locus of care, irrespective of the socio-economic status of their families, and until they or their parents died. The poor relief carers received was often minimal although this varied according to the difficulty of the patient. It is unlikely that the care bestowed on the congenital 'insane' came from anything other than emotional attachment and responsibility. As noted above, the often rapid change in behaviour of the congenitally insane once long-term carers had died or become incapacitated could well have been a way of expressing loss and dislocation. Even when we come to analyse those whose experience of insanity came on in later life, it is not safe to assume that their rapid admission to the asylum was simply a response to the pressures of household economics, although it is fair to assume that the presence of an insane family member could have a devastating effect on the household economy. At times this was clearly too difficult to bear. When a parent of a young family fell mentally ill, their spouse had to consider the interests of the family. Such concerns were also apparent when a child became ill. When the elderly became carers, income could become a crucial consideration and maybe, as with young families, sometimes hard decisions had to be made. Recognizing the impact of life-cycle poverty does not mean, however, that such decisions were taken lightly or that they reflected a decline in familial bonds. It is clear, as Wright has shown, that families used asylums strategically and for some they genuinely seem to have offered the hope of cure.[103] Husbands and wives used savings and borrowed to try and ensure the best terms of admission. Friends and employers lent them money by way of support. The letters written to the NGLA Finance Committee rarely spoke of the 'lunatic' relative in emotional terms; instead they focused on the difficulties faced, economically and domestically, when insanity hit a family. It might perhaps have been considered irrelevant or inappropriate to talk emotionally about a friend or relative when the aim of the letter was to solicit financial support. It was certainly the household economy that those who sat on the NGLA's Finance Committee were interested in, and rarely did they enquire about anything other than income. But reading between the lines and evaluating the endeavour of husbands and wives, friends, employers and local men of note in trying to secure appropriate funds or a reduction in weekly asylum costs, even the rapid rate of asylum admission could tell another story. While living with insanity had severe economic implications, it often elicited from family and community members a response that was suggestive of care, support and, in terms of asylum admission, even hope for a swift recovery.

Notes

* A Wellcome Trust Research Leave Award in 2007 supported the research and writing of this article.

1 *The Derby Mercury*, 12 September 1838 p. 2, col. 1.

2 *The Morning Chronicle*, (London) 11 July 1845, p. 6, col. 2.

3 *The Pall Mall Gazette*, 21 November 1868, p. 10, col. 2.

4 Ellis, W. C. (1838), *A Treatise on the Nature, Symptoms, Causes, and Treatment of Insanity*. London: Samuel Holdsworth, pp. 57–8.

5 Tuke, D. H. (1878), *Insanity in Ancient and Modern Life*. London: Macmillan, p. 95.

6 Bartlett, P. (1999), *The Poor Law of Lunacy. The Administration of Pauper Lunatics in Mid-Nineteenth-Century England*. London: Leicester University Press, p. 262, Appendix 1, Fig. 1.

7 Michael, P. (2004), 'Class, gender and insanity in nineteenth-century Wales' in Andrews, J. and Digby, A. (eds), *Sex and Seclusion, Class and Custody: Perspectives on Gender and Class in the History of British and Irish Psychiatry*. Amsterdam: Rodopi, pp. 95–122, p. 99.

8 Tilly, L. A. and Scott, J. W. (1987), *Women, Work and Family*. London: Methuen.

9 Valenze, D. (1995), *The First Industrial Woman*. Oxford: Oxford University Press.

10 King, S. and Tomkins, A. (eds) (2003), *The Poor in England 1700–1850. An Economy of Makeshifts*. Manchester: Manchester University Press, p. 268.

11 This was certainly what Scull believed; Scull, A. (1982), *Museums of Madness. The Social Organization of Insanity in Nineteenth-Century England*. London: Harmondsworth.

12 Ibid., p. 243.

13 St. Andrew's Hospital Archive (hereafter SAHA) Annual Report of the NGLA, 1858: ll.

14 Walton, J. K. (1979), 'Lunacy in the Industrial Revolution: a study of asylum admissions in Lancashire, 1848–50', *Journal of Social History*, 13, 1–22, p. 16.

15 Anderson, M. (1976), 'Sociological history and the working-class family: Smelser revisited', *Social History*, 3, 317–34, p. 328.

16 Suzuki, A. (2006), *Madness at Home. The Psychiatrist, the Patient and the Family in England, 1820–60*. Berkeley: University of California Press.

17 Wright, D. (2001), *Mental Disability in Victorian England: The Earlswood Asylum, 1847–1901*. Oxford: Clarendon Press; Wright, D. (1997), 'Getting out of the asylum: understanding the confinement of the insane in the nineteenth century', *Social History of Medicine*, 10, 22–46.

18 Bartlett, P. (1998), 'The asylum, the workhouse and the voice of the insane poor in nineteenth-century England', *International Journal of Law and Psychiatry*, 21, 421–32, pp. 431–2.

19 Coleborne, C. (2006), 'Families, patients and emotions: asylums for the insane in colonial Australia and New Zealand, c. 1880–1910', *Social History of Medicine*, 19; Kelm, M. (1994), 'Women, families and the provincial hospital for the insane, British Columbia, 1905–15', *Journal of Family History*, 19.

20 Wannell, L. (2007), 'Patients' relatives and psychiatric doctors: letter writing in the York Retreat, 1875–1910', *Social History of Medicine*, 20, 297–314.

21 Porter, R. (1985), 'The patient's view. Doing medical history from below', *Theory and Society*, 14, 175.

22 Smith, C. A. (2006), 'Family, community and the Victorian asylum: a case study of the Northampton General Lunatic Asylum and its pauper lunatics', *Family and Community History*, 9, 109–24.

23 Tomes, N. (1984), *A Generous Confidence: Thomas Story Kirkbride and the Art of Asylum Keeping, 1840–83*. Cambridge: Cambridge University Press.

24 It was also common for those of wealthier backgrounds to write querying financial arrangements; Wannell, 'Patients' relatives', 303.

25 King, S. (2007), 'Regional patterns in the experiences and treatment of the sick poor, 1800–40: rights, obligations and duties in the rhetoric of paupers', *Family and Community History*, 10, 61–75; Sokoll, T. (2006), 'Writing for relief: rhetoric in English pauper letters, 1800–34', in Gestrich, A., King, S. and Raphael, L. (eds) *Being Poor in Modern Europe: Historical Perspectives 1800–1940*. Frankfurt: Peter Lang, pp. 91–111; Sokoll, T. (2001), *Essex Pauper Letters, 1731–1837*. Oxford: Oxford University Press.

26 Wannell, 'Patients' relatives'.

27 Smith, C. A. (2007), 'Parsimony, power and prescriptive legislation: the politics of pauper lunacy in Northamptonshire 1845–76', *Bulletin of the History of Medicine*, 81, 359–85.

28 SAHA, MIN 1, Minutes of the proceedings relating to the General Lunatic Asylum at Northampton, 14 April 1835.

29 Smith, L. D. (1995), 'Levelled to the same common standard'? Social class in the lunatic asylum, 1780–1860', in Ashton, O., Fyson, R. and Roberts, S. (eds), *The Duty of the Discontent. Essays for Dorothy Thompson*. London: Mansell, p. 147.

30 SAHA NGLA Annual Report 1859: 7.

31 Hirst, D. (2005), 'A ticklish sort of affair': Charles Mott, Haydock Lodge and the economics of asylumdom', *History of Psychiatry*, 13, 31; MacKenzie, C. (1992), *Psychiatry for the Rich. A History of Ticehurst Private Asylum*. London: Routledge, p. 97; Hunter, R. and Macalpine, I. (1974), *Psychiatry for the Poor: 1851 Colney Hatch Asylum, Friern Hospital 1973*. London: Dawsons.

32 Smith, C. A. (2007), 'Insanity and the "civilising process": violence, the insane and asylums in the nineteenth century', in Watson, K. (ed.), *Assaulting the Past: Violence in Historical Context*. Newcastle: Scholars Press, 250–68.

33 Wright, D. (1999), 'The discharge of pauper lunatics from county asylums in mid-Victorian England. The case of Buckinghamshire, 1853 –1872', in Melling, J. and Forsythe, B. (eds), *Insanity, Institutions and Society, 1800–1914: A Social History of Madness in Comparative Perspective*. London: Routledge, pp. 93–112; Ray, L. (1981), 'Models of madness in Victorian asylum practice', *European Journal of Sociology*, 22.

34 Michael, P. (2003), *Care and Treatment of the Mentally Ill in North Wales 1800–2000*. Cardiff: University of Wales Press, p. 14.

35 Houston, R. (1999), '"Not simple boarding": care of the mentally incapacitated in Scotland during the long eighteenth century', in Bartlett, P. and Wright, D. (eds), *Outside the Walls of the Asylum. The History of Care in the Community 1750–2000*. London: Athlone Press; Wright, D. (1998), 'Family strategies and the institutional confinement of "idiot" children in Victorian England', *Journal of Family History*, 23, 190–208; Wright, D. '"Childlike in his innocence": lay attitudes to "idiots" and "imbeciles" in Victorian England', in Wright, D. and Digby, A. (eds), *From Idiocy to Mental Deficiency: Historical Perspectives on People with Learning Disabilities*. London: Routledge, pp. 118–33.
36 SAHA CL3 Admission No. 1390.
37 Houston, '"Not simple boarding"', p. 21.
38 SAHA: R1 and CL3 Admission No. 900.
39 Northamptonshire Records Office (hereafter NRO): HO107/0798.
40 NRO: QSLR 1845, Daventry Union.
41 SAHA: R1 and CL3 Admission No. 900.
42 NRO: HO107/0804.
43 Ibid., HO107/1735/F389.
44 BMDIndex.co.uk.
45 NRO: QSLR 1853 and 1860, Banbury Union.
46 Ibid., QSLR 1845–63, Kettering Union.
47 Ibid., 1855.
48 SAHA: CL 2 Admission No. 2510.
49 Ibid., R2 Admission No. 2595 (although also recorded as 2596).
50 Ibid., CL 6 Admission No. 2595: 33.
51 Bartlett and Wright, *Outside the Walls*, p. 3.
52 SAHA: CL6 Admission No. 2592: 27.
53 Ibid.
54 NRO: RG9/0949.
55 Tomes, *A Generous Confidence*, pp. 108–9.
56 SAHA: CL7 Admission No. 2798: 9.
57 Ibid., CL4 Admission No. 2736: 323.
58 Marland, H. (1999), 'At home with puerperal mania: the domestic treatment of the insanity of childbirth in the nineteenth century', in Bartlett and Wright, *Outside the Walls*, pp. 45–65.
59 Bartlett, *The Poor Law of Lunacy*, p. 270, Table 5.
60 Ibid., p. 217, Table 6.
61 Prior, P. (1997), 'Mad not bad: crime, mental disorder and gender in nineteenth-century Ireland', *History of Psychiatry*, 8, 502; Walsh, O. (2004), 'Gender and insanity in nineteenth-century Ireland', in Andrews and Digby, *Sex and Seclusion*, p. 82.
62 Walton, 'Lunacy'.
63 Andrews and Digby, *Sex and Seclusion*, pp. 14–18.
64 Scull, *Museums of Madness*, pp. 223 and 232, Table 9.
65 Tomes, *A Generous Confidence*, p.109.
66 Melling, J., Forsythe, B. and Adair, R. (1999), 'Families, communities and the legal regulation of lunacy in Victorian England: assessments of crime, violence and welfare in admissions to the Devon Asylum, 1845–1914', in Bartlett and Wright, *Outside the Walls*, p. 172.
67 SAHA: R2 Admission No. 2804.

68 Ibid., CL7 Admission No. 2804.

69 Wright, 'Family strategies', pp. 203–4.

70 Blaikie, A. (2005), 'Accounting for poverty: conflicting constructions of family survival in Scotland, 1855–1925', *Journal of Historical Sociology*, 18, 202–26; Snell, K. D. M. (1985), *Annals of the Labouring Poor: Social Change and Agrarian England, 1660–1900*. Cambridge: Cambridge University Press; Thane, P. (2000), *Old Age in English History: Past Experiences, Present Issues*. Oxford: Oxford University Press; Sokoll, T. (1993), *Household and Family Among the Poor: The Case of two Essex Communities in the Late Eighteenth and Early Nineteenth Centuries*. Bochum: Brockmeyer.

71 Henderson, J. and Wall, R. (eds) (1994), *Poor Women and Children in the European Past*. London: Routledge.

72 Farr, W. (1837), 'Vital Statistics' in McCulloch, J. R. (ed.), *Statistics of the British Empire*. London: Black.

73 PP27: Report of the Metropolitan Commissioners in Lunacy 1844.

74 Cherry, S. (2003), *Mental Health Care in Modern England. The Norfolk Lunatic Asylum St Andrew's Hospital, 1810–1998*. Woodbridge: Boydell, p. 39.

75 Walton, 'Lunacy in the Industrial Revolution', p. 12.

76 Hunter and MacAlpine, *Psychiatry for the Poor*, pp. 172–3.

77 SAHA: RG2 Admission No. 2499.

78 Ibid., MIN 27, 21 July 1862.

79 Ibid.

80 SAHA: CL 4: 7.

81 Ibid., MIN27: 300.

82 SAHA: R3 Admission No. 2986. As the letter indicates, Catherine had been admitted before, first entering NGLA in December 1858 at the age of 22. This first admission lasted only a month before she was discharged recovered.

83 Pamela Michael argues that 'recurrent child-bearing was specially burdensome for women who were vulnerable to mental afflictions following pregnancies'. Michael, 'Class, gender and insanity', p. 108.

84 NRO: RG9/0939.

85 SAHA: CL4 Admission No. 2986.

86 SAHA: MIN27: 301–2.

87 Ibid., 338.

88 Ibid., MIN 28, 19 April 1871: 99–100.

89 Ibid., R2 Admission No. 2703.

90 Ibid., MIN27: 125.

91 Ibid., CL4 Admission No. 2703: 301.

92 Ibid., MIN 26 19 March 1861.

93 Wright, 'Family strategies', pp. 197–8.

94 SAHA: R3 Admission No. 2985.

95 Ibid., R3 Admission No. 2985.

96 Ibid., MIN 27, 24 October 1866: 276.

97 Ibid., CL 4: 450.

98 Ibid.

99 Ibid., 134–5.
100 Ibid., R3 Admission No. 3761.
101 Ibid., MIN 27, 23 November 1864: 163.
102 Ibid., 23 August 1864:198.
103 Wright, 'Family strategies'.

7

Narratives of poverty in Irish suicides between the Great Famine and the First World War, 1845–1914

Georgina Laragy

Introduction

At the beginning of 1847, in the midst of Ireland's Great Famine, Dublin newspaper the *Freeman's Journal* reported the 'melancholy suicide' of Mr Patrick Barden. Barden was a water bailiff in the city and had recently worked on the relief committee in his parish, St Nicholas Without. Dr John Ryan, who had known the dead man for some time, was called to Barden's house on the morning of 17 January where he 'found deceased stretched in the stable with his throat cut'.[1] At the subsequent inquest, witnesses revealed that Barden was a 'sober, steady and well-conducted' man. In the days prior to his death he appeared to 'be labouring under some slight mental derangement but his bodily health was good'. The local clergyman stated that although Barden's business had failed he was not 'embarrassed in his circumstances' and that 'no man could be more happy with a wife and children'. His situation was vastly different to the thousands of starving men, women and children then living in Dublin city and throughout the countryside; Barden killed himself at the beginning of 'Black '47', believed by many to be the worst year of the Irish Famine.[2] He did not believe such misery could be witnessed in any part of the world and had described the inhabitants of Walker's Alley in Dublin's inner city as 'walking corpses . . . it [is] a disgrace to a civilised country to witness such scenes'.[3] Friends believed that witnessing such poverty had unhinged his mind and drove him to suicide.

We return to Barden later in the chapter, but it will be clear from his story that legal records and newspaper accounts of inquests on suicides comprise an accessible means of discovering how, why and who committed suicide in Victorian and Edwardian Ireland. These records reveal the reactions of families, friends and communities to the tragedy of self-inflicted death and explore a wide variety of explanations for suicide, as well as providing evidence of the circumstances in which the deceased had taken their own lives. Poverty and sickness in their myriad forms featured consistently in witness testimony and through this we can examine the popular understanding of how poverty and suicide intersected. We can glimpse different sections of 'poor' Irish people – the destitute and homeless, the sick poor, the working poor and those who were 'embarrassed' – and weave together competing and complementary narratives about them.

This said, poverty in the nineteenth century was a relative concept, and while we attempt to identify the poor as a social group it is important to understand what we mean by poverty. Historians argue that definitions of poverty and the poor are necessarily shifting because 'the boundaries between working class, indigent and destitute were fluid'.[4] Being poor depended on a number of variables including stage of life, gender, geographic location, employment status and family circumstance; and individual experiences of poverty could range from indebtedness and the loss of property, to unemployment, homelessness and starvation. This chapter will thus look at different categories of the poor in order to construct narratives of poverty in the context of suicide. For the most part it focuses on suicides that occurred outside public institutions including workhouses. Studying the poor beyond the workhouse walls enables us to explore a broader experience of poverty, including the initial stages of downward social mobility which often led to workhouse admission. Moreover, in common with inquests on suicides in lunatic asylums in nineteenth-century Ireland, the investigation of pauper suicides in workhouses tended to ignore the individual's circumstances and focus only on the failure of the institution to ensure the safety of inmates.

While newspaper reports, witness statements and suicide notes – the stock-in-trade of the chapter – are not akin to pauper narratives of the sort explored elsewhere in this volume, more of their potential for understanding experiences of both poverty and sickness is revealed through further elaboration of Barden's case. The inquest on his body rejected the 'usual' markers of a suicidal life – insanity, alcohol problems, sickness, financial or family difficulties – as possible explanations for his death. In the absence of any obvious personal problem, it was believed that 'mental derangement' – perhaps akin to the melancholic feelings explored for England and an earlier period by Alannah Tomkins elsewhere in this volume – lay at the heart of Barden's suicide. Contemporaries believed, as we have already hinted, that his peace of mind had been destroyed by the 'harrowing scenes of misery and distress which he saw' as he worked with the parish relief committee in St Nicholas Without.[5] According to a neighbour, Barden only became despondent after 'he came into contact with the scenes of misery which he encountered in the parish'. The medical witness Dr Ryan, who also worked on the relief committee, 'thought [he had] expressed an unwillingness to undertake the painful duty . . . [Barden] . . . acted for one day and then tendered his resignation saying, that from the scenes of misery he had witnessed he could not act'. The local pastor stated that

> . . . from the state of [Barden's] mind, witness had no doubt the melancholy scenes might have so operated on a person of his sensibility as to induce a peculiar hallucination of mind on these subjects, and that under the influence of such alienation of intellect, he might have committed the rash deed . . .[6]

In these intersecting narratives of Barden's suicide, the poverty of Dublin had two functions for the newspaper that reported it: first it helped the editor 'call the attention of the public to the state of things in which this painful circumstance had its origin'.[7] The significance of Barden's suffering and tragic death was extended beyond the confines of his private turmoil and the misery of those who lived in Walker's Alley. Poverty was stalking 'civilised' Irish cities and towns, unhinging the sanity of sensitive and altruistic men and challenging the existing social and political order of laissez faire economics. Secondly, and ironically, poverty lent an air of respectability to the tragic, and at this time criminal, death by suicide of Barden.[8] Responsibility fell not on Barden himself, whose sensitivity made him vulnerable to such misery, but rather the wider system which allowed this suffering to persist. The middle-class readership of the *Freeman's Journal*, much as was the case with readers of the Spanish newspapers cited elsewhere in this volume by Beate Althammer, was confronted with the dark underbelly of their city and the threat that such misery posed for members of their own class. For historians, these competing and complementary, mediated and unmediated, official and semi-official, narratives provide an intriguing way into an understanding of the relationship between poverty and mental affliction in one of Europe's more peripheral societies, as well as underpinning the intertwining of broad quantitative perspectives with detailed case studies.

Suicide during the Famine

Individual cases reveal that contemporaries saw chronic poverty as part of the broader context of the lives of those who killed themselves; but did Irish Victorians believe that poverty itself caused suicide? Certainly during the Famine individual suicides were attributed to starvation and want. In

September 1846 the editor of the *Freeman's Journal* described how 'death seizes the poor in various and appalling forms. One in Galway terminates his sufferings by suicide.'[9] The same issue contained the excerpt of a letter from a parish priest, Fr. O'Brien originally printed in the *Tipperary Vindicator*. He described how

> . . . a man named Evans, being out of employment, pennyless and in a state of extreme destitution, put a period to his sufferings by hanging himself. I fear, ere long, many such tragical [sic] events will occur here, for the people are starving and there is no employment.[10]

The reports of suicide from want were less frequent in the earlier years of the Famine. In December 1846 a Sligo correspondent for the *Freeman's Journal* reported that a poor woman had died in the parish of Clooncall from starvation and that 'her sister drowned herself the same day to avoid a like fate'.[11] Though such reports also cited disappointment in love, drink and physical and mental illness as causative factors during this period,[12] by the late 1840s examples of suicide as a result of famine, destitution and want were proliferating in line with the sharp increase in suicide generally in these years. Various official sources record that the rate of suicide increased between 1831 and 1914. For the period 1833–41, before the outbreak of Famine, the average annual rate was 1.0003 per 100,000. Between the years 1842–51 it rose by over a quarter to 1.26 per 100,000 and in the following decade it rose slightly to 1.27.[13] Recorded suicide rose from 60 in 1845 to 120 in 1848 (Figure 7.1).

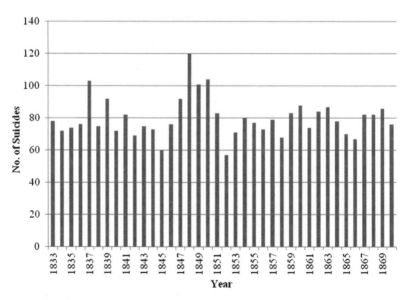

FIGURE 7.1 Numbers of suicides in Ireland, 1833–70.
Source: Census of Ireland, 1841, 1851, 1861 & 1871.

This reported rise is significant given the time and circumstances in which it was recorded. Before the creation of the Office of the Registrar General in 1863 the Census Commissioners under the direction of ophthalmologist Sir William Wilde included in the Census a 'Report on deaths and diseases' which required heads of households to record details of all those who had died in the previous ten years, their names, date of death, age and cause of death.[14] This information was returned at the end of each given ten-year period. The overall rise for the decade in which the Great Famine occurred is all the more startling given that there were far fewer people making returns to the Census Commissioners; the Census of 1851 revealed that the population had dropped by over two million since 1841.

The weekly discussions of the 'state of the country' in the *Freeman's Journal* add meat to the bare bones provided by those numbers. It becomes clear from these narratives that many lived in abject poverty but that there were distinctions between the poor and those who, through famine, were 'becoming poor'. The reports noted that those who last year had 'enjoy[ed] ...comparative wealth', or who had at least 'the means to keep the wolf from the door', had now descended into pauperism. In comparison to the 'want and destitution' in which they now found themselves they had been wealthy. Strategies of survival were no match for persistent potato blight and a famine that raged for years. Even the state's Poor Law system, established in 1838 and administered locally by boards of guardians, fell foul of the extreme conditions of 1840s Ireland. A man living in Tomgrany, Co. Cork 'attempted suicide from distress' on 8 December 1847.[15] Along with his wife and six children he had been refused admission to the Scariff workhouse because it was overcrowded, having 740 inmates.[16] Public works were introduced in 1846 by Robert Peel's government but were deemed anathema to the free market economics of new Prime Minister Lord John Russell in late 1846. He reorganized the public works scheme to the detriment of many individuals. The cumulative effect of famine and chaotic public relief systems was devastating; 'it is extraordinary to witness the peaceable conduct of the people up to the present, and their resignation to the will of Providence. Till now they had hope. The delusion has vanished. They are yielding to despair.'[17] In May 1847 the parish priest of Ballymachugh and Drumlumman in County Cavan, Fr R. Murray, an equivalent to the epistolary advocates that one finds corresponding with so many English parishes on behalf of the poor, wrote that between 1 October 1846 and 1 April 1847, 76 people died from starvation in his parish. Since the beginning of May (at that point only five days old) another 15 had been added to the list.

Two of the number died on their return from the public works. One of the others, fearing that he would not be able to 'bring round' his family, as they say, got into a gloomy state of mind and poisoned himself by taking arsenic. The wife of a small farmer named Denny had her throat cut by her husband who got into a state of phrenzy [sic] from a similar cause.[18]

The government under Russell eventually passed the Poor Law Extension Act in 1847 which transformed the system by providing outdoor relief on certain conditions and to certain types of individuals (e.g. the permanently disabled and poor widows).[19] However, even the provision of outdoor relief did nothing to stem despair for some. In February 1848 an unknown man 'whose appearance indicated that . . . [he] . . . must have suffered from the most abject poverty' was found hanged. He had a recommendation for outdoor relief in the pocket of his coat.[20]

Post-Famine: Family, 'Friends' and the importance of social support

After the Famine, the situation began to improve but there remained a section of Irish society which continued to require public and private assistance since economic progress was neither unbroken nor universal. Not only did admissions to workhouses begin to increase from the 1870s onwards, but the number of Irish paupers who received outdoor relief also rose.[21] Despite the increasing acceptance of public welfare from the boards of guardians, poverty remained a cause of distress for many individuals, and wider socio-economic changes – rural and urban – impinged strongly on the mindsets of individuals who contemplated suicide.

In economic terms, the consolidation of farms and a shift to pastoral production boosted the Irish economy but it also led to personal crises for some individuals. Clearances which had begun before the Famine were enacted to consolidate farms and observers were clear as to the effects of this process: 'Landlords here [County Down] are now actively pursuing the clearance-out system with a vengeance against all tenants who are unable to pay all rent and arrears of rent up to November last. The unfortunate tenants-at-will have become maddened.' This led to malicious burnings and suicides according to the reporter.[22] The clearances ensured greater productivity, and more generally persistent emigration and population decline relieved pressure on finite resources. Nonetheless, Irish Catholics in particular continued to produce large families and the majority of those children were disinherited as parents moved away from customary partible inheritance to practices which concentrated heritable wealth and resources.[23] As Joe Lee describes it, 'the integrity of the family was ruthlessly sacrificed, generation after generation, to the priority of economic man, to the rationale of economic calculus'.[24] Rehabilitation of the Irish economy, then, brought its own human and emotional costs and added to them in terms of a latent pressure to secure and maintain improved economic circumstances, an issue that we revisit below.

Social changes, too, influenced the backdrop against which we must interpret suicide. Emile Durkheim argued in 1897, 50 years after 'Black

'47', that 'there is very little suicide in Ireland, where the peasantry leads so wretched a life . . . poverty may even be considered a protection'.[25] Along with endemic poverty, low rates of Irish suicide were also attributed to its Catholic and largely rural population. Being accustomed to their 'wretched' life and with the support of close-knit agricultural communities and the influential presence of a religion that prided itself on communal practices and rituals, the Irish were viewed as highly socially integrated and less prone to suicide.[26] For Durkheim, the family was a protective institution and one of the mechanisms by which emotional stability was to be achieved: 'However poor one is, and even solely from the point of view of personal interest, it is the worst of investments to substitute wealth for a portion of one's feelings.'[27] From this viewpoint, poverty was preferable to prosperity achieved at the expense of emotional contentment. The Irish family, then, contributed to distinctively low suicide rates.

Durkheim was wrong in at least two respects. First, in his understanding of suicide levels. The Office of the Registrar General was established in 1863 and its annual reports reveal the rise in suicide rates from that year onwards (Figure 7.2).[28] Suicide rates doubled between 1864 and 1892 and continued to increase until 1912. This period witnessed years of significant economic distress including 1879–82, 1886 and 1891,[29] though the relationship between distress and suicide is not unilinear. If we take the overall national rate of suicide as an indicator, suicide rose between 1879 and 1883 but it dropped both in 1886 and again in 1891.[30] Overall, though the period covered by this chart was one of increasing stability and prosperity for many, the rising rate of suicide reveals that the 'moral danger involved in every growth of prosperity . . . should not be forgotten'.[31] Durkheim was also wrong in his understanding of the character and role of the later nineteenth-century Irish family. Kushner has criticized Durkheim's 'sentimental visions of the family and . . . ambivalence to social change',[32] and it is certainly true that

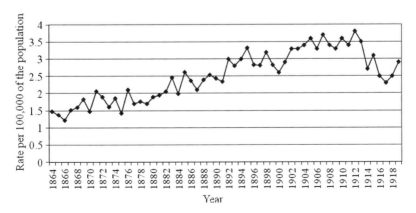

FIGURE 7.2 Rate of suicide in Ireland, 1864–1919.
Source: Annual reports of the Registrar General.

post-Famine demography saw radical change in this area. Marriage rates were on the decline before the outbreak of Famine but the drop accelerated afterwards. High fertility remained but levels of celibacy increased as did emigration. In short, the nuptial and familial situation for young people was transformed and adhered little to Durkheim's understanding. As one historian has noted, when celibacy increased so too did lunacy.[33] And so too did suicide, for, as we shall see, family circumstances often appear in suicide narratives as a factor in drawing the individual low, as was the case for the men analysed by Alannah Tomkins elsewhere in this volume.

Within the sociological discourse of the late nineteenth century it was not poverty per se which led to suicide, but rather the social circumstances in which poverty had emerged. Rising levels of suicide alongside improvements in the standard of living of many Irish people – 'the Famine's part in improving the lot of most people who survived is indisputable'[34] – were compatible where the socio-economic, institutional and familial mechanisms for maintaining economic progress were themselves fragile. The importance of this observation can be measured by turning once again to individual cases of suicide. These reveal that single people in particular were often disappointed when it came to calling on family and friends in times of need. Moreover, and at least for women, both society and family were willing to apply moral yardsticks which heightened the probability of suicide.

Thus, Anastasia Mulhall's body was found in the River Barrow in Carlow in March 1904 and the inquest heard her landlady relate that, 'She paid me for her lodging and was not as far as I knew destitute.'[35] However, Anastasia 'had no friends . . . and complained of not being very well and not being able to work'. Another particularly revealing case occurred in Cork in 1896. Susan Fagan was 25 years old when she was convicted in April of attempting to kill herself. In comparison with the criminal records of other women convicted of attempted suicide, Fagan's record was quite short. Since January of that year she had been convicted on four occasions for being drunk and disorderly.[36] Judge Neligan, the Recorder of Cork, had sentenced her to two years' hard labour, which was the maximum sentence available in such cases, and unusually harsh.[37] However, Neligan was motivated by concern for the girl in sentencing. When she was put to the bar to plead, the judge was struck 'by [Susan's] miserably wretched appearance – she seemed young – very haggard and emaciated'; she was also 'stone deaf'. The judge communicated with her through writing (revealing that she was literate), and discovered that she was a native of Dublin who had been turned out by her father having been seduced. She ended up on the streets and somehow made her way south to Cork. The judge in his sympathy wished 'to have something done for this unfortunate creature'. He communicated with the Roman Catholic chaplain in the prison who then contacted a community of nuns willing to 'take charge of this poor girl as an act of charity and to treat her with special consideration'. The petition for release was made by the judge and she was legally transferred over to the custody of nuns at the Good Shepherd convent in Cork. He promised 'I shall myself see to her removal and will occasionally make enquiry at the convent about her.'

After being thrown out of home Susan Fagan had found herself homeless in a strange city. Although we do not know why she attempted to kill herself, it is clear that her disability and the failure of her family to support her ensured that she was vulnerable. Through chance and perhaps good luck she came to the attention of a sympathetic state in the person of Judge Neligan who viewed her offence as a cry for help from a desperate and destitute young woman with nowhere else to turn, rather than the action of a career criminal. The poverty in which Fagan had found herself was not entirely of her own making; her disability ensured her status as a member of the 'deserving poor'. The issue of 'deserving' and 'undeserving' poor highlights the Victorian concern with respectability and moral behaviour and the importance of distinguishing between those unable to work through health or disability, and those unwilling to work through idleness, dissipation and disinclination. These concepts of poverty were steeped in Victorian notions of proper behaviour and gender roles.[38] The welfare system in both England and Ireland was based on conceptions of who deserved state support and who did not. However, it was not only within the purview of the state to provide support to the poor. The first port of call in times of crises tended to be the family. But like the boards of guardians, they were not averse to making judgements based on respectability and moral behaviour. Susan Fagan had been deemed unworthy of continued support by her father; she ended up far from home, emaciated and suicidal.

Another young lady, Margaret Cowley, found herself in a similar situation in 1900, in a case that highlighted, as Fagan's does, that women's domestic security and emotional stability were dependent on adherence to a certain code of behaviour. Cowley was accused of having a relationship with a married man, and, having been dismissed from her position as a domestic servant, drowned herself in August 1900 in the Royal Canal in Dublin. Alongside her hat on the bank of the canal she left two notes in which she protested her innocence. After her dismissal she had returned home to her father who then threatened to throw her out. Among the working poor, Fuchs has argued that 'people's private lives were community concerns . . . communities policed courtships'.[39] In Victorian Dublin the honour and reputation of a young woman was important, it determined her employment opportunities and her right to support from within the family network.

Both women, through their socio-economic status and in Fagan's case, disability, were vulnerable. More generally, members of the working classes and the sick poor were in an exposed position; the descent into homelessness and poverty rested on subjective but powerful judgements of an individual's respectability and worthiness. For women in particular, the lack of a significant manufacturing base meant that the employment opportunities that may have provided an alternative means of support were limited, with a particular focus on domestic service.[40] In this area, however, the replication of the family system meant that domestic harmony and respectability was as important to employers as parents. Single women, dependent on family or employment to keep poverty at bay, were particularly vulnerable; separated and widowed women lived under the shadow of poverty. Jane Boylan tied two 16-pound stones in an apron and fastened it to her body before she drowned in Monaghan town in 1858. She was separated from her husband and had recently admitted stealing from her brother. Her husband only days before her death had agreed to pay for board and supply her with a shilling a week, 'being as much as he could afford'.[41] This did not alleviate Jane's worries and she killed herself. Becoming a widow also lent itself to financial worries, and when Bridget McKenny's husband died by hanging in March 1907 she began to 'fail'; over a year later at the inquest into her death her son recounted that she 'was in debt and this used to worry her and I do believe it was the most cause of her annoyance'.[42]

In the case of single or widowed men, illness and a lack of family support were themes in suicide inquests but rarely was there mention of the moral concerns present in the cases of female suicide above. John Carroll, an unemployed tramp with no family had been injured in the course of a robbery; in 1909 he complained that 'my foot is hurt. I can't look for a living and must.'[43] At the inquest on the body of William Dickson who had been found dead on 6 March 1912 in Ballybay, Co. Monaghan, the coroner and his jury heard the story of a twice-widowed man who was homeless and down on his luck. The local publican described how he had lent the deceased money as 'he had no means', while the local shoemaker testified that Dickson had stayed in his house for the two nights before his death: 'he didn't pay me for his accommodation; as he had no money'. His brother, who had not seen him in 12 months, described him as having 'no fixed abode' and being 'financially embarrassed'. The man had been sober the night before he died although he was known to be 'peculiar' when he had taken drink.[44] It is quite clear that Dickson was destitute but in the absence of any word from the man himself it is not clear that his destitution was the cause of his suicide. Being homeless and without money were part of the fabric of Dickson's life, and they were significant in the eyes of those who testified.

More widely, sociological studies considered single men more likely to commit suicide because 'on men the hurtful influence of celibacy and widowhood is lasting'.[45] The lack of family support for poor Irish men is evident when we examine the pauper inmates of Irish workhouses, revealing that it was not only women who were vulnerable to poverty in the broader context of a single life. Men as a proportion of all adults comprised the greater number of inmates admitted in both the North Dublin Union and Thurles but there was a significantly higher proportion of men in the workhouse in Thurles; by 1911 men accounted for 69 per cent of all adults admitted; in Dublin the figure was 56 percent.[46] By 1871 approximately 59 per cent of all adult males admitted to the provincial workhouse of Thurles were single;

this figure had risen to 75 per cent in 1911.[47] The pattern was reversed in the North Dublin Union where just half of all adult males admitted in 1871 were single, a figure that dropped to 46 per cent only in 1911.

Financial difficulties, anxiety and the 'revolution of rising expectations'

Yet our focus on the poor should not be confined to those who bore the traditional markers of poverty. It was not only those who entered workhouses, became homeless, experienced hunger pangs and were without means to support themselves who can be considered 'poor'. The working and lower-middle classes and professionals in Ireland were all vulnerable to swift changes of fortune, as we have seen above. In 1862 an unknown elderly man of 'gentlemanly' appearance was found dead. A note found beside his body revealed; 'I have been sleeping on the rocks these two nights.'[48] His appearance and literacy suggest an educated middle-class man but his sleeping arrangements point to a very sharp decline in his fortunes which he may not have wished to reveal to anyone in his circle. This may account for his suicide far from where he was known. An inquest from the early twentieth century also included a record from the deceased himself – the illuminating diary entries of Dr John Jones revealed that he was 'hopeless – soon homeless – helpless – friendless . . . awful temptation – debts on every side – no way of escape – save one which greatly tempts'.[49] Dr Jones was in the process of 'becoming poor' and this propelled him towards suicide.

Across the post-Famine period there is evidence to suggest that anxieties about financial difficulties were viewed as understandable reasons for someone to kill themselves, even if in comparison to the inmates of a workhouse they were well-off. In August 1863 Patrick Prunty hanged himself after a period in which he 'was greatly depressed in mind, from various causes – loss of one of his farms [and] the death of some cattle'.[50] James McDonnell was a 'respectable farmer' with 25 acres from Sligo, but he was worrying about bad crops in 1878, which came in the middle of a particularly difficult period.[51] Although living comfortably with his family, he had some notion that his farm did not belong to him. This insecurity was also apparent in the context in which another Sligo man Patrick Brennan shot into a neighbour's house before he turned the gun on himself. Brennan's wife revealed that 'he was afraid that his cattle could be seized by the Sheriff and Police and there was no reason for he [sic] believing this. He also thought the bog was also taken from him.'

These middle-aged men who committed suicide in the 1860s and 1870s had survived the Famine and earlier subsistence crises when farms, crops and livestock had been lost. Insecurity of tenure was not just an imaginary problem; it prompted decades of agitation by labourers and farmers who participated in the 'Land War'. The initial phase of this 'war' began in 1878 when Michael Davitt and Charles Stewart Parnell formed the Irish Land League. That was the same year Patrick Brennan, fearing his cattle and bog would be seized, turned a gun on himself. It is not surprising that anxious thoughts plagued the minds of these men who had only recently achieved success. Its fragile nature ensured that none rested easy[52] against the backdrop of what J. J. Lee describes as a 'revolution of rising expectations'.[53] This revolution highlights the fluidity of ideas about poverty and financial security over time as well as between the classes at any given time. Engels' experience of 'Little Ireland' in Manchester made him 'conscious . . . that human needs are not uniform: an Englishman could not subsist on as little as an Irishman'. Similarly, within Ireland men who before the Famine might have been happy with a small-holding of four acres now worried about the loss of one of their two farms. Impressionistic evidence taken from inquests suggests that in the second half of the nineteenth century, particularly from the 1870s on, men were preoccupied with the loss of financial security which denoted that they had achieved a degree of comfort. Descriptions of 'destitution' did not apply to these men; for some 'becoming poor' in the later part of the nineteenth century meant experiencing far greater losses than those who had faced famine.

Conclusion

Did poverty cause suicides? Or rather, did nineteenth-century Victorians living in Ireland believe that poverty caused suicides? The answer to such a question is largely unknowable; the clues that have survived for historians' inspection rest chiefly in the words of those who were left behind to explain suicidal deaths – families, friends, neighbours, doctors and police. The specific suicide narratives included here are representative of a particular group of people who mentioned financial difficulties but not poverty per se; levels of literacy as well as access to pen and paper might explain the lack of suicide notes left by poor people. However generated, these notes reveal that people began to consider suicide on 'becoming poor'. This corroborates Durkheim's argument that chronic financial problems were not as detrimental as 'crises of prosperity'. When poverty is endemic it becomes the established 'collective order . . . [and] wherever serious readjustments take place in the social order whether or not due to a sudden growth or to an unexpected catastrophe, men are more inclined to self-destruction'. The Irish Famine of 1845–50 qualified as such a catastrophe though Durkheim failed to include it in his discussion.

During this time the newly created public welfare system collapsed under the weight of thousands of starving bodies; shared suffering and private despair are evident in the newspapers and official statistics that recorded an increase in suicides. Contemporaries made a causal link between poverty and suicide and in doing so highlighted the lack of mechanisms to help the hungry. The importance of networks of support was underlined by the response of those who had none. In the absence of social support networks – either familial or communal – the state, in the form of the courts, welfare institutions and lunatic asylums, stepped in to assist troubled individuals during times of personal crises. Yet despite the increasing intervention of the state in private lives suicide continued to increase. Equally, notwithstanding general improvement in social and economic conditions in Ireland during the post-Famine period, suicide rose. While there are numerous practical explanations for this pattern it must be considered that informal networks of support provided more than just practical assistance. They were also an emotional buffer when times were tough. As suicide narratives reveal, however, for many Irish people the family and its support was a double-edged sword. Against this backdrop, disability, illness, economic downturn and the threat of the loss of social respectability led many – the single in particular – to contemplate committing suicide.

Stitching together several narrative forms – from witness testimonies, through diaries and to newspaper reporting of inquests – does more, however, than just tell us something new about Irish suicide patterns. Various dimensions of 'the troubled mind' that led Irish men and women to commit suicide were common themes in unmediated pauper narratives and petitions across Europe. The language of the witnesses before Irish inquests has distinct resonance with that of the epistolary advocates who wrote in support of the destitute to their parishes of settlement in Germany and England. Similarly, the moral undertones that we can detect in the narratives relating to Irish female suicide coincides neatly with similar concerns expressed in relation to the Swedish venereal disease patients analysed elsewhere in this volume by Anna Lundberg. And like all of the narratives by or about the poor underpinning the different chapters in this volume, those employed here provide at least an oblique window onto the everyday experiences of the poorest sections of society who might otherwise remain submerged in the historical record. At the same time, and importantly, studying Irish suicides as one aspect of the European sick poor calls our attention to something less often highlighted in the secondary literature: that the process of becoming poor, whether real or imagined, was as disabling and fundamental as the status of destitution itself.

Notes

1 *Freeman's Journal*, 18 January 1847.
2 Gray, P. (1999), *Famine, Land and Politics: British Government and Irish Society, 1843–50*. Dublin: Irish Academic Press; Hoppen, K. T. (1998), *The Mid-Victorian Generation*. Oxford: Clarendon Press; Ó'Gráda, C. (2000), *Black '47 and Beyond: The Great Irish Famine in History, Economy and Memory*. Princeton: Princeton

University Press; McLean, S. (2004), *The Event and Its Terrors: Ireland, Famine, Modernity*. Stanford: Stanford University Press; Kinneally, C. (2002), *The Great Irish Famine: Impact, Ideology and Rebellion*. New York: Palgrave; Miller, D. W. (1978), 'Irish Catholicism and the Great Famine', *Journal of Social History*, 9, 81–98.

3 *Freeman's Journal*, 18 January 1847.

4 Fuchs, R. (2005), *Gender and Poverty in Nineteenth Century Europe*. Cambridge: Cambridge University Press, p. 14. See also Koven, S. (2006), *Slumming: Sexual and Social Politics in Victorian London*. Princeton: Princeton University Press, pp. 10–11; Strange, J.-M. (2005), *Death, Grief and Poverty in Britain, 1870–1914*. Cambridge: Cambridge University Press, p. 22.

5 According to various articles in the *Freeman's Journal* in late 1846 and throughout 1847 the inhabitants of the civil parish of St Nicholas Without came together in December 1846 to address the issue of destitution in their parish and do something for their parishioners (23 December 1846). A meeting held in January of 1847 mentioned the attendance of the Catholic Rector Rev. Dr Flanagan, the Protestant Rector Rev. Mr Hallahan and a variety of other local officials including Town Commissioners and other local notables. Patrick Barden was listed as one of the secretaries (9 January 1847). Over 3,000 individuals were receiving assistance by the end of January (1 February 1847). At the end of March the committee of St Nicholas Without had come together with other local parish-based relief committees in Dublin to seek assistance from the government under the umbrella of the 'South City Relief Committee' (27 March 1847).

6 *Freeman's Journal*, 18 January 1847.

7 Ibid.

8 Suicide was a criminal offence under common law. Since the medieval period those found guilty (or felo de se) were punished through ignominious burial and confiscation of property. The law on ignominious burial had changed in 1823 following the death by suicide of the Lord Castlereagh the previous year (4 Geo. IV.cap.52. (U.K.), Felo de Se Act). In 1872 the forfeiture of goods of felons became illegal (33 & 34 Vict.cap.23 Forfeiture Act) and in 1880 and 1882 further legislation was passed prescribing the means of burial for suicides (43 & 44 Vict. cap. 41.[Eng.] Internment Act; 45 & 46 Vict.cap.19. [Eng.] Internments (Felo de se) Act). The legislation of 1880 and 1882 dictating burial applied in England and Wales only, not Ireland or Scotland. When Barden committed suicide in 1847 he was found innocent of the crime of self-murder by the verdict of temporary insanity; this meant he was free to be buried in consecrated ground. See Gates, B. T. (1988), *Victorian Suicides: Mad Crimes and Sad Histories*. Princeton: Princeton University Press, chapter one. For further information on the history of suicide, see Anderson, O. (1987), *Suicide in Victorian and Edwardian England*. Oxford: Clarendon Press; Minois, G. (1999), *History of Suicide: Voluntary Death in Western Culture*. Baltimore: Johns Hopkins University Press; Bailey, V. (1998), *This Rash Act: Suicide Across the Life-cycle in the Victorian City*. Stanford: Stanford University Press; Lederer, D. (2006), *Madness, Religion and the State in Early Modern Europe: A Bavarian Beacon*. Cambridge: Cambridge University Press; Watt, J. R. (2001), *Choosing Death: Suicide and Calvinism in Early Modern Geneva*. Kirksville: Truman State University Press.

9 *Freeman's Journal*, 28 September 1846.

10 Ibid.

11 *Freeman's Journal*, 1 December 1846.

12 *Freeman's Journal*, 23 January 1847, 3 April 1847, 23 July 1847, 20 January 1847, 1 September 1847, 5 December 1848, 6 April 1848.

13 These figures are based on the 'Reports of deaths and disease' compiled by the Census Commissioners for the decennial census in 1841, 1851 and 1861 in conjunction with the population figures found in Vaughan, W. E. and Fitzpatrick, D. (eds) (1978), *Irish Historical Statistics*. Dublin: Royal Irish Academy. A similar report was included in 1871 but as the annual reports of the Registrar General began to be published in 1864 this was the final census in which such a report was included: House of Commons Parliamentary Papers *Census Returns*, 1841, 1851, 1861 and 1871. There are numerous problems with both the Census 'Report on deaths and diseases' and the Annual Reports of the Registrar General. See Laragy, G. (2010), 'Suicide and insanity in post-Famine Ireland' in Cox, C. and Luddy, M. (eds), *Cultures of Care in Irish Medical History, 1750–1970*. London: Palgrave Macmillan, pp. 82–3. In comparison with other European countries at this time, Ireland's rate of suicide was quite low. In France during the period 1851 to 1855 the annual average rate of suicide per 100,000 was 10. The rate in Scotland between 1856 and 1860 was 3.4 per 100,000.

14 *Census of Ireland, 1851, part V, 'Report, tables of pestilences, and analysis of the tables of deaths'* H.C. 1856 [2087–1], xxix. See also Crawford, E. M. (2003), *Counting the People: A Survey of the Irish Censuses, 1831–1911*. Dublin: Four Courts Press, pp. 73–9.

15 *Freeman's Journal*, 8 December 1847. Another case of attempted suicide from distress can be found in *Freeman's Journal*, 19 March 1847, 'Famine – Attempt at Self-Destruction'. A man named McEntire caught stealing from a house 'while labouring under the cravings of hunger, made an attempt on his own life, by cutting his throat'. The article did not state whether it was in the house that he made this attempt, it certainly was not jail, as he was only committed to jail after being found to have committed this second offence.

16 *Freeman's Journal*, 8 December 1847.

17 *Freeman's Journal*, 5 April 1847.

18 Ibid.

19 Burke, H. (1987), *The People and the Poor Law in Nineteenth Century Ireland*. Littlehampton: The Women's Education Bureau, pp. 130–9.

20 *Freeman's Journal*, 15 February 1848.

21 Crossman, V. (2006), *Politics, Pauperism and Power in late Nineteenth-century Ireland*. Manchester: Manchester University Press, pp. 12–15.

22 *Freeman's Journal*, 16 January 1849.

23 Hynes, E. (2008), *Knock: The Virgin's Apparition in Nineteenth Century Ireland*. Cork: Cork University Press, p. 130.

24 Lee, J. J. (1973), *The Modernisation of Irish Society, 1848–1918*. Dublin: Gill and Macmillan, p. 5.

25 Durkheim, E. (2000), *Suicide: A Study in Sociology*. London: Routledge, p. 345.

26 Ibid., p. 288.

27 Ibid., p. 201.

28 General Registry Office (1995), *Registering the People: 150 years of Civil Registration*. Dublin: General Registry Office.

29 Lucey, D. S. (2011), 'Poor relief in the west of Ireland, 1861–1911', in Crossman, V. and Gray, P. (eds) (2011), *Poverty and Welfare in Ireland, 1838–1948*. Dublin: Irish Academic Press, p. 41.

30 Regional disparities in terms of wealth and poverty as well as the bureaucracy which gathered the data on mortality are important to remember here. Evidence from Mayo reveals that geographical location played a significant role in whether or not inquests were held. See Laragy, 'Suicide and insanity', pp. 82–3. There was also a regional aspect to the experience of poverty and the provision of poor relief in Ireland during this period.

31 Durkheim, *Suicide*, p. 254.

32 Kushner, H. I. (1999), 'Suicide, gender and the fear of modernity in nineteenth century medical and social thought', *Journal of Social History*, 33, p. 461.

33 Lee, *The Modernisation*, p. 6. There is little current scholarship on the history of marriage in Ireland, but see Cosgrove, A. (ed.) (1985), *Marriage in Ireland*. Dublin: College Press; Ferriter, D. (2009), *Occasions of Sin: Sex and Society in Modern Ireland*. London: Profile Books. For a literary treatment of the relationship between poverty, marriage and land (with suicidal thoughts thrown in), see Lawless, E. (1892), *Grania: The Story of an Island*. London: No publisher.

34 Ó'Gráda, C. (1994), *Ireland: A New Economic History, 1780–1939*. Oxford: Clarendon Press, pp. 236, 250.

35 National Archives of Ireland (hereafter NAI), Inquest Records, Carlow, 1886–1905, IC. 12.55

36 NAI, Convict Reference Files, 1892/D/68 Kathleen Dolan and 1915/C/62 Catherine Cunningham. Dolan had 85 previous convictions for a variety of crimes including prostitution.

37 Sentences usually ranged between four and twelve months.

38 Fuchs, *Gender and Poverty*, p. 198.

39 Ibid., pp. 162–3.

40 Hearn, M. (1990), 'Life for domestic servants in Dublin, 1880–1920', in Luddy, M. and Murphy, C. (eds), *Women Surviving: Studies in Irish Women's History in the Nineteenth and Twentieth Centuries*. Dublin: Poolbeg, p. 149.

41 McGoff-McCann, M. (2003), *Melancholy Madness: A Coroners' Casebook*. Cork: Mercier Press, pp. 126–7.

42 NAI, Inquest records, Leitrim, 1905–19, ID.47.73. Widow pensions were not introduced in Ireland until 1935. Ferriter, D. (2004), *The Transformation of Ireland, 1900–2000*. London: Profile Books, p. 402.

43 NAI, Inquest Records, Wexford, IC.12.19.

44 NAI, Inquest Records, Monaghan, Monaghan IC.59.28. 6 March 1912.

45 Morselli, E. (1881), *Suicide: An Essay on Comparative Moral Statistics*. London: Kegan Paul, Trench and Co., p. 232.

46 Laragy, 'Suicide and insanity', p. 59.

47 Laragy, G. (2011), 'Poor relief in the south of Ireland, 1851–1921', in Crossman and Gray, *Poverty and Welfare*, pp. 58–9.

48 *Cork Examiner*, 1 August 1862

49 NAI, Inquest Records, Meath, IC.27.84.

50 McGoff-McCann, *Melancholy Madness*, p.129.

51 Downpatrick Recorder, 2 June 1878

52 Boyce, D. G. (2005), *Nineteenth Century Ireland: The Search for Stability*. Dublin: Gill and Macmillan, rev. edn, pp. 175–9.

53 Lee, *The Modernisation*, p. 94.

8

Stories of care and coercion: Narratives of poverty and suffering among patients with venereal disease in Sweden, 1860–1920

Anna Lundberg

Introduction

Theresa went under many aliases trying to support herself and her son in a mining town in the north of Sweden.[1] Her life was characterized by poverty; female employment was scarce in a mining town and she supported herself by selling food and by making and selling illegal cigarettes, an activity which brought her into constant contact with the police. In February 1919 Theresa suffered from an ulcer that had become infected and went to see a doctor, who diagnosed her with second-stage syphilis but was unable to admit her to medical care because the local hospital was filled to capacity. Instead she went to another town, leaving her son behind, but was refused help there as well. Trying to get medical attention at a third hospital, and still pursued by the police, she eventually ended up in Stockholm hospital, more than 700 miles away from her home. Professor Johan Almkvist answered police requests for her release into their custody by stating that Theresa needed many more months of medical care. Once out of the hospital, she faced more trouble. Starting her new life as a seamstress in the town where her son lived she found she had no time to go back and see the physician for repeated medical examinations. He wrote to her on many occasions stating that if she did not attend she would be arrested by the police and taken to these examinations. Since the professor in Stockholm had stated that she was free from syphilis Theresa argued against this, stating, 'I will report this [a recurrence of syphilis], like I have before.'[2]

For vagrants like Theresa, Swedish laws on venereal disease became part of a raft of social legislation that aimed to create more orderly citizens. Her story is, as we shall see, shared by many ordinary Swedes. Such, for instance, was the syphilitic baker Mattias Jonson. He was contacted by his doctor because he had missed an appointment and told that he would be taken into custody if he did not prove that he was under the supervision of another physician. Mattias wrote back, proving that he had contacted the hospital in Stockholm by sending an extract of his chart from the hospital. 'I hope you will no longer bother me with this' he opined in his letter.[3]

Poverty has always been closely interwoven with venereal disease. When men and women of some prominence were affected by these diseases they were treated by private physicians under the strictest discretion. Poor men and women, unable to pay for privacy, soon became entangled in the network of civil servants and coercion that characterized Swedish measures against venereal disease. Medical care was available free of charge, but its provision implied behavioural rules and, in the case of non-compliance, total loss of freedom. Discourse on this issue changed significantly during the nineteenth century, becoming more public and significantly more gendered, and the overarching aim of this chapter is to analyse the nature and impact of measures taken by Swedish society in order to try and curb the spread of venereal disease.[4] In particular, it will be concerned with the experiences and life-chances of poor men and women suffering from syphilis and gonorrhoea. Being a Swedish citizen has long implied a strong interface between rights and obligations,[5] and Peter Baldwin, in his extensive study on health and public policy in Europe, characterizes measures against venereal disease in Sweden, Norway and Denmark as the 'Scandinavian Sonderweg'.[6] He clearly believes that more decisive measures were taken in Sweden than elsewhere and this chapter will investigate the nature and impact of such decisive action.

The Demographic Database at Umeå University[7] holds unique historical material for this project. Parish registers from 60 parishes in different regions have been transcribed for the period 1700–1900, constituting about 5 per cent of the nation's population. The catechetical registers for these parishes have also been digitized. This material enables us to study the socio-demographic life-course of ordinary Swedes, building life-biographies that outline what happened to men and women before and after they had been treated for venereal disease. Patient records from two hospitals in the county of Västernorrland in northern Sweden have been transcribed into computer files by the Demographic Database to facilitate the identification of venereal life-cycles. Some 6,837 patient records from the hospital in Härnösand, over the period 1814–46, and 20,180 patients from the hospital in Sundsvall, between 1844 and 1900,[8] constitute the basic material for this study. The electronic record incorporates name, age, gender, social position, geographical origin, disease profile, the number of days a person spent in the hospital and the result of treatment, as well as narratives by or about patients.

Of course, reconstructing disease and life-histories on such a scale is impossible for a chapter of this length. Thus, 230 venereal patients from the hospital in Härnösand and 704 venereal patients from the hospital in Sundsvall have been selected for more detailed life-cycle and family reconstruction. A control sample of non-venereal patients (comprising 415 men and women from Härnösand and 1,451 from Sundsvall) corresponding as closely as possible in age, gender, social position and geographical origin to the venereal patients has also been constructed, allowing us to analyse whether the migration, marriage, family formation or mortality patterns of venereal patients differed from the 'norm'.[9]

Venereal disease as an historical problem

The intimacy between venereal diseases and the histories of sexuality, sin, disease and poverty percolates the secondary literature. Thus, Siena showed that venereal diseases were treated differently depending on whom the disease had struck. When the sufferers belonged to the upper classes, syphilis was thought of as easily treated. Physicians did not mind taking care of those that could pay good money for their treatment. When syphilis spread among the poor it was thought to be caused by their crude living conditions, brought on by loose sexuality and worsened by their poverty and squalor.[10] Similarly, Boehrer has shown that venereal disease among the rich was thought of as a sign of life at the court. Poor prostitutes were judged very differently from the wealthy, promiscuous ladies among the gentry, as we will see.[11]

European states adopted overlapping but discrete responses to the threat of venereal disease. Quetel traces how the sick in Paris were told either to receive medical care or be removed from the city. In the countryside suffering from syphilis meant being thrown out from the village where one had lived and roaming from place to place trying to find medical help.[12] In Britain voluntary hospitals financed by private donations shied away from providing treatment and specialist Lock hospitals had to be founded to incarcerate poor sufferers.[13] In some countries, venereal disease became a matter for voluntary medical care while in others policy was orientated towards preventing carriers from spreading disease. Certainly, the regulation and suppression of prostitution became a stock-in-trade response. Originating from the thoughts of French intellectual Alexandre Jean Baptiste Parent-Duchalet, a new French regulatory system of the nineteenth century categorized prostitutes according to whether they solicited customers in the street or worked in brothels. In Paris this system meant that each woman was registered as belonging to one specific category and were expected to behave according to strict regulation, including enforced medical care.[14] This system quickly spread across Europe to Italy, Great Britain, The Netherlands and the Scandinavian countries.[15] However, opposition to regulation could be strong. In Great Britain, such legislation was only enforced between 1864 and 1886 and the movement to abolish the regulation of prostitution, founded by Judith Butler, influenced opposition around Europe.

In this context, the experiences of the Scandinavian countries were relatively distinctive. For Sweden, strong rules were set in motion early to protect the nation and population from contagion, with the regulation and suppression of prostitution, for instance, continuing until 1919.[16] At the heart of the Swedish system lay a balancing of care, as in free medical care, and coercion, as in the surveillance and control of the sick.[17] As Baldwin explains, 'preventive strategies against contagious diseases go to the heart of the social contract, requiring a determination of where the line runs between the interests of the individual and those of the community'.[18] One might extend this argument to the rights and duties of the sick poor more generally. In Sweden, the interest of the collective was considered much more important than that of the individual and Beronius shows how the judicial means to impede venereal disease increased knowledge of those afflicted as well as vectors of disease.[19] Women were targeted especially hard as being responsible for the upkeep of the health of the population. As such the history of venereal disease also tangents issues of citizenship, with legislation on venereal disease helping to shape opinions on what being a good citizen implied. For women, subject to increasingly intrusive regulation of their sexuality, citizenship came with a high socio-cultural price if they did not have the means to pay for the physician's services and discretion. It is this core theme to which we move in the rest of the chapter.

Early measures against venereal disease: Enhancing the state of the population

During the second half of the eighteenth century, provincial physicians in Sweden began reporting an increased incidence of venereal disease. Syphilis had spread in the countryside when soldiers returned home from the early eighteenth-century wars with Russia. By the 1770s most provincial physicians, apart from those in the northernmost parts of the country, had become increasingly concerned about the disease. Sufferers were mostly poor, in the advanced stage of the disease, and laboured under fevers, aches and large sores on the face and extremities. In some parts of the country the situation was particularly problematic since there were no hospitals and the physician lacked the resources to take care of all the patients.[20]

However, a policy change was about to take place. Work to improve the health of citizens had long since been carried out by the government, and by the late eighteenth century policy measures increasingly became targeted at patients with venereal diseases. Mercantilist ideas had prompted societal reforms that increased the significance of the state and church. Thus, the new Church Act (1689) gave each parish more responsibilities and duties towards the poor. It also legislated that every minister in the country was to keep notes on every parishioner and their families as well as their skills in reading, writing and catechism. This reform took some time to enforce, but by 1749 these parish records formed the basis of a nationwide collection of statistics – the *Tabellverket* – instigated because of increased state interest in its population, especially since the large epidemic of plague in 1709–10 and the war against Russia.[21] Numbers from the *Tabellverket* pointed to problems such as high infant mortality and seemed to point to the need for wider societal action. Publications, including advice on infant care and the importance of breastfeeding young children, were circulated among the poorer classes.[22] The importance of midwives was also debated, and a systematic education programme for midwives was begun so as to increase their number and their skill, a measure that took more than a century to come to ultimate fruition.[23]

Analogous debates about the education of physicians and the state of the population led to the opening of the *Serafimerlasarettet* in Stockholm in 1753. Initially conceived as a national hospital, a lack of beds and the impracticality of transporting patients to Stockholm meant that several provincial hospitals were subsequently founded. This said, the hospitals differed greatly from each other. The hospital in Stockholm soon grew to become a significant institution, ready to take care of a large number of patients. The county hospitals in the north of Sweden were often no more than a small wooden house for 10–20 patients at once.[24] Such foundations coincided with the upsurge in venereal disease and many patients were treated at these hospitals.[25] They were frequently impoverished and vagrant, unable to pay for the physicians to come to their home. Whether the hospital was large or small, and whatever the composition of the patients, they symbolized the government's ability to provide medical care. As the patients were treated until the physician thought them healthy – and notwithstanding the fact that physicians often complained about patients running away before medical care was finished – the hospitals also symbolized the coercion that the government could subject its people to.[26]

However, the county hospitals in particular were expensive to run and the responsible body of government, *Serafimerordensgillet*, saw its financial means drained within a couple of decades. After the last war on Swedish soil, that between Russia and Sweden in 1809–10, the fate of orphans and impoverished children and the lack of treatment for the mentally ill came to be tied up with the wider issue of funding for medical care and a poll tax, with the proceeds hypothecated to finance treatment for patients with venereal disease, among others, was suggested. The poll tax – to be set at 3 *skillingar* per adult – was debated in parliament during 1815. The peasantry was worried that being heads of large households would bring heavy burdens and this estate of the parliament considered the mandatory tax unnecessary. Rather, they thought the previous voluntary efforts to collect means for medical care were sufficient. They also argued that venereal diseases were uncommon in their districts. The nobility, clergy and bourgeoisie were more positive towards the tax, considering it a good thing to provide free medical care for those impoverished. The county governor of Stockholm believed that no more 'patriotic contributions' were to be expected from private donations and that the revenue would provide protection for the nation. Another member of the nobility, A. J. Hagströmer, believed that a stronger enforcement of social legislation and the opening of more county hospitals would curb venereal disease. Thus, by 1817 a definite decision was taken by parliament (75 members for, 44 against) to implement a mandatory poll tax to be collected by the county governor and used to provide medical care for those impoverished and suffering from venereal disease.[27] Hammarström considers the revenue a philanthropic piece of legislation that was aimed as insurance against the diseases.[28]

Such measures also went hand-in-hand with surveillance. Already in 1785 suggestions had been made that certain groups should be subjected to examinations. Prejudice against men and women of low incomes and different ethnicity characterized the categories that were to be inspected. These were Jews, women that worked in coffeehouses, peddlers, travelling journeymen, servants, glassblowers and the men and women that travelled from the fisheries on the West coast. A similar suggestion was made by Anders Nordenstolpe, a member of the nobility, in the parliament of 1809–10, and a committee was formed. This group also suggested that other groups, such as sailors and soldiers, should be inspected and carry a health certificate with them when travelling. A proposal was brought before the four chambers in parliament in 1811, but the peasantry protested once more. They stated that it was offensive to compare 'prominent sailors' and orderly tradesmen to promiscuous rascals and feared that restrictions on movement would destroy these groups financially. Those who felt themselves affected by potential legislation also protested violently against it, though noble and other groupings, who knew that they could circumvent any potential provisions, were more sanguine.[29] Thus, in 1812 a new piece of legislation enabled authorities to control those believed to be dangerous to public health. Early nineteenth-century Sweden enforced strong coercive measures against venereal disease in order to protect the collective and prevent those afflicted from spreading the diseases further. A moral citizenship implied strong behavioural rules and regulations that were to be followed.

Venereal disease among the agrarian poor: Early nineteenth-century social narratives

Most Swedes lived in the countryside in the early nineteenth century and their work was hard and seasonal. The men fished and hunted, and in summer they took care of the farm animals and the harvest. In the winter men worked in the forest while the women continued to take care of the household and the children.[30] Marriage was closely intertwined with the ownership of land, and the age at first marriage was already comparatively high in Sweden.[31] This situation was not, however, static. Significant population increase allied with land reforms during the early nineteenth century uprooted a large number of families who came to form a large underemployed agrarian proletariat.[32] Much effort was put into controlling this newly emergent group, which was often characterized as dangerous and feckless.[33] Against this backdrop, policies on venereal disease (framed in 1812) were enforced in very different ways. Thus, in Stockholm activity was centred on identifying vagrant women, who were subsequently sent to hospitals.[34] In the countryside the law was difficult to enforce because there were so few officials and physicians that could carry out the inspections. The vast distances between the villages and towns in the north of Sweden also made it difficult to monitor and control travellers. Yet, and perhaps unsurprisingly given frequent migration, the disjuncture between town and country, and between disease experiences in town and country, was by no means complete. Thus, the orphan Carl Carlson came from Stockholm to Härnösand as an infant and was transferred between different families during his childhood. Eventually he ended up in the family of a policeman, where he stayed for ten years until he was a young adult. As a 13-year-old he was treated for degenerative venereal disease, which he might have had since infancy or been infected with in one of his families. Carl lived to marry three times, losing his first wife only a month into the marriage but having four children with his second wife. Carl's last wife was also an orphan and he died in 1868 from something the minister chose to call 'brainfever'. Catharina Johansdotter lost her only son to drowning a couple of years before she lost her first husband in Stockholm where he had probably moved to find employment. She remarried another man 17 years her junior, a man that was noted down in the registers as being a criminal. When she died from 'old age' (at 56 years of age) in 1841, she had just finished a period of treatment at the hospital for degenerative venereal disease.

While there were clearly many urban–rural connections of this sort, a county hospital had opened up in Härnösand as early as 1788. It was an inconspicuous wooden building with nine settled beds. During the first half of the nineteenth century the hospital expanded and mental patients were moved to another building. Previously situated on the outskirts of the town, urban expansion in Härnösand meant it was swallowed up and located close to the only inland entrance to the town which was considered noisy and heavily trafficked.[35] During an inspection of 1838 the hospital was found to be 'spacious and joyful'. Patient records suggest that venereal disease was epidemic in agrarian Sweden, often striking villages and then never returning. Thus, between 1814 and 1844, 20 patients were brought to the hospital in Härnösand from Forse foundry in Långsele parish (Västernorrland). Eleven of them were admitted during the years 1835 and 1836 when debates were also running high about the violence and drunkenness that took place in the foundry. Ingeborg, Catharina, Sara Brita, Inga-Märta, Anna-Stina and Hans were all children under the age of 11 and they were accompanied by an elderly couple in their 70s and two maids who were also affected by venereal disease. Ten patients from the village Lästa were also admitted in the mid-1830s, and nine of them (consisting of a 33-year-old man and a number of children) came from the same household.[36]

Patients with venereal disease represented between 20 and 70 per cent of the inmates at Härnösand hospital between 1814 and 1844. Although most patients in the hospital were men, the majority of those suffering from venereal disease were young women. Over the whole period, 500 males and 791 females were diagnosed with venereal disease. While 20 per cent of all female patients were aged 15–24, some 29 per cent of the female patients suffering from venereal disease could be found in the same age category. This difference was smaller among men with 26 per cent of male hospital patients aged 15–24, while 29 per cent of men with venereal disease belonged to the same age category. There is prima facie evidence here that measures against venereal disease were particularly targeted at young women in agrarian Sweden,[37] with young single mothers particularly prevalent in this group.

Two further patient characteristics are also worthy of comment. First, the patient cohort with venereal disease was disproportionately poor. Some 39 per cent of female patients could not define themselves as having any kind of profession, while 48 per cent worked as maids. Among men, 21 per cent could not leave a profession to their name in the records and 25 per cent of them worked as farmhands. Other groups among the male patients were sailors, fishermen, farmers and crofters. A very small proportion of patients defined themselves as lodgers. Second, very few patients (less than 1 per cent) came from Härnösand itself. A further 18 per cent did not reveal where they came from, while 77 per cent came from the county of Västernorrland.[38]

Within the framework of this study we have been able to identify 97 male and 118 female patients whose origin was in parishes whose catechetical registers have been registered by the Demographic Database and for whom we can reconstruct fuller life-stories. Thus, Olof Olsson had been in the hospital in Härnösand for 52 days in 1826. Together with his wife, a maid and two girls he had been treated for degenerative venereal disease. At the same time as the Olsson family was admitted to the hospital, the physician also cured a young woman, Anna Njurenius, of severe venereal disease. For Olof, life continued on the farm. When identifying him in the catechetical registers we find that the maid that accompanied him to the hospital was married to his son and continued to stay with the family. One of the girls turned out to be Olof's granddaughter and the other had been taken into the household as a step-daughter. All of them remained on the farm. His wife died from consumption three years later while Olof died seven years later from a similar disease. His daughter-in-law was able to remarry when her husband died and the two girls also married eventually. Clearly, venereal disease did not imply that they were shunned from society. For Anna life ended in 1827 when she died from 'longterm venereal illness'. She was 42, had never married and had worked as a maid her entire life.[39]

Several observations about the life chances of the entire patient cohort might also be made. Thus, quantitative evidence from the linked patient records weighed against that for the comparative cohort suggests that mortality was higher among those who had been admitted to the hospital for venereal disease. Mortality was high among infants, with 30 per cent of the cohort dying, and children, with 25 per cent of those admitted in childhood also dying in childhood or young adulthood. In the comparative cohort, only 16 per cent of children died. The cohort difference is even clearer among those who were admitted as young adults or adults. Only 51 per cent of those who were treated against venereal disease as young adults survived until old age, while 78 per cent of the men and women in the comparative cohort survived until this point.[40]

There were also differences between in the two cohorts in terms of migratory status. While young adults in Sweden frequently migrated to find employment,[41] some 53 per cent of the traceable patients treated for venereal disease had a migratory history compared to 38 per cent of the comparative cohort. A larger percentage of venereal patients would also go on to move, either to other parts of the parish they had lived in before they sought medical attention or further afield, after treatment had finished.[42] Anna Njurenius was one of the patients who had to move many times during her lifetime, and this may indicate that individuals were forced away from the household where they lived when they became ill. Eva Wulf was 32 when she was admitted to hospital and she appears to have moved around the region too much for the minister to keep her under control. She married at 41 years of age, but does not seem to have given birth to any children or stayed in any of the parishes in the region for any significant time. Christian was 51, unmarried and noted as being of 'feeble mind and slow memory' when admitted for treatment. He died nine years later, alone and having spent most of his life moving from one place to another.

Interestingly, however, there were no significant differences in marriage rates between the two cohorts. Some 20 per cent of the men in both cohorts had married five years after their discharge from the hospital and 35 per cent of women in both cohorts had married within the same time frame.[43] The patients that were married when they were discharged generally remained married until one of the spouses died and these couples tended to be the least mobile elements of the patient cohort. The girls that accompanied Olof to the hospital could remain on his farm, marry and settle down to a more regular family life. An opposite case, but one very much to prove the rule, is Christian Billström, a 23-year-old farmhand from the parish of Indahl. He had spent 46 days in the hospital with a case of 'primitive venereal disease' and after treatment he returned home to his parish, where he married two years later. Since he was poor and unable to find steady employment he frequently moved from one village to another. In 1845 his first child was born, a daughter named Anna. A second child was born in 1848. Eleven years later the family settled in Indahl again. It becomes obvious that patients with some sort of attachment to the parish, such as ownership of land, more easily adapted themselves back to the life they had lived previous to their medical treatment. The impoverished, like Christian, could elaborate no such belonging and normality.

Regulating the urban poor – measures against venereal disease in the second half of the nineteenth century

Sweden slowly industrialized during the second half of the nineteenth century. In Västernorrland, the first steam sawmill opened in Tuna parish in 1849 and industrialization accelerated thereafter. This implied much increased migration. The town Sundsvall, north of Härnösand, was soon to become, for instance, one of the biggest sawmill and shipbuilding areas of northern Scandinavia.[44] There were important consequent effects for Sundsvall's demographic patterns: infant mortality, falling since the 1810, increased in the 1870s;[45] marriage ages decreased; and population growth came to depend more on fertility than immigration in the 1890s.[46] By the later nineteenth century, Sundsvall was a bustling community of 15,000 inhabitants, one of the largest towns in the north of Sweden.

Similar patterns can be observed elsewhere, and it is no surprise that venereal disease became much more an urban problem during the second half of the century. According to statistics on the number of patients in Swedish hospitals issued by the Board of Medicine (*Medicinalstyrelsen*), venereal disease decreased in the countryside and increased in the cities such as Stockholm and Gothenburg. The diseases also became more common in towns like Sundsvall and the surrounding sawmill districts. The local provincial physician blamed the migrant workers and argued that 'syphilis and gonorrhoea was second only to alcoholism and maybe more common than tuberculosis'.[47] Once again, poor men and women were blamed for the spread of these diseases and were the focus for wide-ranging social reforms.[48] In Stockholm the regulation of prostitution was introduced in 1847, building on previous powers to detain, inspect and treat vagrant women from the 1810s, after long debate over increased rates of venereal disease in the capital. Such measures proved insufficient and by 1859 a new regulation was enforced under which 'vagrant' women were subjected to weekly inspections, with those who refused confined to the workhouse for between two months and one year. The women were also prohibited from frequenting public places and had to ply their trade within the framework that society had set up for them. There was little debate over this later legislation, reflecting contemporary consensus that venereal diseases required social regulation and that being a 'proper' Swedish citizen implied conforming.

Despite this regulation, venereal disease continued to increase, and in 1868 the question about how to stop the diseases from spreading further was once again raised among Swedish physicians. A stronger and more coercive system was introduced in 1875 to regulate the behaviour of prostitutes and poor and vagrant women. They were not permitted to sit in lit windows, call out to men in the street or frequent certain parts of Stockholm. They were only allowed to sit in special seats at the theatre and they were not allowed to leave Stockholm without notifying the police. Yvonne Svanström points out that a special citizenship was presented to these women, strictly limited to what society thought would prevent the spread of illicit sexuality and venereal disease.[49] This notwithstanding, no significant objections were raised against these regulations until 1878,[50] when Hugo Tamm, also a member of the First Chamber of parliament, began to use medical, ethical and statistical evidence to argue that regulation was inefficient, that it did not protect the population against venereal disease, that it left more than 500 girls unregulated and that it did nothing to prevent disease from spreading among men. Tamm also challenged Swedish physicians, stating that they were the only ones in Europe who still believed that solely controlling women would curb the spread of disease and contending that Edvard Welander, a leading physician among those who got involved in the debate over venereal disease, had exaggerated the consequences of venereal diseases.[51] Tamm faced severe criticism for these views, especially from the chairman of the Board of Medicine, Theodore Almén, who argued that if Stockholm city was forced to repeal the control regulations they would simply enforce the much more draconian 1812 Act. Neither did Almén agree that the regulation of prostitution made men in Stockholm feel safe from venereal disease; he thought the men highly aware of the dangers they subjected themselves to if they visited these girls.[52]

Conservative members of parliament also considered it obvious that the government should be allowed to prevent women from soliciting men, on the same grounds as they were allowed to prevent begging and vagrancy. Conservative county governor Curry Treffenberg argued that it was beneath the members of the First Chamber even to discuss these things: the women should be sent to prison. Later changes put prostitution on a par with suicide, forgery, public singing, coffee-shops, birth-control, variety-shows and theatres, and presented venereal disease as tangent to different sorts of immoral behaviours. Being a proper healthy citizen meant avoiding all of these vices.[53]

The motions that Tamm filed with the parliament were sent out to different bodies for comments. In *Svenska Läkarsällskapet*, the Swedish Medical Association, Edvard Welander argued forcefully against the repeal of regulation. He did not worry about the exchange of money for sexual services or single women living with men, but he was concerned about the hardened women who entertained numerous men every day and night. The 'professional' prostitute was the greatest danger to society and needed to be controlled and inspected regularly.[54] He flatly denied that medical care for venereal disease in the hospital would be embarrassing and stigmatizing, although he admitted that the private clinics were crowded with such cases when employment rose in the summer months. He also argued that the poor showed up at the hospital during unemployment simply to find food and shelter, blaming their medical conditions on the most insignificant ailment.[55] The argument for repeal was lost and surveillance and forced treatment of women continued to be the primary measure against venereal disease. The foundation of the Swedish Purity Movement in 1888 reinforced opposition to repeal by physicians and others.[56] These measures also generate a considerable body of mediated and unmediated narratives through which we can understand and analyse the nature of sickness, its relationship to poverty and the relative balance of subjection and agency for the sick poor. This is particularly true of the Swedish provinces.

Social narratives of the urban immoral – caring and coercing

Against this 'national' backdrop, the number of patients suffering from venereal disease in Västernorrland expanded during the great famine of the late 1860s, when migration increased significantly as people came to Sundsvall in particular attempting to find employment,[57] and during a general strike of 1879.[58] A significant increase in the numbers of patients with venereal disease can also be found after a great fire in 1888, when large numbers of workers came to Sundsvall in order to find employment during the rebuilding of the town.[59] Mattias was one of those migrant workers. He moved from Stockholm in 1865 and stayed on until 1869 when (aged 29, and single) he moved to Kalmar, another town in southern Sweden, some seven months after his discharge from hospital where he had been treated for venereal disease.

By the time Mattias left, the increased frequency of venereal disease was causing local consternation and in 1880 the Sundsvall authorities instigated a similar control and surveillance regime to their counterparts in Stockholm. Women considered as prostitutes were registered by the police and apprehended for medical inspection. They were subsequently treated at the same hospital as the generality of patients, but can be found in the patients records as '*fille publiques*' since the term prostitute was used only after 1890. The crackdown caused debate in the town not least because it was difficult to find a place were the inspections could take place. Physician Emil Falk had been appointed in 1882 but at one point threatened to stop carrying out the inspections because the town could not provide adequate rooms. In 1885, a year after his objections, a house owned by the authorities was turned into a morgue and the inspections took place there. During the 1890s the inspections were carried out in the hospital for epidemic diseases and later in the city hall.[60] The rich records of this period afford us a window onto the range of womens' experiences under such regulations. Twenty-six-year-old Erika moved to Sundsvall in 1885 and spent several periods in the hospital, registered as a '*fille publique*', being treated for venereal disease. Nonetheless she remained in the town and married a younger travelling salesman after a two year engagement. At marriage, when she was living in the household of a postmaster, Erika's status had risen to that of housekeeper. Hedvig, by contrast, was reported as a prostitute in the patient records of 1880 (when she was 29 years old), and retained this status until the records cease. Young Malin, only 20 years old, moved just a couple of months after treatment and discharge and disappears from the records.

Stories such as these slightly mask the fact that by the second half of the nineteenth century the epidemiological pattern of venereal disease had changed. A much larger proportion of the men and women at the hospital came from the town than during the first half of the century, but a significant proportion of the patients came from other parts of the county or country. Some 56 per cent of men and 31 per cent of women came from other parts of Västernorrland or Sweden. Only 10 per cent of male patients claimed to live in surrounding sawmill parishes, perhaps indicating their desire to keep ill-health secret from present or future employers. The women most likely tried to avoid letting their families know that they suffered from venereal disease, and might also have told lies about where they came from.[61]

The diagnoses made in the hospital also changed. Syphilis was no longer labelled degenerative venereal disease but was called secondary syphilis, an indicator that the physicians at the hospital in Sundsvall were up to date with the new medical knowledge and terminology of the later nineteenth century. Some 44 per cent of male patients were diagnosed in this way, as were 64 per cent of women. Gonorrhoea also became a disease label in its own right, with 29 per cent of male patients and 12 per cent of female patients diagnosed with the disease. Mercury also became more common as a therapeutic measure, either via injection or salve, and an ever larger number of people were treated as out-patients. Sailors who needed to go back to work, or women who needed to go back to the farm, could get jars of 'grey-ointment' prescribed to take with them.

While 60 per cent of the patient discharge records fail to indicate whether patients were restored to health or not, those that did indicate a significant cure rate: 72 per cent were discharged as 'cured' and 23 per cent as 'improved'.[62] Christian Billström's daughter, Anna, was one patient who did not secure benefit. At the age of 22 she had been diagnosed with *ulcus molle* and treated for 12 days. In 1871 her first illegitimate child died and she continued to have illegitimate children in 1872 and 1873. None of them lived longer then three months, and in 1875 Anna herself died from consumption aggravated by venereal disease. More generally, Sundsvall and its surrounding parishes did not experience infant mortality below 200 per thousand live births until the late 1880s. This partly reflected the lack of proper housing and poor sanitation in the town.[63] It also reflected the fact that children born within nine months of their parents' discharge from the venereal wards suffered the highest infant mortality. For these parents, infant mortality rose to 362 per thousand live births, while among the men and women in the control cohort the analogous figure was just 135 per thousand. Among children that were born two years after their parents discharge infant mortality was rather lower although still above the control cohort at 273 per thousand live births. Mortality was considerably higher for children born between two and five years after their parents discharge, a reflection of the intense legacy of venereal disease in northern Sweden.[64]

More generally, however, the demographic characteristics of venereal patients were little different to their non-afflicted peers. Those who could be linked from the patient records to the parish registers within five years of their discharge from the hospital showed no significant differences in adult mortality to the comparative cohort. Migration rates were very similar between the two cohorts, and the same can be said about marriage rates and ages.[65] Thus, most venereal patients married in their mid-20s, the same marriage experience as those in the comparative cohort. Even the prostitutes that could be linked to the parish registers tended to marry eventually.[66] Lovisa, for instance, had migrated from Finland to Sundsvall and married when she was 34, after having suffered from venereal disease and given birth to an illegitimate child.[67] The widespread poverty in town made stigmatization less prominent and enabled men and women to stay on and form a life to the best of their abilities. If the patients were married when they were admitted to the hospital they generally returned home to their spouses and children. Carolina was the wife of a restaurant owner in Sundsvall. She returned home to her husband and gave birth to a child that died a year after her discharge. After that she had four more children until her husband died from heart paralysis at the age of 48, when she moved with her children and at least one maid to Stockholm. Ownership and status made it easy for Carolina to stay in the town until widowhood. For poorer patients, lodgers being very common in Sundsvall, it is likely that opportunities arose to find new living arrangements when returning from the hospital, in a house where no one knew about the medical treatment one had just undergone. In town, then, life was different for the returning patients than it had been in the countryside.

Conclusion

Care and coercion characterized the way Swedish society faced the spread of venereal disease. Categories of poor men and women were singled out as specifically dangerous to society, persuaded or coerced into medical care and subjected to strong behavioural norms. The force of this policy developed across the period. In the early nineteenth century a protective political discourse against venereal disease progressed congruent to other measures that aimed at enclosing the poor in a societal network to deal with a problem with a relatively distinctive rural flavour. Poverty was not only a signifier of laziness, indulgence and bad morals it also came to suggest poor health and sexual promiscuity. Swedish citizenship implied that medical care was available but at the cost of integrity and personal freedom. In the later nineteenth century, when venereal disease was rife in urban areas, intense stigmatization of the sick poor can be observed, with coercive legislation, singling out travellers, those in low-income employment and vagrants as especially dangerous. Women came to be seen as the primary vector for venereal disease and thus the main focus of corrective and coercive measures. Their narratives – or rather narratives about them – litter the archival records at the level of the hospital and other institutions.

This much has been broadly known. What is new here is the exercise in this chapter to link patient records from two hospitals in the north of Sweden to parish registers digitalized by the Demographic Database at Umeå University. Such linkage provides the means whereby we can look at the histories and future life stories of those afflicted with venereal disease compared to those who were sick but did not have a sexually transmitted disease. These are not exactly narratives but analogous in form and intent. These life stories suggest that in rural areas social control of the poor, and of the female poor in particular, was strong. Annual collections to fund medical care for those afflicted with venereal disease were a reminder of syphilis and gonorrhoea and their association with the poor. Stigmatization of this group certainly worsened when venereal disease struck. Whereas those linked with the parish by ownership of land or marriage could much more easily stay on at the farm or in the village where they had resided when struck with disease, vagrants, single women, sailors and farm hands were easily disposed of if suffering from poor health.

In an urban environment, life was probably slightly easier for poor men and women. Despite the increased gendering of poor health, the bustling environment of Sundsvall proved more beneficial for the recuperating patients among the labouring poor. Adult mortality was lower among these people and re-migration rates were lower (indeed, resembling those of the comparative cohort), indicating that the patients could find employment in the town or the surrounding sawmills and shipyards. Marriage rates were very similar in both cohorts, even among the prostitutes. The fate of urban vagrants is harder to pin down. Female vagrants such as the woman Theresa with whom we started this analysis, were often hounded by the police and the physicians because they were considered dangerous and lecherous. Communities themselves were little better. Families were asked about their teenage children's whereabouts and neighbours gossiped about the mail that the family received, looking for teenagers who had moved to disguise their afflictions. Neighbours sometimes even reported other neighbours if their sexual conduct was ill-thought of. Women reported other women who had affairs with their husbands and had passed on a venereal disease; their illicit sexuality made these women a threat to honourable families and to society in general. While the narratives of Swedish plebian life might be rare, this chapter has suggested that we can reconstruct the sentiments of such narratives through multiple source record linkage so as to reach a compelling picture of the scale and experience of sickness and poverty.

Notes

1 All names have been changed to protect anonymity.

2 Härnösands landsarkiv, (hereafter HLA) Förste provinsialläkaren i Norrbottens län, CIIIa: 5.

3 Lunds landsarkiv, (hereafter LLA); Karlskrona Kommunarkiv; Karlskrona stad; Stadsläkarens arkiv, F1C:1 och F1C:2, Karlskrona I upphörda myndigheter, stadsläkarens arkiv, Lex Veneris anmälan, 1919–27, 1928–38.

4 This article is based on my doctoral thesis, Lundberg, A. (1999), *Care and Coercion, Medical Knowledge, Social Policy and Patients with Venereal Disease in Sweden 1785–1903*. Umeå: Demographic Database Report Number 14.

5 Olsson, S. (1990), *Social Policy and Welfare in Sweden*. Lund: Arkiv.

6 Baldwin, P. (1999), *Contagion and the State in Europe 1830–1930*. Cambridge: Cambridge University Press, pp. 400–18.

7 See www.ddb.umu.se for information on the database and a bibliography.

8 The names of patients were not registered after 1889, and therefore no linkages have been possible after this year.

9 Lundberg, *Care and Coercion*, pp. 46–9.

10 Siena, K. (1998), 'Pollution, promiscuity and the pox: English venereology and the early modern medical discourse on social and sexual danger', *Journal of the History of Sexuality*, 8. Analogous narratives were used to characterize the German poor at risk of cholera, as Beate Althammer shows in her chapter for this volume.

11 Boehrer, B. T. (1990), 'Early modern syphilis', *Journal of the History of Sexuality*, 1, 197–214.

12 Quetel, C. (1990), *Syphilis*. Padstow: Polity Press, pp. 24–5, 64–6.

13 Williams, D. (1995), *The London Lock – a Charitable Hospital for Venereal Disease 1746–1952*. London: Royal Society of Medicine Press. For perspectives on European histories of venereal disease, see Davidson, R. and Hall, L. (2001), *Sex, Sin and Suffering: Venereal Disease and European Society Since 1870*. London: Routledge.

14 Corbin, A. (1990), *Women for Hire: Prostitution and Sexuality in France after 1850*. Cambridge, MA: Harvard University Press.

15 The literature on prostitution is vast; see, for instance, Walkowitz, J. (1980), *Prostitution and Victorian Society: Women, Class and the State*. Cambridge: Cambridge University Press; Spongberg, M. (1997), *Feminizing Venereal Disease: The Body of the Prostitute in Nineteenth Century Medical Discourse*. Basingstoke: Macmillan, 1997.

16 Svanström, Y. (2001), *Policing Public Women – the Regulation of Prostitution in Sweden 1812–80*. Stockholm: Atlas Akademi, pp. 69–112.

17 Baldwin, P. (2005), *Disease and Democracy: The State Faces AIDS in the Industrialized World*. Ewing: University of California Press, pp. 42, 45.

18 Baldwin, *Contagion and the State*, p. 563.

19 Beronius, M. (1994), *Bidrag till de sociala undersökningarnas histori,a*. Stockholm: Brutus Östlings bokförlag.

20 See, for instance, Hagström, J. O. (1997), *Brev från Johan Otto Hagström, provincial medicus I Östergötland till Kungl. Collegium Medicum, åren 1755–85*. Linköping: Östergötlands Medicinhistoriska sällskap.

21 Sköld, P. (2001), *Kunskap och kontroll. Den svenska befolkningsstatistikens historia*. Umeå: Demographic Database Report Number 17, pp. 13–29.

22 Brändström, A. (1990), 'Från förebild till motbild. Spädbarnsvård och spädbarnsdödlighet i Jokkmokk', in Åkerman, S. and Lundholm, K. (eds), *Älvdal i norr*. Stockholm: Almqvist & Wiksell International, pp. 307–52.

23 Brändström, A. (1984), *'De kärlekslösa mödrarna' – spädbarnsdödligheten i Sverige under 1800-talet med särskild hänsyn till Nedertorneå*. Umeå: Umeå Studies in the Humanities, Vol. 62, pp. 56–60.

24 Thyresson, N. (1991), *Från fransoser till AIDS*. Stockholm: Carlssons, pp. 40–8.

25 Åhman, A. (1976), *Om den offentliga vården*. Uddevalla: Sveriges arkitekturmuseum.

26 Lundberg, A. (1997), 'I detta mest nordliga luftstreck – veneriska sjukdomarnas härjningar i Dalarna och Norrland 1755–1838', *Oknytt*, 1, 63–86.

27 Lundberg, *Care and Coercion*, pp. 98–9.

28 Hammarström, I. (1979), 'Ideology and social policy in the mid-nineteenth century', *Scandinavian Journal of History*, 180–1, 184.

29 Lundberg, *Care and Coercion*, pp. 95–7.

30 Hellspong, M. and Löfgren, O (1974), *Land och stad – svenska samhällstyper och livsformer från medeltid till nutid*. Malmö: Gleerups, pp. 63–73, 232–63.

31 Göransson. A. (ed.) (2000), *Sekelskiften och kön – strukturella och kulturella övergångar år 1800, 1900 och 2000*. Stockholm: Prisma, pp. 17–23. Also

Hedenborg, S. and Wikander, U. (2003), *Makt och försörjning*. Lund: Studentlitteratur, on the development of the Swedish family.

32 Winberg, C. (1977), *Folkökning och proletarisering. Kring den sociala strukturomvandlingen på Sveriges landsbygd under den agrara revolutionen.* Lund: Berlingska Boktryckeriet.

33 Persson, B. (1983), *Den farliga underklassen – studier i fattigdom och brottslighet i 1800-talets Sverige*. Umeå: Umeå University.

34 Svanström, *Policing Public Women*, p. 313.

35 Wawrinsky, R. (1906), *Sveriges lasarettsväsende förr och nu. Ett stycke svensk kulturhistoria*. Stockholm: Författarens förlag, pp. 873–4.

36 Lundberg, *Care and Coercion*, pp. 124–5.

37 Ibid., pp. 120–1.

38 Ibid., p. 123.

39 DDB, Umeå University, Sweden. www.ddb.umu.se.

40 Lundberg, *Care and Coercion*, p. 134.

41 Lundh, C. (1999), 'Servant migration in Sweden in the early nineteenth century', *Journal of Family History*, 24, 53–73.

42 Lundberg, *Care and Coercion*, p. 137.

43 Ibid., p. 138. Previous research on convicts shows that marriage was a significant part of their lives; if they married they mostly stayed out of trouble. Taussi-Sjöberg, M. (1986), *Dufvans fångar: brottet, straffet och människan i 1800-talets Sverige*. Stockholm: Författarförlaget, pp. 150–2.

44 Björklund, J. (1997), 'Tillväxt och differentiering – näringslivet 1870–1940', in Tedebrand, L.-G. (ed.), *Sundsvalls historia, Volume 2*. Sundsvall: Sundsvalls kommun; Olsson, R. (1949), *Norrländskt sågverksliv under ett sekel*. Stockholm: Nordiska museet, pp. 56, 68–70.

45 Edvinsson, S. (1992), *Den osunda staden – social skillnader i dödlighet i 1800-talets Sundsvall*. Umeå: Demographic Database Report Number 7, pp. 163–4.

46 Tedebrand, L.-G. (1977), 'Demografisk stabilitet och förändring under det industriella genombrottet', in Tedebrand, L.G. (ed.), *Historieforskning på nya vägar – studier tillägnade Sten Carlsson*. Lund: Studentlitteratur.

47 Riksarkivet, Stockholm, Medicinalstyrelsens arkiv: Reports from the provincial physicians in 1888, E 5:A.

48 Matsson, H. (1991), *Den gode förmyndaren. Om samhällets behandling av fattig*. Stockholm: Allmänna förlaget, pp. 60–4. On the practice of Swedish poor law, see Engberg, E. (2005), *I fattiga omständigheter. Fattigvårdens former och understödstagare i Skellefteå socken under 1800-talet*. Umeå: Demographic Database Report Number 25 and Engberg, E. (2004), 'Boarded out by auction: poor children and their families in nineteenth-century northern Sweden', *Continuity and Change*, 19, 202–26.

49 Svanström, *Policing Public Women*, chapters 8 and 10.

50 Boëthius, U. (1969), *Strindberg och kvinnofrågan till och med Giftas*. Stockholm: Prisma, pp. 63–5.

51 Printed Acts from the parliament, motion number 27, 1889, and motion number 15, 1893.

52 Minutes from the parliament, from the First Chamber, 20 March 1889.

53 Minutes from the parliament, from the First Chamber, 6 May 1893, and from the Second Chamber, 26 April 1893.

54 Welander, E. (1889), 'Till belysning av prostitutionsfrågan', *Hygiea – medicinsk och pharmaceutisk månadsskrift*.

55 Welander, E. (1890), 'Några ord i prostitutionsfrågan', *Hygiea – medicinsk och pharmaceutisk månadsskrift*.

56 Lundberg, *Care and Coercion*, pp. 198–212; Gay, P. (1984), *The Bourgeois Experience: Education of the Senses*. Oxford: Oxford University Press; Gay, P. (1986), *The Bourgeois Experience: Victoria to Freud*. Oxford: Oxford University Press; Mason, M. (1994), *The Making of Victorian Sexual Attitudes*. Oxford: Oxford University Press.

57 Häger, O. (1978), *Ett satans år – Norrland 1867*. Stockholm: Sveriges Radio.

58 Norberg, A. (1978), 'Sundsvallsstrejken 1879 – ett startskott för den stora Amerikautvandringen', *Historisk Tidskrift*, 98.

59 BiSOS, Annual reports from Kungl. Sundhetskollegium and Medicinalstyrelsen.

60 Lundberg, *Care and Coercion*, p. 226.

61 Ibid., pp. 235–6.

62 Ibid., pp. 238–40.

63 Edvinsson, *Den osunda staden*, pp. 161–78.

64 Lundberg, *Care and Coercion*, p. 255.

65 Ibid.

66 Ibid., pp. 251–2.

67 Brändström, A. (2004), 'Påterbesök i Nedertorneå. Spädbarnsdödlighet, utomäktenskaplighet och sociala närverk', in Brändström, A., Edvinsson, S., Ericsson, T. and Sköld, P. (eds), *Befolkningshistoriska perspektiv. Festskrift till Lars-Göran Tedebrand*. Umeå: Demographic Database Report Number 14, pp. 35–58.

9

From unemployment to sickness and poverty: The narratives and experiences of the unemployed in Trier and surroundings, 1918–33

Tamara Stazic-Wendt

Introduction – the 'welfare unemployed'[1]

Unemployment was an ingrained facet of the Weimar Republic. Even before the Depression, millions of people experienced unemployment, the character of which had basically changed after World War I.[2] The risk of unemployment was no longer restricted to a clear-cut group of the labouring population – the unskilled and casual workers – but also encompassed new groups such as skilled and white-collar workers and even academics. In practice, analysis of the '(un)employment biographies' and 'biographies of relief' which can be traced in the individual case files of local poor relief and unemployment assistance bodies shows that from the mid-1920s a large number of workers experienced long-term unemployment, albeit often interrupted by short phases of employment.[3] In the post-war era, labour market structures changed and with them the character and stability of 'employment biographies'. Employment contracts became shorter and companies related employment to demand much more systematically. For those who had lost their job it was difficult to find a new regular employment; such people often eked out a living wandering from one precarious employment to the next. People who had formerly worked for the *Reichsbahn* found themselves working as casual labourers on construction sites, as 'paper boys', door-to-door salesmen or pedlars. Examples of 'downward mobility' in the archives are numerous.[4]

The unemployment support system (*Erwerbslosenfürsorge*) introduced in Germany after World War I took little cognizance of such developments, being orientated chiefly towards combating short-time unemployment and resting on the principle of indigence.[5] Besides the large group of the long-term unemployed falling through the safety net, various other branches of trades or professions (agricultural workers, domestic personnel, the self-employed, apprentices, unskilled workers) and whole population groups (women and young people) were excluded from relief or received only limited support.[6] Moreover, flexible definitions of 'unemployment' allied with the potentially arbitrary qualifications demanded to establish welfare entitlement ('need' (*Bedürftigkeit*) or 'willingness to work') meant that the total number of benefit recipients could be further reduced at any time. Entitlement was more firmly established with the enactment of an unemployment insurance scheme in the autumn of 1927, but the scheme had little longevity. It was incrementally revoked for ever wider swathes of the unemployed people, and after a series of emergency decrees virtually fell apart during the Depression.

A look at the case files of poor relief shows best how employment policy failed to sufficiently protect most of the labouring population from the material and social consequences of unemployment. In Trier and its suburban communities the unemployed and their relatives became an increasingly common subgroup of recipients. This group of mostly young and able-bodied people, which did not 'fit' properly into the local welfare system, and indeed was rare prior to 1923, became, by the middle of the decade, the main clientele of poor relief. In the suburb of Euren 15 per cent out of the 3,500 inhabitants were temporarily forced to turn to local poor relief because of unemployment.[7] In Trier, the 'welfare unemployed' made up more than 30 per cent of the supported unemployed in 1928 and more than 40 per cent the following year. This development drastically intensified during the Depression. In June 1930, more unemployed people were being supported by the welfare office than the labour office.

Since poor relief[8] never lost its stigmatizing character, going to the welfare office was not only a completely new but also an exceedingly difficult experience for most unemployed people. Moreover, their situation deteriorated through the 1920s and 1930s as debt-ridden parishes reacted to the increasing pressure and the transference of costs for unemployment

from the national to the local level with cuts in social welfare spending. Long
before the *Deutsche Städtetag*[9] embraced the slogan 'cuts everywhere',[10]
the city council of Trier, and still earlier the rural communities, turned to
a radical economy drive. The subsequent 'individualization' of the burden
of economic crisis took place at different levels. It ranged from cuts in
benefit payments to an intensified rejection of applications, which led to
the complete exclusion of many unemployed people from the public welfare
system.[11] Parallel measures primarily aimed at pushing more and more
existing unemployed recipients out of poor relief also developed. In Trier,
compulsory labour was comprehensively established as early as June 1929.[12]
Five days a week, hundreds of the 'welfare unemployed' had to prove that
they were not 'work-shy' but 'deserving' by helping to build stadia, public
swimming pools, playgrounds or by doing street cleaning and archaeological
excavations. In Trier, this strategy of shifting the burden of costs went so far
as to spatially exclude and displace unemployed people and their relatives.
Hundreds of unemployed from Trier were put into a camp outside the gates
of the city, and neither the city council nor the *Landkreis* (rural district),
on whose ground the wooden shacks were standing, felt responsible for
its inhabitants.[13] While such developments failed to contain costs given
deteriorating economic conditions, they certainly shaped the applicants'
attitude towards poor relief as well as the 'atmosphere' at the relief office.
Conflicts between the unemployed and the officials were fuelled by feelings
of injustice, humiliation and shame on the part of the welfare clients, and
most unemployed people tried to avoid going to the welfare office for as long
as possible. Only when all other possibilities were exhausted, when material
need grew so acute that the family's existence seemed to be endangered and
in particular when their children fell ill, did the unemployed turn to the
welfare office.

This micro-level of interaction and negotiation between the (often sick)
unemployed and the local welfare officials will be at the centre of the current
chapter. Drawing on pauper letters and petitions from the rural hinterland of
Trier, the chapter examines the disputed boundaries of 'legitimate' poverty
and locates the relevance of sickness in the negotiation processes between the
unemployed and the local authorities.[14] For the largely agrarian suburbs of
Trier the case files of the local poor relief authorities are completely preserved
for the Weimar Republic.[15] The dossiers contain letters from the applicants,
recorded oral requests, relief bills and official correspondence like records
of the clients' circumstances based on investigations, resolutions, or medical
certificates for individual cases. The case files show which population groups
were primarily affected by poverty and unemployment as well as who received
and who was denied relief. They provide insight into the welfare recipients'
living conditions and strategies of negotiation, an important addition to
a literature on German unemployment which has often concentrated on
the aggregate and policy level. Although, during the 1920s, the applicants'
personal data was usually recorded in a form, the form had by no means

replaced the 'narrative' for either officials or paupers. The surviving letters, which for the most part had been written by the applicants themselves, allow us to approach the issue of poverty, unemployment and ill-health from the perspective of the poor and the unemployed. Contrary to sources like diaries or autobiographies, which in recent years have increasingly been used to (re) construct experiences of the sick,[16] in pauper letters the lower classes – those who lived in poverty or on the margins of society – express themselves.

The first part of the chapter sketches the unemployed people's room for strategic manoeuvring in the system of local poor relief, as well as the welfare practices in rural regions. This attempt at defining the 'place' of the unemployed within the relief system is necessary to locate the experiences and actions of the sick unemployed within a wider context. The chapter then moves on to deal with the welfare authorities' perceptions of the sick unemployed, with the 'status' they assigned to them and the ways in which ill-health and 'deservingness' were interconnected. The last and most substantial part of the chapter investigates the significance of ill-health in everyday processes of negotiation between (sick) unemployed and local administrators about material support. Within this context the chapter will focus on the language used by the sick unemployed to describe their condition. What did they mention and what did they withhold? And last but not least their views on poor relief and a 'regular' life as they can be found in their letters will be examined.

The 'place' of the unemployed within local poor relief

How the poor and the unemployed acted and negotiated at the welfare office, what they reported on their life, poverty and sickness, how they argued and what they demanded is not only to do with personal abilities and preferences. It is also to do with their view on poor relief, whether they knew the decision-maker with whom they had to communicate, how acute their momentary distress was and how far they were integrated into the social structure of the village or marginalized. The surviving letters and oral applications allow us to explore the *'Raum des historisch Möglichen'*[17] (the space of the historically possible) and provide insight into the different strategies of negotiation.

At the beginning of the twentieth century, then, most poor and unemployed people from rural regions had little trouble in articulating their interests either in writing or orally.[18] The majority of the unemployed wrote very polite but sometimes also demanding, accusing or even menacing letters, in common with the broad spectrum of types established in England and Wales for a rather earlier period by Steven King elsewhere in this volume. Some applicants tried to describe their destitution without emotional gestures in a concise and objective way. They stated little or nothing about their everyday life, their fears and sorrows, they did not appeal to the officials' sympathy, but tried to be convincing by giving 'verifiable' information.[19] Others, though, wrote quite openly about their poverty and distress, motivated no doubt by an implicit understanding of the extent to which emotional openness was necessary to persuade the authorities. Many applicants combined emotional and reserved, offensive and defensive, gestures in one single letter. The language and style of the surviving writing ranges from stylized letters showing solid knowledge of orthography and grammar, to clumsy ones written with difficulty and which are difficult to read. Most applications were clearly structured and contained the information relevant to the assessment of the case, for example information on income and family, the causes of distress and why the family was no longer capable of surviving without public assistance. The communication between the poor and officials could take various forms. Many unemployed people presented their request for poor relief orally. They went to see the municipal council or the mayor, who was responsible for the administration of poor relief in rural regions, depicted their difficulties and demanded or asked for material support. Others made their applications mostly in writing (sometimes without exception) although they might as easily have gone to see the municipal council on foot. Obviously they wanted to avoid having direct contact. It was probably easier for them to write about their destitution than to talk about it at the welfare office.[20] The distinction between these letters – written largely from within a settlement – and equivalent English narratives – largely written from outside settlements – is striking.

The relationship between the unemployed and the local welfare authorities was often tense and laden with conflict. This is not particularly surprising, since the everyday welfare practices were not just about granting or denying material support, but also encompassed moral instruction and 'normalizing' judgements. With the receipt of poor relief complex processes of inclusion and exclusion were connected. These were often experienced as unjust and humiliating, especially by able-bodied people. The applications of unemployed families were frequently rejected and if support was granted the unemployed usually faced higher demands than the classic clientele.[21] The 'welfare unemployed' from Trier, for example, were the only ones who had to ask for relief at the police station instead of the welfare office, who had to endure investigations by police officers in uniform and who had to carry out compulsory labour in return for the benefits they received.

Unsurprisingly, in the poor relief files various forms of non-conformity and protest can be located. While collective protest may have been rare in rural areas, there were persistent individual attempts at self-assertion, which could occasionally be offensive and 'loud', but also subtle and careful. The unemployed objected to the communal administrator's decision and called into question their authority and competence. They fought against the permanent doubts over their 'willingness to work', the authorities' interference in their private lives, the peremptory tone of the official in charge, Mr Alt, and the stigmatizing name of 'New-Morocco' (*Neu-Marokko*) for the camp of the unemployed in Euren.[22] The unemployed also rebelled against the measure that police officers in uniform intruded into their apartments in front of the whole neighbourhood,[23] writing letters to the Prussian Minister of Welfare or to Hindenburg himself asking for help or complaining about the behaviour of local administrators. They wrote letters to the editor of the local press in which they publicly expressed their discontent about the treatment at the welfare office; and they organized advocates like the parish priest or the headmaster, who testified their 'deservingness' in a couple of lines enclosed with the application.[24] These sorts of epistolary advocates are a common feature of welfare systems that generated narratives, as several of the contributors to this volume show.

The reactions of the unemployed to their experiences with the local administrators can neither be reduced to a common denominator nor simply to heuristic models such as 'compliance' or 'resistance'. The unemployed and the poor acted and reacted in different ways, and partly contradictorily. And their attempts to assert their interests and their identities were not only directed against those in charge, but also against each other.[25] The surviving letters and oral applications show that the poor were not just passive objects of a public administration, but that they became active of their own accord, that they knew how to appropriately formulate their interests and how to use the scope offered by the communal poor relief. At the same time the poor relief files clearly show that the balance of power between officials and their clientele was unequal and that the scope for the unemployed and the poor to enforce their interests was limited.[26]

Welfare practices in rural regions

While in urban areas during the 1920s a differentiated welfare system had been established and trained social workers were looking after the needy, the local practices of poor relief in the rural communities in the region of Trier maintained their traditional patterns.[27] Even after national guidelines were issued in 1924, the decisions on the granting of poor relief were still made by the municipal council. As a rule, men with a low risk of becoming poor and who were often not only ignorant of the new guidelines but sometimes even hostile towards the Reich's welfare initiatives decided on applications for relief.[28]

The communities were officially obliged to support everybody who could not make an independent living and therefore were regarded as 'needy' (*bedürftig*). However, the legal regulations were lacking in objective criteria (such as income-minima) to exactly define 'neediness' and an absolute legal entitlement to poor relief did not exist. Applicants turned down for poor relief could only appeal to the supervisory authority, itself part of the administrative apparatus and which often lay behind welfare retrenchment,[29] leaving the unemployed limited room to contest the 'official narrative' of 'their case'. The local administrators were free to decide who to relieve, what kind and amount of support to give and who to exclude from public assistance. This wide scope made for a patchwork of different local welfare practices, these often having little to do with the actual extent of poverty in a community and more to do with the prevailing financial situation, the local infrastructure of welfare and the socio-political constellation in a village.

This patchwork notwithstanding, harsh welfare practices were very common in rural areas, as officials sought to cap the number of recipients and the expenses of poor relief. As theoretically able-bodied paupers the unemployed were in a particularly difficult position. Although the local authorities knew about the structural causes of unemployment, their dealings with the individual unemployed in the concrete practices of poor relief were heavily laden with moral agendas and a great discomfort with granting public allowances to this group. Unaffected by advances in national thinking on the causes of poverty, the behaviour of local administrators towards the unemployed remained highly dominated by distrust and fear of abuse. There were also ideological reasons for these harsh attitudes. Communities often could not, and sometimes were unwilling, to take financial responsibility for the burden of unemployment, which the Reich increasingly shifted onto the local level through cutbacks in the system of unemployment insurance. In the concrete interactions with the individual unemployed at the welfare office, material and moral motives were overlapping and with the mass unemployment during the Depression financial matters became more important still.

Unsurprisingly, perhaps, the unemployed from the Trier hinterland keenly appreciated that poor relief intervened only in case of extreme emergency and then with considerable stigma. Thus, as a rule only those without any income and little or no property applied for public assistance. Against this backdrop, 'neediness', meaning the material situation of the applicant, played a minor role when applications from unemployed people were assessed. Indeed, the applications of the unemployed were most commonly not turned down because the applicant had too much income to qualify,[30] but because of moral criteria such as doubts about their 'willingness to work'.[31] The internal official statements show how important the traditional concept of 'deservingness', besides the primacy of economy, still was in the practices of poor relief in rural areas.[32] Whether applicants received support, the form of payments, the regularity of relief, the nature of clothing given to applicants and the respect (or otherwise) with which they were treated at the welfare office, often depended on how the officials judged their personality. That is, was the applicant a work-shy malingerer, did they spend their money wisely, did they smoke, drink in the local pub, attend fairs or just generally 'hang about' in the streets? With women there were frequent judgements on housekeeping and sexual behaviour. Moreover, the authorities' picture of an applicant was not only based on their own observations, but also comprised the statements of other villagers, who often turned voluntarily to the officials supplying them with information on individual recipients. The network of social control in rural regions was rigid and the able-bodied poor on public assistance were, as can be seen from the surviving letters of denunciation, in a difficult position. They could count on less solidarity than for example old people, who rather lived in a kind of 'integrated poverty'.[33]

Depending on how the poor and the unemployed behaved and acted at the welfare office, depending on their reputation and social status, whether they had advocates or ill-disposed neighbours, the officials generated totally different judgements in spite of similar living conditions. While one unemployed office worker and his family were even granted kindergarten fees for their children besides their regular benefits, others in a similar material situation were completely thrown back on their own resources. Vague legal guidelines left the authorities with plenty of room to manoeuvre in the individual case and the dividing line between inclusion and exclusion was a fine one. A 'respectable citizen' found deserving of support could quickly turn into a 'professional complainer' in the officials' perception. One application too many or a request presented too offensively could be decisive. The local administrators quite naturally, without thinking about their practices complying with the new regulations or being 'just', linked the access to poor relief with moral criteria reflecting their personal views and being part of an age-long tradition concerning the treatment of able-bodied poor.

From unemployment to sickness

Unemployment and poverty were inextricably interwoven, especially since the benefits provided by unemployment support (and even more so by poor relief), often consisting only of food ration cards, were not sufficient to make ends meet. Individual case files allow insights into a complex economy of makeshifts and a difficult, sometimes even desperate, daily struggle to ensure survival.[34] All the patchy strategies and alternative resources that unemployed persons exploited were essential in times of crisis, and even the 'deserving poor' were expected to make use of them.[35] Yet, the case files also reveal the limits and fragility of this daily 'muddling through', and the way in which prolonged unemployment or sickness rapidly brought families to their knees.[36] Events of sickness in particular – whether affecting oneself or a family member – usually pushed people into 'neediness'. The financial burdens that were caused by illness could outreach the amount of several monthly incomes, and even in normal times the majority of the rural population could hardly master these costs without (public) support. This is all the more so in times of long-term unemployment. Even those unemployed who received unemployment benefits, and thereby were covered under health insurance, often depended on additional poor relief payments in cases of illness. In practice, health insurance paid for only a part of the resultant medical expenses and – what was even worse – family members were usually excluded from coverage. For the unemployed standing outside the public welfare system, ill-health and the compromised ability to work often led to a complete breakdown of the economy of makeshifts. Risks of falling ill accumulated with the duration of unemployment, affecting families with children in particular, and such sickness was a core reason why unemployed people 'crossed the threshold' and requested local poor relief.

The status of the sick unemployed was, however, problematic for poor relief authorities. Sickness and the restricted ability to work had been considered as central criteria of the 'deserving poor' since the Middle Ages.[37] The sick poor could not earn their living. Their poverty was not stained with 'unwillingness to work' and it bore 'no fault of their own'. From a theological viewpoint a sick person was always considered deserving of support. In the practices of poor relief, however, things were more complex, a theme that was central to the introduction to this volume. Not every sick applicant was granted relief. Ill-health confronted the officials with moral dilemmas in a special way, counterposing custom and moral obligation with the decisive paradigm of the need to minimize costs. The strategies that were used to minimize the expenditure on health care ranged from shifting the costs onto other institutions – health insurance or former employers – to the granting of credits which had to be paid back by the sick, through to attempts at restraining the free choice of doctors for the recipients of poor relief. This said, the sick poor still had a better chance of receiving relief than other groups among the poor; the number of rejected applications in the Trier hinterland was lower for requests because of illness than for any other cause, while expenditures on medical fees, medication and hospital treatment always represented the most important entry of costs for local poor relief.[38] During the 1920s, most requests for poor relief to meet the costs of illness were only made after the medical treatment had been completed, suggesting in fact that it had become 'normal' for the poor to consult a doctor in case of illness. The letters in the case files clearly show that they subsequently expected the bills for such treatment to be met.

In turn, the poor had a clear appreciation of the importance of sickness vis-à-vis unemployment when seeking relief. The unemployed who turned to poor relief as sick petitioners and asked for the cost of their illness to be met usually had far better chances of receiving support than those acting as 'unemployed' and asking for a one-off payment or long-term poor relief. Usually, the welfare authorities at least granted financial support for medical visits or medication. In case of hospitalization and severe illness the officials often paid for the entire costs. In urgent cases the mayor sometimes decided in favour of the applicant without waiting for the usual statement made by the municipal council. But as a rule, requests linked to ill-health were also passed to the municipal council who decided on them in a meeting. Those turning to poor relief for other reasons than illness usually had to wait for several weeks, in some cases even up to three months, for the resolution as local administrators prevaricated. Things were different for requests related to sickness, where the mayor required, and usually obtained, a fast resolution by setting a time limit. Case files suggest that the outcome of this decision-making process depended in part on the nature of the illness, the social status, gender and age of the sick. Families with children had particularly good chances to receive support. When children fell ill, local administrators often reacted with a certain sensitivity and sometimes even generosity. The families' requests to meet the costs of illness were immediately dealt with and usually granted. Besides paying the costs of medical treatment, the welfare officials often granted additional benefits like milk or food ration cards. In some cases, poor relief financed costly health cures for children. The physical suffering of children, but also of mothers and pregnant women was obviously touching and even in the practices of poor relief in rural areas their well-being was highly valued. Others, unmarried mothers for example, were judged differently. The latter group were often labelled as 'sluts', or even linked to prostitution, and their chances of receiving poor relief in case of sickness were just as bad as for unmarried men. Even children coming from families which the officials stigmatized as 'anti-social' were deprived of the minimum level of solidarity that was usually granted in case of illness.[39]

Thus, local welfare practices ranged from generosity and sensitivity towards the situation of some of the sick, to granting the 'minimum benefit' for most petitioners, and a certain indifference towards some groups. On balance, however, the case files of poor relief demonstrate that even in the 1920s illness was generally still considered a 'legitimate' reason for poverty and a classic characteristic of the 'deserving poor'. Besides old people, the sick generally had better chances to receive poor relief than any other group. This also applies to unemployed people who turned to poor relief for help because of sickness. In the official perception, they were often categorized as 'sick' while their unemployment faded into the background. That the poor had a keen appreciation of the negotiating value of sickness can be seen in their narratives, to which we now turn.

Narratives of sickness and poverty – sickness in the negotiating process

Pauper letters are strategic writings, though they can by no means be reduced exclusively to strategy and rhetoric.[40] Most petitioners seem to have planned very neatly how their case might best be put and which arguments to present in order to make sure their petition would appear 'legitimate'. What they chose to reveal or to omit is to a certain degree related to what they thought the authorities would want to hear; pauper letters reflect the socio-institutional contexts of their origin rather than necessarily revealing feelings and 'authentic' experiences of ill-health, fear and pain. Nonetheless, the narratives and self-portrayals of unemployed and sick people provide at least some insight into their own ideas and their views on poverty and sickness.

Of course, pauper letters are not patient records of the sort used by Cathy Smith elsewhere in this volume, where the description of ill-health and being ill is at the core and which often contain detailed accounts of symptoms and ailments. In pauper letters descriptions of illness often covered only a few lines or consist of isolated references, with the applicants instead focused on the concrete costs of medical treatment and the financial problems of coping with sickness. The unemployed merchant Peter W. from Biewer, for example, first turned to poor relief after two years of unemployment, when his wife fell ill. In his letter to the municipal council he asked for financial support to cover the costs of hospitalization, as the health insurance paid only parts of the expenditures and he felt unable to pay the remainder:

> My wife had to be admitted to the 'Herz-Jesu-Hospital' on 26 September. The local health insurance fund for the county of Trier-Land pays a share of the costs of hospitalisation that amounts to 1,80 RM daily . . . The daily rate for hospitalisation amounts to 3,50 RM. I have been out of work over a longer period and receive crisis relief [*Krisenfürsorge*] that amounts to 20,45 RM per week. This support hardly allows me to supply my family of four with the most essential food. This is why I lack all means to meet the remaining costs for hospitalisation and I plead for public welfare to bear these expenses.[41]

During the 1920s a large number of unemployed persons turned to poor relief with similar petitions. Many unemployed families were in an even more precarious situation than Peter Ws, since family members of unemployment benefits recipients were usually excluded from health insurance and had to bear the costs of illness themselves. For the unemployed who were outside the system of unemployment insurance and who had to secure their livelihood through a mix of alternative resources, even much smaller items like the cost of medication or prescribed food were unattainable without (public) help. The applicants' focusing on the financial consequences of sickness was imperative, since they wanted to be reimbursed for exactly these expenditures. Such pleading demonstrates how closely poverty was linked to illness from the perspective of the sick poor and unemployed.

Yet, if pauper letters shared the basic characteristic that descriptions of ill-health were rather short, in other respects the narratives of sickness differed considerably according to the individual rhetorical skills, the nature of the illness, on whether the applicants were reporting their own condition or an event of sickness in the family and whether they intended to achieve the reimbursement of costs for medical treatment or other benefits. When describing their condition, the petitioners often used general terms like 'ill' and 'ailing' or 'sickness' and 'suffering', without ever specifying the illness. Mrs Peter Sch., for example, submitted a request for her 'sick daughter', for whom she could not care any longer as she herself was out of work and 'sick' on top of that.[42] In his letter to the mayor of Ehrang, Nikolaus G. spoke about a 'war-affliction' (*Kriegsleiden*) which caused him 'considerable costs' and prevented him from 'doing hard work'.[43] Similarly vague are the statements by Johann Sch. from Euren regarding his illness: 'Due to my illness and my wife's illness I find myself in a desperate plight, so that I am not able to pay off the debts I had to incur while I was out of work.'[44] When women and children were affected, sickness was often described with terms like 'ailing' (*kränklich*) and 'weakly' (*schwächlich*) indicating a person's prolonged illness or increased susceptibility to ill-health.[45]

The general statement of 'illness' or 'suffering' was often extended by additional attributes like 'serious' or 'long-lasting', thereby intending to reinforce the description of the personal plight. The unemployed worker Gertrud M., for example, turned to poor relief for help because of her husband's 'serious illness'.[46] Josef H. gave 'the permanent illness of [his] wife, who has been seriously suffering for six years' as a reason for his 'difficult situation' (*zerrüttete Verhältnisse*).[47] Anna G. gave a more detailed account of her husband's state of health when she mentioned that he had been sick for a long time and also that he was bedridden: 'In recent years my husband has been ill a lot and bedridden for longer periods of time. Only a fortnight ago he had to stay in bed for five days.'[48] Variations in the motif of being bedridden constantly reappear in descriptions of ill-health in the letters to the welfare authorities, emphasizing not only the seriousness of the illness, but also an inability to work. A letter from the rag-and-bone man, Johann Sch., illustrates this well:

> Due to his illness, which has been medically certified and which may last up to four weeks, the undersigned is in extreme need. Being bedridden I cannot pursue my trade and am left without any income. My wife is still ailing, too. Both my sons, which are unemployed and do not receive relief, can neither find work nor income. In view of my situation of great need I most politely plead the welfare-office of the county of Trier-Land to grant me financial support, at least for the duration of my sickness.[49]

Unlike Johann Sch.'s previous requests, in which he explained his neediness as 'due to bad economic circumstances'[50] which did not allow him to earn a livelihood in his trade, this time the mayor approved his request. In a situation where inclusion and exclusion in the local practice of poor relief mainly depended on the assessment of one's ability and 'willingness' to work, it is unsurprising to find the sick unemployed emphasizing their inability to work in their letters. Both the appeal to one's inability to work and the focus on the costs of illness constituted a necessity in the negotiation process. At the same time, the descriptions and the concrete handling of illnesses of the rural poor reveal something about their own perception of ill-health and being ill. In most cases, such paupers only turned to the doctor when they saw their ability to work threatened.[51]

Which specific illnesses hid behind vague descriptions remains mostly unclear. In some cases, the actual illnesses can be tracked down only through drawing on additional sources like medical certificates or the doctor's notes on prescriptions, which can sometimes be found in the files. The fact that the applicants often described their illness in general terms instead of specifying it might, with certain diseases like the contagious pulmonary tuberculosis or syphilis, be due to a feeling of shame or the fear of being stigmatized. According to observations made by Dr Cyranka, the long-time physician responsible for the district of Trier-Land, shame still played an important role in the way diseases like tuberculosis were dealt with in rural areas in the 1920s. Cyranka, who stated that he was not content with holding surgery only, but also visited his patients in their houses in order 'to gain better insight into their entire social situation',[52] reported that people who suffered from pulmonary diseases dreaded applying for poor relief because they were scared that 'one could talk about it behind their back'.[53] Anna Lundberg in her contribution to this volume has noted similar concerns over the way in which reporting syphilis might affect a person's subsequent life chances in early twentieth-century Norway.

Clearly, there were certain diseases about which one did not talk in front of neighbours and other villagers, and least of all in letters to the poor relief administration. Poor and unemployed people from rural areas had to accept that their case was dealt with in public and that the whole village usually knew who was on poor relief.[54] Irrespective of social mores, applicants also had to consider exactly how much to reveal about their personal lives in letters to the local officials.[55] Applying for poor relief represented a special situation of communication that shaped the description of illness decisively. Even if a disease was not contagious, the petitioners usually did not say much about their condition because after all the interaction with welfare officials was not a medical consultation between doctor and patient. The applicants just wanted their costs covered and not a doctor's opinion. In some cases, the vague description of the illness was possibly to do with the fact that petitioners simply did not know which disease they suffered from or that they assumed that their condition was known anyway, given the tight social relationships inside small villages.

Yet, pauper letters from the 1920s and early 1930s do sometimes contain quite concrete labelling of sickness. When portraying his medical condition, the unemployed guard Georg D., for example, pointed to his restricted ability to work because 'I am suffering from chronic articulate rheumatism and cardiac insufficiency, so that is why I can only work from time to time.'[56] Anny J.'s description was somewhat more detailed. In her letter to the municipal council of Euren she named the disease and also said how long she has been sick and under medical treatment. She even hinted at the physical consequences:

As I came down with pleurisy three weeks ago and I am currently being in a state of debility, hardly being able to keep myself upright, I am unfortunately unable to call on personally. I have been under medical treatment with Mr Frings for the last two weeks. Taking into consideration my great distress, I hope my request has not been made in vain.[57]

Most petitioners used more or less common names of diseases, like *Gliedwasser* (swollen legs), gallstone or *Offenes Bein* (chronic leg wound), and often referred to previous medical consultations or the medical diagnosis. The pauper letters even sometimes contained medical terminology which was more or less obviously copied from the medical certificates. In his letter to the welfare authorities, Christian K., for example, asked for coverage of costs for a '*Datermiebehandlung*' (diathermic therapy) in hospital. He copied the medical term including its spelling mistake from the medical certificate which he presented to the welfare authorities.[58] The unemployed mainly turned to poor relief in case of physical illness. Only three times do the case files of poor relief include references to mental illness of the sort discussed by Alannah Tomkins, Cathy Smith and Georgina Laragy. In his request, the unemployed Valentin T. referred to the fact that his wife, due to 'all the deprivations of the past years', had turned 'emotionally disturbed' (*gemütskrank*), but he avoided further details.[59] The two remaining cases also reveal only a brief hint to a 'nervous affliction' (*Nervenleiden*), without further description.[60]

Experiences of pain or mental burdens related to illness hardly ever appear in letters to local poor relief officials. Suffering and pain were at the most insinuated, for example by referring to the 'seriousness' of the sickness, but explicit or extensive descriptions are completely absent. The applicants clearly focused their writings on the costs of illness and tried to prove their 'neediness'. The welfare office was not the place to communicate, at least voluntarily, individual feelings and physical or even mental sufferings. In their letters to the local officials, unemployed mothers and fathers again and again expressed their concern for the well-being of their children. They often neglected their own concerns – including their health. Being tied up in the daily struggle for survival, they probably did not even have the time or peace of mind to deal with their own illness, to look at their own body, or even to put these observations into words.

Sickness, inability to work and 'outside-help'

Just as sickness played a key part in the letters of paupers, so in connection with a limited ability to work sickness was very often the central argument for the recognition of need in official statements. The application of Christian Q., an unemployed electrician from Euren, was approved by the mayor on the grounds that, 'Considering the fact that, in recent weeks, the applicant has been almost constantly without income due to a serious injury and the fact that he and his family had to endure several cases of illness, which made them slip into destitution, I approve of a one-off payment of 30 RM.'[61] The way in which the authorities acted and argued in the case of Christian Q. was in many respects typical of their dealings with the (sick) unemployed. In this case the applicant's long-term unemployment was not mentioned at all. Rather it was Christian Q.'s injured hand, as well as his wife's and his daughter's unspecified illnesses, that, from the authorities' point of view, brought about the family's distress. Previous applications had all been turned down with a note saying that the unemployed electrician should try harder to find employment.[62] The officials intervened – as they did in plenty of other cases – only after the family's health situation had declined seriously and poverty could be seen as definitively not the fault of the applicant.

Further evidence of this tendency can be seen in a statement made by the mayor in the case of Barbara M. from Euren: 'Due to grave cases of illness – Mrs. M. for example had to have medical treatment in hospital over a longer period of time – the M.'s got into serious difficulties through no fault of their own, which, in my eyes, is also due to arrears with the rent.'[63] The mayor subsequently intervened to prevent eviction. This was not necessarily altruistic, as presumably he saw the cost of an imminent homelessness bearing down on poor relief, but nevertheless the close connection of ill-health with a plight 'through no fault of one's own' is clearly evident in this statement. Significantly, the mayor did not mention at all that Josef M. had been unemployed for over two years, which – also from the family's point of view[64] – was the real reason for their distress.

In turn, and as we have already seen elsewhere in this volume, those writing pauper letters often co-opted official language and phraseology, as well as employing external interlocutors to help bolster the impression that poverty was an inevitable consequence of illness, the costs of its treatment and the consequences of its incidence, rather than the fault of the applicant. Thus, on 15 July 1929, the wife of the unemployed Johann B. asked for her husband's referral to a specialist:

My husband has been suffering from a serious hardening of the arteries for three years now. Because of that he was dismissed from his post with Loeser last year. Although – according to a report from Dr. Poggemann – the hardening of the arteries is put down to the influence of war, an entitlement to benefits was turned down even after an appeal. For quite a time now his condition has been deteriorating in such a way that my husband can hardly stand straight. Something special has to be done in order to prevent a constant aggravation and to preserve my husband. Therefore I plead for specialist treatment and for a health cure in an appropriate hospital.[65]

Katharina B. portrayed her husband's state of health more thoroughly than was usual in pauper letters. She also mentioned, though only vaguely, her husband's physical pain and that his condition had deteriorated considerably.[66] By writing 'in order to preserve my husband'[67] and calling on the expert testimony of Dr Poggemann, Katharina tied up her requests for aid with the gendered space of family life and responsibilities, the status of the doctor and the moral duties of the poor law officials. We see this intersection again in the case of Nikolaus B., an unemployed mason from Pfalzel who, having previously been turned down for relief but having subsequently been to hospital because of an accident, applied for long-term relief on 17 September 1929.[68] The request was turned down by the local officials with a note saying that his wife was able to earn a living for the family by carrying out casual work.[69] On 11 November 1929 Nikolaus B. filed another application in which he depicted his wife's ill-health and inability to work more precisely:

> It is impossible for my wife to take up a job as an hourly employee because after suffering a relapse she has again been ill for 8 weeks now and is being medically treated. She has water in her limbs and there is a danger that her suffering turns into tuberculosis. Following medical instructions, she is not allowed to carry out any strenuous work, not even cleaning and the like . . .[70]

Whereas Nikolaus B. had described his wife merely as being 'in poor health' (*kränklich*) in his first letter, he concretely gives her medical condition in the application he made in November, referring to the doctor's opinion, an external interlocutor, when depicting his wife's inability to work. The phrase 'there is a danger that her suffering turns into tuberculosis'[71] was most likely borrowed from the medical consultation.

More widely, references to medical competence and authority are commonplace in negotiation processes with the welfare office. The sick unemployed tried in varied ways to include a doctor as an external authority into the decision-making and thus to apply pressure on the local officials. They got themselves medical certificates revealing their state of health, their inability to work or the medical necessity of 'tonics'. They showed these statements to the welfare administration, which was forced to at least take notice of this external authority. The applicants borrowed medical terminology along with the phrasing and whole sentences from medical reports and consultations with their doctor. By means of this borrowed scientific terminology and authority they were hoping for their own case to be more convincing and credible. This 'borrowing of authority' is shown when applicants referred to the doctor's diagnosis or 'order' as in the letter from Nikolaus B. above. In a letter to the District Administrator (*Landrat*) the unemployed rag-and-bone man Jakob Sch. even wrote that he applied for welfare benefits 'on doctor Losen's recommendation'.[72]

At the beginning of the 1920s the recipients of poor relief could choose their doctor freely. This regulation had been introduced within the framework of poor relief and it replaced the institution of the relief physician (*Armenarzt*), giving more agency for the poor and unemployed. The needy could decide for themselves which doctor to see, and the possibility of choice presented new potential for the negotiations with the welfare office. Which doctor to choose depended on various factors, including medical competence and trust. For welfare clients the choice apparently also depended on the extent to which the medical man in question would support their negotiations with the welfare office. At any rate, when browsing the files of the poor relief, it catches one's eye that the needy chose particular doctors rather than necessarily the ones who were nearest. Moreover, there are a strikingly large number of medical reports issued by these 'preferred' doctors that suited their patients, for example medical certificates on the necessity of milk. In some cases doctors strongly advocated their patients' needs by issuing milk orders over a longer period of time, or by stressing the necessity of 'better food' for recovery. In doing so they supported their patients' application for food ration cards or higher poor relief payments. Besides medical considerations, social reasons and sympathy might have played a role in this extraordinary commitment to their patients. Often, the doctors had already known their patients over a longer period and had lived through their social decline.

While the free choice of a doctor strengthened the position of the sick poor in many ways – sometimes even creating the impression of a partnership between patient and doctor – for the poor relief administration the loss of the relief physician meant a loss of control.[73] The doctor's opinion was hardly ever welcomed by the authorities as can be seen from efforts made by the city parliament of Trier during the Great Depression to limit the free choice of doctor for welfare clients. On the other hand, the poor relief administration was dependent on medical certificates. Often the local authorities demanded a doctor's opinion since they did not see themselves in the position to decide a case without one.[74] Moreover, and despite their ambivalent view, in most cases welfare officials attended the doctor's orders and recommendations. Through this help 'from outside', which challenged the welfare administration's exclusive authority over 'one's case', the destitute often managed to strengthen their position in the negotiation process and to enforce their agency. The attitudes of local officials, to which we now turn, were complex in the face of often quite sophisticated pauper appeals.

Sickness, 'deservingness' and attitudes to the relief system

Most of the unemployed and poor people who turned to local poor relief were acquainted with the inherent principles of the relief system. They were aware of the fact that besides their material situation, specific moral preconceptions, tied into the construction of 'deservingness', were a central access criterion. Descriptions of the material predicament, the family background and the cause(s) of poverty were at the core of the letters to the welfare office. Apart from that, the narratives were characterized by attempts to demonstrate one's 'deservingness' and moral integrity.[75] Unemployed applicants were automatically in a position of having to work doubly hard to justify their claims, as we have seen. Thus, letters from this group often apologized for applying and becoming 'a burden to the community'. Not only did unemployed people try to demonstrate their willingness to work, but they also thought it necessary to point out that they were no 'drunkards', 'squanderers' or 'criminals', suggesting that they expected the authorities to picture them in this fashion.[76] The unemployed from the camp in Euren experienced the displacement from Trier to the wooden shacks on the outskirts of the town often as a difficult social decline. In their interactions with the local administrators they repeatedly stressed that even though they were unemployed and living in a bad area, they were still 'upright' (rechtschaffen). Hence, 'Even if I have to live in the old shacks, which already means great distress . . . one can still be considered an upright citizen.'[77]

Within this rhetoric of deservingness, ill-health was an important element. References to illness can be found not only in letters in which the unemployed pleaded for direct medical care, but often also in requests for other forms of support like long-term poor relief, one-off payments, linen or clothes and shoes. In these letters, illness appears as a part of the personal plight and sometimes as the strongest evidence and expression of neediness and destitution 'through no fault of one's own'. In his request for a 'winter allowance', Nikolaus S. from Euren wrote: 'The current situation of my family of eleven proves the great need we are in: six members are ill, two of them seriously.'[78] The numerous references to sickness in the letters to the poor relief administration primarily reflect the social reality of the poor and the unemployed, their experiences of material privations and increasing risks of falling ill. At the same time, the applicants used the rhetoric of sickness to demonstrate their personal integrity, assert their identities and to tell their own version of events. They referred to the same implications of sickness as the authorities did in their internal communication about individual cases. In her request, unemployed worker Maria M. pointed to her miscarriage and 'abdominal pain' and pleaded with the municipal council of Euren: 'In the light of these special circumstances would you kindly grant me support so that I can get out of the distress which is no fault of my own.'[79] Unemployed Christian Q. from Euren made a similar statement. In his petition from April 1926 he asked for the costs of his wife's hospitalization to be met as well as for a one-off payment, since his family had got into great need through his unemployment and his wife's long-lasting illness. In his letter he emphasized that he and his family had 'not the slightest responsibility for [his] wife's long-lasting suffering and the entire misery'.[80] Rather, the 'difficult situation' (*zerrütete Verhältnisse*) was to blame for all the destitution.[81] His letter closed with the following affirmation:

> So far, I have eked out a living in an honest and upright manner and have never made a claim on public welfare. But now, it is not possible any longer, everything is over. If I could not borrow food, my family and I would have to starve . . . That is why I kindly plead once more to be lenient with me so that my sick wife may not be thrown out of the hospital and the mischief aggravated.[82]

Of course, while references to sickness might increase one's chances of receiving support, this link was by no means automatic. The requests by Maria M. and Christian Q. were rejected, not because of a lack of willingness to work, as was often the case with applications by the unemployed, but because of the community's 'extremely tense financial situation'.[83] The fact that the officials did not question the applicants' 'uprightness' in their negative reply did little to alleviate the material want of either family, but at least rejection did not increase the moral pressure that weighed particularly heavily upon unemployed persons in rural areas and that multiplied the burdens of their personal distress.

These pictures that the unemployed sketched of their poverty, illness and of their personality, show how seriously they saw their moral integrity questioned. Furthermore, their narratives reveal how much their image of local poor relief was linked to questions of morality and 'deservingness'. By actively (rather than defensively) using the rhetoric of morality and 'deservingness', pauper letter writers adapted to the inherent principles of poor relief and the practices of the local officials. At the same time however, these rhetorical episodes reflect the poor's own concepts of society and these resonate strongly with officials' attitudes. Statements such as 'So far, I have eked out a living in an honest an upright manner and have never made a claim on public welfare',[84] 'I have never been a burden to the community so far'[85] or 'I have never lived at the expense of the community'[86] appear in variations in numerous letters and can to some extent certainly be classified as rhetoric and strategy. All the same, they do reflect the applicants' predominant perspective on poor relief and their personal conceptions of a 'righteous' life.

Attempts at self-assertion and numerous descriptions of despair show the extent to which unemployed people were affected and hurt in their pride by the permanent doubts about their personality and by the reproach that their unemployment and poverty were self-induced. Petitioners connected their feelings of despair and resignation not only to the material predicament surrounding them, but also explicitly to experiences of exclusion and stigmatization. The unemployed locksmith Jakob L. and his family, being forced by the Trier city council to move to the camp in the 'no man's land' between Trier and Euren, wrote the following letter to the governor of the Rhine Province in order to describe his experiences as an inhabitant of 'New Morocco':

> ... So, between Trier and Euren, expelled from Trier and assigned to the outskirts, one has no rights anywhere and is placed under disability ... There is nothing left to do, despair soon carries one to extremes. Also I have been to the [administrations of] suburbs to get a credit, therefore I would have given my written agreement to renounce any support, but I was rejected. I have the opportunity to build my own existence through some trading. But one is left to rot and die in this place called Neu-Marokko (camp) by the public of Trier and the officials. Because only poor people from Trier have been planted here, one does not obtain any rights anywhere. The papers often write about the conditions that prevail here. In order not to digress, I, the undersigned, send some examples taken from the papers ... Sincerely waiting for your early reply, Jakob L.[87]

Jakob L. never received a response to his letter. As was common practice with pauper letters addressed to higher authorities, his letter was passed on to lower levels without any comment and presumably without ever being read.

Some letters from unemployed applicants in the 1920s evidence definite attempts to break out of the position of justification and to disconnect poor relief from questions of morality and 'deservingness'. Applicants rather tried to claim a 'right' to which every citizen in need should be entitled, irrespective of personality or reputation. References to legal arguments or the provisions of the new welfare laws can rarely be found in letters from the rural hinterland of Trier but do occur in some cases. In these statements, however rare they are, a different understanding of the state's duties towards its citizens shines through.[88] This said, the majority of unemployed people in rural communities did not know about the new welfare provisions, the social rights that the constitution of Weimar guaranteed to them, and mostly not even the applicable public welfare rates of their community. The rural poor and unemployed who applied for public welfare usually referred to a language of the moral and thus moved within traditional circles.

Conclusion

The letters of the unemployed – to local officials, the governor of the Rhine Province, the Prussian Minister of Welfare or even Hindenburg himself – reveal rhetorical skills, self-reliance and strength. At the same time they show feelings of powerlessness and sometimes a certain speechlessness in the face of the applicant's despair. However progressive the contemporary experts' discourse on poverty, unemployment and welfare was, the traditional concept of 'deservingness', with its moral undertones, remained the main criterion for inclusion and exclusion at the micro-level. Paradoxically, even during the time of mass unemployment the division into deserving and undeserving poor was maintained. Faced with such a negotiating framework, the unemployed were forced to shift their claims-making from structural crisis towards themselves. In a system without any legal entitlement to support and which was traditionally directed towards a temporary safeguard for old and disabled people, the unemployed were in a particularly difficult position.

The 'place' of the unemployed in the rural poor relief system was, even in the Weimar welfare state, an exceedingly fragile one. Their chances of receiving support were usually better if they turned to poor relief for help because of illness rather than merely because of unemployment. To the authorities' eye they often slipped into the category of 'the sick', while their unemployment took a back seat. In the 1920s, ill-health was still considered as a classic characteristic of the 'deserving poor'. Even in the practice of rural poor relief, which was traditionally directed towards economy, the sick's exclusion was limited. However, these limits were variable and subject to negotiation processes. The numerous references to sickness in the letters of the unemployed principally reflect their social and health reality. At the same time these references show the applicants' endeavour to display their moral integrity and to exercise their agency. In their letters they referred to the same implications of illness as did the officials in their statements. Through various means, such as reference to a doctor's authority, they tried to strengthen their position in the everyday negotiations with the local welfare officials. Against this backdrop it is insufficient to judge the continual emphasis on 'deservingness' and destitution 'through no fault of one's own' as a simple rhetorical strategy. By using a language of sickness and morality, unemployed applicants attempted to contest the official narratives of their 'case' and to assert their identities.

Notes

1 The contemporary term '*Wohlfahrtserwerbsloser*' (welfare unemployed) refers to unemployed people who were supported within local poor relief. For the negative connotations of this term, see Homburg, H. (1985), 'Vom arbeitslosen zum zwangsarbeiter. arbeitslosenpolitik und fraktionierung der arbeiterschaft in Deutschland 1930–33 am beispiel der wohlfahrtserwerbslosen und der kommunalen wohlfahrtshilfe', *Archiv für Sozialgeschichte*, 25, 251–98.

2 For the development of unemployment at the national level during the 1920s, see Führer, K. C. (1990), *Arbeitslosigkeit und die Entstehung der Arbeitslosenversicherung in Deutschland: 1902–27*. Berlin: Colloquium-Verlag; Lewek, P. (1992), *Arbeitslosigkeit und Arbeitslosenversicherung in der Weimarer Republik 1918–27 (VSWG; Beiheft 104)*. Stuttgart: Steiner. For the time of the Great Depression, see Berringer, C. (1999), *Sozialpolitik in der Weltwirtschaftskrise: die Arbeitslosenversicherungspolitik in Deutschland und Großbritannien im Vergleich 1928–34*. Berlin: Duncker & Humbolt.

3 For the biographies of relief of the unemployed from the suburbs of Trier, see Stazic, T. (2003), 'Arbeitslosigkeit und Arbeitslosenunterstützung im Raum Trier 1918–30', Unpublished MA thesis, University of Trier, pp. 22–42.

4 Not until the Depression did experts perceive this change in employment structures and the erosion of permanent employment as problematic. See, for example, Gaebel, K. (1932), *Die deutsche Wirtschaft und das Berufsschicksal der Frau*. Berlin: Hower, p. 5ff.

5 On the genesis of unemployment assistance in the Weimar Republic see Führer, *Arbeitslosigkeit* and Lewek, *Arbeitslosigkeit*. Berringer, *Arbeitslosenversicherungspolitik*, examines the unemployment insurance policy in Germany and Great Britain during the Depression. Up to now, the issue of unemployment and unemployment assistance has almost exclusively been described from the perspective of the state and of politics. In particular about unemployment and poverty in rural areas and the correlations between national insurance, local welfare and other traditional forms of support like family networks we still know almost nothing. Detailed community level analysis of the practical efficacy of unemployment assistance and social policy as well as studies on the living conditions of the unemployed and the poor are still missing for the twentieth century. For the current state of research in the fields of poverty and poor relief, see Marx, K. (2005), 'Armut und Armenfürsorge auf dem Land. Die Kreise Bernkastel und Wittlich von den 1880er Jahren bis 1933', Unpublished PhD, University of Trier. Presenting a slightly older state of research, but still current, Rudloff, W. (2002), 'Im souterrain des sozialstaates. Neuere forschungen zur geschichte von fürsorge und wohlfahrtspflege im 20. jahrhundert', *Archiv für Sozialgeschichte*, 42, 474–520.

6 These restrictions and exclusions reflect predominant views on the rights of youth, the employment of women, concepts of 'work', and considerations to the interests of (agrarian) employers.

7 The figures are taken from Stazic, 'Arbeitslosigkeit', 27–31.

8 Still central for the history of German poor relief is Sachße, C. and Tennstedt, F. (1988), *Geschichte der Armenfürsorge in Deutschland, Fürsorge und Wohlfahrtspflege 1871 bis 1929*. Stuttgart: Kohlhammer. For the discussion of Weimar welfare policy at a national level, see Hong, Y.-S. (1998), *Welfare, Modernity, and the Weimar State, 1919–33*. Princeton: Princeton University Press. The Weimar welfare state from its clientele's point of view is analysed in Crew, D. F. (1998), *Germans on Welfare. From Weimar to Hitler*. Oxford: Oxford University Press. For the practices of poor relief as well as the living conditions and experiences of the poor and the unemployed in rural areas from 1860 to 1975, see the research of the project B5 (Poverty in Rural Regions between Welfare Politics, Charity and Self-Help during the Industrial Age, 1860–1975). For detailed information and a listing of publications within the project, part of the CRC 600 'Strangers and Poor People. Changing Patterns of Inclusion and Exclusion from Classical Antiquity to the Present Day' at the University of Trier, see http://www.sfb600.uni-trier.de.

9 The umbrella organization of German municipal administrations.

10 *Mitteilungen des Deutschen Städtetages*, No. 9, 25 (1931): 1.

11 The official unemployment statistics do not reveal this extent of exclusion. National recording of the 'welfare unemployed' did not occur until the summer of 1930. In spite of the community's complaints about skyrocketing welfare

costs, the Reich had been turning a blind eye to this issue until then. Even then, official statistics on the 'welfare unemployed' are anything but trustworthy. They include – as the analysis of case files shows – only a part of the supported unemployed. See Stazic, 'Arbeitslosigkeit', p. 23ff.

12 Reflecting different political constellations, compulsory labour was more extensively ordered in rural and small-town areas than in urban contexts. Wolfgang Ayaß points out that a comprehensive implementation of compulsory labour for the unemployed in German cities was not in train until after 1933. See Ayaß, W. (1998), 'Pflichtarbeit und fürsorgearbeit. Zur geschichte der "Hilfe zur Arbeit" außerhalb von anstalten', in *Arbeitsdienst – wieder salonfähig? Zwang zur Arbeit in Geschichte und Sozialstaat*. Frankfurt: Frankfurter Arbeitslosenzentrum – FALZ, pp. 56–79.

13 For the situation of the inhabitants of the camp between Trier and Euren, their living conditions and experiences, see Stazic, 'Arbeitslosigkeit', pp. 133–7.

14 For the methodological problems and the potential of pauper letters, see Sokoll, T. (2001), *Essex Pauper Letters, 1731–1837*. Oxford: Oxford University Press. For Germany, where pauper letters have only been gradually discovered as sources 'from below', see Marx, 'Armut', 137–49.

15 This chapter draws on records of the poor relief of the suburbs' mayor's office (*Bürgermeisterei der Vororte Trier*) as well as other communities of the rural district of Trier (*Kreis Trier-Land*). Well into the twentieth century a good portion of the people from the economically underdeveloped region of Trier were dependent on small-scale subsistence farming. In order to survive smallholders often had to work as day labourers on large-scale farms or in the industries of the Saarland or Lorraine in addition to their regular work. In the suburbs of Trier there had been a mixed employment structure. While in Kürenz most inhabitants were industrial workers, most people from Euren, Olewig and Zewen were living on agriculture and a part of the inhabitants were working in the crafts, in trade or industry. Women were frequently working for the cigarette factories of Trier or as domestic workers.

16 For the state of research with regard to ill-health and poverty, see Krieger, M. (2007), 'Arme und Ärzte, Kranke und Kassen. Ländliche Gesundheitsversorgung und kranke Arme in der südlichen Rheinprovinz 1869 bis 1930', Unpublished PhD, University Trier, pp. 31–9.

17 On the question of how representative microhistorical studies are, see Ammerer, G. (2003), *Heimat Straße. Vaganten im Österreich des Ancien Régime*. Vienna: Verlag für Geschichte und Politik, pp. 23–4.

18 Reflecting the compulsory schooling established in nineteenth-century Prussia, the degree of literacy at the beginning of the twentieth century was quite advanced.

19 Implicit here is the 'correct way' to communicate with authorities. The formal, official tone of many letters allowed the poor not to expose themselves too much, but to keep a certain distance and to preserve personal and emotional matters for themselves.

20 When browsing the case files it is noticeable that applicants, in particular when first making contact with poor relief, preferred the written form of application. Many applicants also combined written and oral requests.

21 Young unemployed, unmarried applicants and childless couples had the least chance of being relieved. Families with children had better chances, though even their applications were frequently denied or only partly granted. Depending

on the social and professional status of the applicants, their age and sex, their appearance, etc. the numbers of refusals and the granted allowances vary considerably. See Stazic, 'Arbeitslosigkeit', pp. 76–90.

22 The applicants' criticism was not directed towards the system of poor relief, but rather towards the acts and behaviour of the individual welfare official, who was perceived as responsible for their destitution. For this observation, also see Crew, *Germans*, p. 85.

23 See, for example, the letter of protest from the 'makeshift alliance of unemployed office workers' (*Notgemeinschaft der erwerbslosen Angestellten*): Stadtarchiv Trier (hereafter STAT) Tb12/139, 10 February 1929.

24 See, for example, STAT Tb14/482: Letter from the parish priest of Euren to the mayor of the suburbs, 18 November 1929: 'I would absolutely recommend to approve of this application. As far as I know the applicant is a decent young man, who deserves support.'

25 Besides various forms of solidarity and mutual help, there are also many cases of whistle-blowing. See, for example, STAT Tb14/482: recorded oral request made by Johann E., 30 April 1927: 'I certainly do know that Mrs Heinrich B. has already been working for two months in the French laundry for a weekly salary of about 30 Mark. Additionally, her husband receives long-term poor relief.' The motives of informers are difficult to discern but presumably personal conflicts and perhaps the hope of ameliorating one's own situation at the office through this kind of cooperation with the authorities, were important.

26 Occasionally there are examples in the poor relief files of the unemployed negotiating very successfully with the officials, enforcing their interests and even virtuously navigating the system. But these were singular cases. Examining the huge volume of files and trying to quantify success and failure of these negotiation processes (by concretely counting how many petitions and appeals had been granted and how many denied; see Stazic, 'Arbeitslosigkeit') it becomes evident that the scope for pauper agency was lopsided, with the poor only rarely able to communicate at eye level with officials.

27 See Marx, 'Armut'.

28 See, for example, 'Verwaltungsbericht Trier-Land', 1920–2: 33ff.

29 Contemporary observers criticized the fact 'that welfare authorities sat in judgement on their own decisions' (Crew, *Germans*, p. 77). A legal entitlement to public support was not been established in Germany until the *Bundessozialhilfegesetz* of 1961.

30 The material situation of applicants was intimately entwined with 'deservingness', since even a low income or little property could be sufficient for denial of relief.

31 The judgement of 'unwillingness to work' used by the authorities in negative replies was often rather a rhetorical strategy than an expression of 'sincere' moral doubts. In times of mass unemployment, this short phrase, being used quasi-automatically with the unemployed, allowed poor relief administrators to casually turn down applicants without having to consider their situation or take much time for a more detailed explanation.

32 See Stazic, 'Arbeitslosigkeit', 63–103; Marx, 'Armut'.

33 For the term '*pauvreté intégrée*', which describes an ideal-type of poverty, see Paugam, S. (2001), 'Les formes contemporaines de la pauvreté et de l'exclusion en Europe', *Etudes Rurales*, 159–160, 73–96.

34 For the term 'economy of makeshifts' and the current state of research, see King, S. and Tomkins, A. (2003), 'Introduction', in King, S. and Tomkins, A. (eds),

The Poor in England 1700–1850. An Economy of Makeshifts. Manchester: Manchester University Press, pp. 1–38.

35 See Marx, 'Armut', 283; Rudloff, W. (1995), *Die Wohlfahrtsstadt. Kommunale Ernährungs-, Fürsorge- und Wohnungspolitik am Beispiel Münchens 1910–33*. Göttingen: Vandenhoeck and Ruprecht, p. 629.

36 'Muddling through' and similar terms were used by unemployed and poor people themselves in their letters to describe their daily struggle for survival. See, for example, STAT Tb14/482: Letter from Nikolaus S. to the mayor of the suburbs of Trier, 4 April 1926.

37 See, for example, Rheinheimer, M. (1993), 'Armut in Großsolt (Angeln) 1700–1900', *Zeitschrift der Gesellschaft für Schleswig-Holsteinische Geschichte*, 118, 54.

38 For the suburbs of Trier, see Stazic, 'Arbeitslosigkeit', pp. 137–46. For an extensive account of other rural districts in the southern Rhine Province, see Krieger, 'Kranke'.

39 The family of the unemployed scrap metal merchant Nikolaus S. had 11 members and represents an extreme case. After several unsuccesful requests, the suburb granted the family long-term support of 40 RM. This was the amount usually allotted to a family of four. The children of the family repeatedly suffered from serious illnesses. Three of them had to be hospitalized during several months because of pneumonia, malnutrition and physical weakness (*Körperschwäche*). Two of the children died in hospital. Without consideration of these cases of serious illness, all requests made by Nikolaus S. to raise his long-term payments and to obtain food, clothes and shoes for his children were denied because of the family's 'anti-social behaviour'. See STAT Tb14/482.

40 See Sokoll, *Essex*, pp. 67–70.

41 STAT Tb14/470: Letter from Peter W. to the municipal council of Pfalzel, 2 October 1929.

42 STAT Tb14/482: Letter from 'Mrs Peter Sch.' to the suburbs' mayor's office, 2 September 1928.

43 STAT Tb14/470: Letter from Nikolaus G. to the municipal council of Pfalzel, 19 February 1925.

44 STAT Tb14/482: Letter from Johann Sch. to the suburbs' mayor's office, 1 November 1928.

45 Jacob L., for example, describes his youngest son merely as 'ailing child' and Gerhard S. describes his wife as 'ailing' and unable to do factory work. STAT Tb14/480: Letter from Jakob L. to the governor of the Rhine Province, 24 September 1926; STAT Tb14/470: Letter from Gerhard S. to the municipal council of Pfalzel, 29 November 1929.

46 STAT Tb14/482: Letter from Gertrud M. to the suburbs' mayor's office, 11 September 1926.

47 STAT Tb14/470: Letter from Josef H. to the municipal council of Pfalzel, 12 July 1927.

48 STAT Tb14/470: Letter from Anna G. to the municipal council of Pfalzel, 4 February 1930.

49 STAT Tb14/482: Letter from Johann Sch. to the mayor of the suburbs of Trier, 11 October 1929.

50 See STAT Tb14/482: Letter from Johann Sch. to the mayor of the suburbs of Trier, 1 August 1928.

51 For a detailed description, see Krieger, 'Kranke'.

52 Verwaltungsbericht Trier Land, 1926–28: 166.

53 Ibid., 167.

54 Petitions for poor relief were decided in the assemblies of the municipal council. These assemblies were often held at the local inn, thus in public. Superior authorities criticized this practice, but the fact that the District Administrator repeatedly saw the need to remind the communities of the county of Trier-Land that they were supposed 'to maintain absolute silence about internals and circumstances of the persons in need' shows that the local administrators did not respect that rule. STAT Tb14/402: Letter from the District Administrator to the mayor of the suburbs of Trier, 8 March 1926.

55 To what extent these attempts could be successful in small villages is difficult to evaluate. Whistle-blowing on welfare recipients by their neighbours or other villagers shows that it was difficult to keep something private. On the other hand, the study of poverty in the *Hunsrück* during the 1990s by Karl August Chassé and Hans Pfaffenberger shows that this 'reduced scale of observation' typical of villages and the feeling of being under permanent social control provoked exceptionally refined strategies of dissimulation. See Pfaffenberger, H. and Chassé, K. A. (eds) (1993), *Armut im ländlichen Raum. Sozialpolitische und sozialpädagogische Perspektiven und Lösungsversuche*. Münster: Lit.

56 STAT Tb14/470: Letter from Georg D. to the municipal council of Pfalzel, 9 August 1927.

57 STAT Tb 14/470: Letter from Anny L. to the mayor of the suburbs of Trier, 7 May 1926.

58 See STAT Tb14/470: Letter from Christian K. to the municipal council of Pfalzel, 17 March 1929.

59 STAT Tb14/482: Letter from Valentin T. to 'President von Hindenburg', 3 June 1927.

60 STAT Tb14/482: Letter from Nikolaus L. to the mayor of the suburbs of Trier, 23 January 1928; and STAT Tb14/482: Letter from Albert D. to the Prussian Minister of Welfare, 6 July 1926.

61 STAT Tb14/482: Letter from the mayor of the suburbs to Christian Q. from Euren, 11 August 1929.

62 See STAT Tb14/482: individual case files, poor relief administration of Euren, family Christian Q.

63 STAT Tb14/482: Letter from the mayor of the suburbs of Trier to the cooperative of *Reichsbahn* employees, 1 August 1929.

64 See, for example, STAT Tb14/482: Barbara M.'s letters to the mayor of the suburbs, 23 July 1927 and 7 January 1929.

65 STAT Tb14/470: Letter from Katharina B. to the municipal council of Pfalzel, 15 July 1929.

66 Ibid.

67 Ibid.

68 STAT Tb14/470: Letter from Nikolaus B. to the municipal council of Pfalzel, 17 October 1929.

69 See STAT Tb14/470: Letter from the chairman of the municipal council of Pfalzel to Nikolaus B., 2 November 1929.

70 STAT Tb14/470: Letter from Nikolaus B. to the municipal council of Pfalzel, 11 November 1929.

71 Ibid.

72 STAT Tb14/482: Letter from Jakob Sch. to the mayor of the suburbs of Trier, 31 July 1929.

73 For a detailed description, see Krieger, 'Kranke'.

74 See, for example, STAT Tb14/482: Letter from the chairman of the municipal council of Euren, 24 May 1927: 'The municipal council is neither able to approve of nor to deny neediness of M. without a medical examination.'

75 The permanent emphasis on one's 'willingness to work' represents more than a rhetorical strategy. It shows the outstanding importance of work and being able to earn one's living in the self-perception of a majority of population. See Sokoll, T. (1997), 'Old age in poverty. The record of Essex pauper letters, 1780–1834', in Hitchcock, T., King, P. and Sharpe, P. (eds), *Chronicling Poverty. The Voices and Strategies of the English Poor, 1640–1840*. Basingstoke: Macmillan, p. 145.

76 See, for example, STAT Tb14/482: Letter from Elisabeth R. to the mayor of Trier, 7 May 1926: 'Would you please be so kind as to lend me your support . . . Because I am not of those who waste their money. And my husband is not a drunkard either.'

77 STAT Tb14/482: Letter from Jakob Sch. to the mayor of the suburbs of Trier, 4 November 1926.

78 STAT Tb14/482: Letter from Nikolaus S. to the mayor of the suburbs of Trier, 14 November 1928.

79 STAT Tb14/482: Letter from Maria M. to the mayor of the suburbs of Trier, 7 September 1926.

80 STAT Tb14/482: Letter from Christian Q. to the mayor of the suburbs of Trier, 20 April 1926.

81 Ibid.

82 Ibid.

83 STAT Tb14/482: Letter from the mayor of the suburbs of Trier to Christian Q., 30 April 1926, and Stazic, 'Arbeitslosigkeit', pp. 146–54.

84 Ibid.

85 STAT Tb14/510: Letter from Maria B. to the municipal council of Kürenz, 17 June 1928.

86 STAT Tb14/470: Letter from Matthias P. to the municipal council of Pfalzel, 25 May 1927.

87 STAT Tb14/482: Letter from Jakob L. to the governor of the Rhine Province, September 1926.

88 War experiences probably played an important role in this shift in perceived responsibilities of the state. Unemployed men who had served in the WWI referred to their actions for their mother country when they had to negotiate with local administrators. See for example STAT Tb14/482: Letter from Friedrich D. to the governor of the Rhine Province, 1 February 1927: 'I request further relief until the economic circumstances change for the better. Thirteen and a half years have I been devoted to serve the Reich, I sacrificed my health during war. I was crowded out of my own house. So many times have I conduced to the passive resistance [*Passiver Widerstand*], but unfortunately only for those who are in employment today. War is ungrateful and it is even sadder that one has to write such lines.'

10

Narratives of ill-health in applicant letters from rural Germany, 1900–30

Katrin Marx-Jaskulski*

Introduction

The 'patient's view' in the social history of medicine has – in both German and English contexts – been largely based on diaries or letters from the middle and upper classes.[1] More recently, there has been a renewed interest in reconstructing the perspective of illness[2] 'from below'. Particularly, but by no means uniquely, in the English context pauper letters have been used as one of the few 'ego-documents' of the lower classes.[3] However, while published analyses of English pauper letters have been largely confined to the early nineteenth century, application letters from German poor relief archives seem to span a longer period and can be used to understand how the poor described, experienced and used illness in a rhetorical sense right up to the early twentieth century. This chapter thus examines such letters from small communities in the rural regions surrounding Bernkastel and Wittlich, situated on the Moselle and in the Eifel, during the period 1900–30.[4] It concentrates first on the nature of illness revealed in pauper narratives and then, using the case study of those applying for relief because of under- or unemployment, on the way in which paupers drew a link between illness in different guises and their poverty. That poverty was and is one of the most important causes of physical and mental sickness is obvious: 'No tightened health prospers in poverty, when poverty is a lasting and exhausting struggle for existence.'[5] Poor living conditions, malnutrition and the lack of financial means to obtain treatment are, and were, major causes for such 'poverty illnesses' as tuberculosis[6] or malaria. In common with the broad agenda for this volume, however, the current chapter turns this linkage on its head, investigating the consequences of ill-health in respect of the poverty and living conditions of indigent people. Although the empirical evidence for the chapter is drawn from a series of small micro-studies of villages, it will offer much wider conclusions about pauper understanding of the links between illness and poverty.

The 'silence' and 'noisiness' of the sources

As others in this volume have suggested, illness, besides and in combination with old age, was one of the most important causes of indigence in early modern and modern Europe. Table 10.1, which provides a summation of 1885 statistics on German poor relief recipients, shows that this observation applies equally keenly to the later-nineteenth-century Prussian Rhine Province and the broad districts analysed in this chapter. To some extent, of course, this is unsurprising and not necessarily related to the underlying incidence of disease; as the literature on England has shown so well, illness, old age and deservingness were firmly yoked together by both pauper applicants and wider communities. The old and the sick were obviously not to blame for their miserable situation, and these conditions were at one and the same time a way of bargaining for relief and a justification for granting relief by officials in the villages examined here.

These observations notwithstanding, answering the question 'How did the poor themselves speak about and characterize their illnesses?' is often a frustrating process. Sometimes applications were obviously written by a third party or were transcribed into poor relief records by the officials, and the mediation of both the pauper voice and the underlying message tends towards narratives that border on the formulaic. Such, for instance, was Jakob F.'s letter to the mayor of Zeltingen on 22 December 1908, in which the hand of the text differed from that of the signature:

> For long suffering from severe illness, I venture to request the laudable municipal council for an illness relief. In my doctor's opinion, I caught the disease during my work as a gravedigger and I hope that I will receive the requested application for this reason. My humble background does not allow a sufficient care, yet apart from the unaffordable costs for physician and medication, of which I sincerely would like to ask for reimbursement.[7]

Yet, even in the letters which were obviously written by the applicants themselves, obtaining an 'authentic' impression of ill-health and sickness through descriptions of, for example, pain symptoms, is very difficult. Precise nosologies of disease are, even at this late date, largely absent from narrative

Table 10.1 Distribution (%) of the causes of indigence according to the national statistics of public poor relief in 1885

		Prussian Rhine-Province		District of Bernkastel		District of Wittlich	
		139 urban communities (1,845,918 inhabitants) 2,852 rural communities (2,495,571 inhabitants altogether) 2 Gutsbezirke (64 EW) 2 mixed associations (2,974 inhabitants) supported persons: 175,346*		1 urban community (2,401 inhabitants) 92 rural communities (41,988 inhabitants altogether) supported persons: 1,072*		one urban community (3,425 inhabitants) 77 rural communities (34,575 inhabitants altogether) supported persons: 492*	
		Absolute	%	Absolute	%	Absolute	%
Injury to the supported person him/herself or to a family member	caused by accident	3,975 (1,882 + 2,093)	2.3%	-	-	4 (4)	0.8%
Injury to the breadwinner		101(35 + 66)	0.05%	-	-	-	-
Death of the breadwinner		1,055 (347 + 708)	0.6%	-	-	6 (5 + 1)	1.2%
Death of the breadwinner	not caused by accident	35,150 (15,247 + 19,903)	20%	266 (109 + 157)	24.9%	123(64 + 59)	25.1%
Illness of the supported person him/herself or of a family member		59,964 (26,435 + 33,529)	34.2%	411 (136 + 275)	38.4%	171(74 + 97)	34.9%
Physical or mental impairment		17,149 (11,437 + 5,712)	9.7%	127 (65 + 56)	11.9%	87(62 + 25)	17.8%

(Continued)

Table 10.1 (Continued) Distribution (%) of the causes of indigence according to the national statistics of public poor relief in 1885

Debility from old age	18,694 (15,712 + 2,982)	10.7%	87 (75 + 12)	8.1%	60(55 + 5)	12.2%
Large number of children	14,073 (2,196 + 11,877)	8%	52(7 + 45)	4.9%	-	-
Unemployment	12,947 (3,373 + 9,574)	7.4%	64(23 + 41)	6%	13(5 + 8)	2.7%
Given to drink (*Trunksucht*)	2,027(760 + 1,267)	1.2%	15(2 + 13)	1.4%	3(3)	0.6%
Work-shyness	772(317 + 455)	0.4%	7(2 + 5)	0.7%	1(1)	0.2%
Other causes	9,434 (4,001 + 5,433)	5.4%	49(21 + 28)	4.6%	24(9 + 15)	4.9%
Not denoted	5(5)	0%	-	-	-	-

* Total 'self-supported' persons and family members (wives, children under the age of 14)

Rhine-Province   81,747 persons   93,599 persons
Bernkastel   440 persons   632 persons
Wittlich   282 persons   210 persons

The figures in bold type elide both the 'self-supported' and family members descriptions.[8] In most cases the terms used to identify diseases tended, as was also the case in early nineteenth-century England, towards simple classifications such as 'illness', 'disease' (*Krankheit*) or 'suffering' (*Leiden*), though as Tamara Stazic-Wendt shows in her chapter, there were exceptions. Thus when the widow of Nikolaus J. wrote to the head of the community of Wehlen on 4 August 1910, she used the same formulaic opening (similar to the form 'honourable gentlemen' in English narratives) as Jakob F., and then described in only the most general terms the nature of the affliction under which she and her eldest child laboured:

> I, the undersigned, am constrained to appeal to the laudable municipal council with the following request. As you know, I got into a burdensome situation by the death of my husband. I've got three children, of which the eldest is even always ill and under medical treatment now, I am myself often restricted in my sole occupation as ironer due to being ill . . .[9]

The letter from the widow of Richard V. to the mayor of Lieser on 18 January 1914 was somewhat less formulaic (itself raising the question of whether there were letter-templates that sick people might utilize, a key concern of the editors in their introduction to this volume) but no more informative regarding the range of severe diseases to which she claimed her mother was subject:

> Dear mayor! On behalf of my mother I write you this letter today. As she is in distress and has a severe illness for a long time, over two months, and furthermore isn't able to help herself in any way, because any property is lacking, and owns only a small pension of 10,95 Mark a month, what is not enough to make a living, certainly not with these diseases, that's why she turns to you with the request to assist her in this distress, dear mayor, and to grant an allowance from the community or the pauper's foundation. We certainly wouldn't have raised the claim if this illness hadn't arisen or if we were able to help ourselves in other ways.[10]

As with earlier English letters, this is a rhetorically complex narrative. However, it is unclear here and in other letters which diseases were encompassed by terms like 'ill', 'very dangerously ill', 'ill during the whole winter', 'ailing', 'fragile', 'infirm' or 'weakly'. Thus the widow of Richard V. describes her mother's illness as a disease that reappears from time to time, has real longevity and restricts or entirely compromises the ability to work. In another letter written by widow V., it is mentioned, that the mother had been bedridden for some time. Such broad symptoms fit with a range of disease patterns and leave little leeway for discussion of pauper knowledge and characterization of individual diseases.

Nor (and in common with many English and Scandinavian narratives) is it easy to classify the suffering of paupers according to useful disease categories such as acute / chronic or external / internal. The term 'suffering' (*Leiden*) occurs relatively often in narratives and appears to have had a precise meaning. It is described in the dictionary as 'persistent illness', a label often borne out by descriptions in series of letters where we can identify continuous illness. As the clientele of general poor relief consisted to a large degree of elderly people, the 'suffering' could also have encompassed forms of infirmity or diseases which appear more often in old age: 'signs of tear' or a wearing out of the body (*Verschleißerscheinungen*) like arthritis, cardiovascular diseases, diminished sight, hearing and motility and so on. Other 'illnesses' coalescing around physical handicap or injury that was visible on the body – 'damage of the body' (*Leibschaden*), 'defect of the body' (*Leibfehler*), or 'crippled' (*krüppelhaft*) – were also dealt with relatively precisely. More general 'catch-all' labels such as 'ill' or 'very ill' are less tractable. Indeed, where the file on a particular applicant for relief contains both a narrative and a medical certificate, we often see that applicants who described themselves just as 'ill', might be malnourished (one female applicant weighed only 48 kilograms), suffering from atonic muscles, experiencing 'moderately accelerated activity of the heart', have scars resulting from gland- and bone-tuberculosis, or be suffering from persistent bronchial catarrh.[11] Thus, while it is a reasonable guess that most poor relief applicants who labelled themselves as sick had either acute or chronic conditions, a definitive picture of the nature of the underlying illnesses experienced by the poor is near impossible to reconstruct in the letters used as evidence for this chapter. The contrast between this observation and the experiences and rhetoric of the paupers of the rural areas around Trier analysed by Tamara Stazic-Wendt – many of whom appear to have copied medical terms from prescriptions, medical certificates and guidance books and in turn quoted them back at officials – is marked. It suggests that even over relatively short distances, the knowledge, nature of agency and rhetorical and strategic abilities of paupers could vary considerably.

In contrast to physical illness, mental illnesses and 'mental weakness'[12] were well denominated in the descriptions of ill-health found in the applicant letters, though mostly with lay terms such as 'mentally weak' (*schwachsinnig*), 'not being in one's right mind' (*nicht recht bei Verstand sein*), 'mentally not normal' (*geistig nicht normal*), 'mentally disturbed' (*geistesgestört*), 'mentally retarded' (*geistig zurückgeblieben*), 'feeble-minded' (*blöd*), 'hysterical' (*hysterisch*) or 'idiotic' (*idiot*). The applicants described their afflictions more precisely when they had to be specified as a reason for lowered ability or inability to work, or where the pauper was seeking relief in the form of reimbursement for the expenses of the illness (hospital, physician, pharmacy) or an accident benefit. For those whose behaviour was encompassed under these labels, and whose conditions were often not deemed curable by local administrators, familial care was the norm. The burden that such mental illnesses placed upon such families can be seen in the narratives where, in at least one case, 'mental weakness' was described as a 'misfortune'.[13] Of course, if familial care broke down or proved inadequate, then the poor relief authorities – in this area not the local general poor relief authorities but the poor relief authority of the Rhine Province – were obliged to intervene. Unsurprisingly, therefore, 'mental weakness' can be found in the files of local general poor relief in various aspects, particularly where such applicants were unable to work for their subsistence and the local poor relief was forced to grant an allowance or to arrange their accommodation, whether in a hospital or by bargaining with kin to provide maintenance. Indeed, in many ways the sorts of mental afflictions described and the way in which these afflictions were used to extend the agency of the sick poor, reflects very strongly the tone and content of the narratives considered by Alannah Tomkins for England (see her chapter in this volume) a full century earlier.

More precision on the nature of the mental illnesses involved – over and above the lay diagnoses mentioned above – is difficult to obtain. Medical certificates involving psychological cases are found only rarely in the case files, though where they do exist the diagnosing physicians (who generally were not psychiatric experts) seem to have used more differentiating labels than the judgements of the authorities or other laymen. In particular, while such certificates rarely named an exact disease, they usually contained precise diagnosis of symptoms like 'nervous excitability' (*nervöse Erregbarkeit*), 'speech disorder' (*Sprachstörungen*), 'filled with fear' (*angsterfüllt*), 'persecution mania' (*Verfolgungsideen*), or 'epilepsy' (*Epilepsie*). In the rare cases where psychiatric doctors testified as to the condition of an individual pauper, the testimonies are thoroughly written in technical and objective diction, containing the precise names of the disease, its course, the therapies that could be or had been applied and a statement about the working ability of the patient or if and to which hospital they should be admitted. Faced with such precise testimony, the poor relief authorities tended to follow the recommendations of the practitioner involved.

The sources that underpin this chapter are thus complex; on the one hand informative about underlying conditions, especially in relation to mental illnesses, and yet on the other strangely silent. To a large extent, the silences of the sources must reflect ignorance of the specific diseases or a limited linguistic range to describe and label the ailments. There may also have been an interlinkage between morality and dignity and particular disease forms, especially in the case of illnesses concerning taboos like sexually transmitted diseases. Venereal diseases, for instance, rarely appear in the letters and diagnoses, reflecting the sorts of moral hazard outlined by Anna Lundberg for Sweden in her chapter for this volume. Moreover, paupers themselves were firmly cemented into a diagnostic and therapeutic culture in which general notions of 'illness' or 'suffering', and more particularly the general weakness or immobility of body, tiredness and other physical conditions associated with malnutrition or old age, were as likely to be used by practitioners as by patients. Nor should we forget that the contents of pauper narratives and case files very much reflect what was at the time considered as sickness, and that some symptoms of disease were so ingrained into ordinary life that they would not have merited a mention. Physical pain, for instance, is barely mentioned in the narratives. And while 'pain and health issues are always hard to express for the person affected',[14] it is clear that the communicational situation implicit in the construction of case files also explains much of their silence. Those sick individuals who wrote appeal narratives were not patients describing their medical condition to the doctor, but primarily paupers who wanted to receive relief for the consequences of illness.[15]

Implications of illness

These observations notwithstanding, pauper letters very often contain poignant descriptions of the implications of illness and complaints about the circumstances that led or could have led to sickness (such as poor working conditions, lack of hygiene, miserable living conditions, deficiency of food, etc.) and which provide an important window onto health and the wider experiences of the poor in early twentieth-century Germany. Thus, one of the most serious consequences of sickness, and in turn the single most important factor in the determination of the indigence and 'deservingness' of the poor,[16] was the inability to work, or at least the compromised ability to do one's normal job. Inability to work in old age was generally accepted and hardly questioned; the work quota that was considered reasonable for elderly people was quite large,[17] but elderly applicants unfit for work were generally supported in early twentieth-century Germany, as was also the case in other European states.[18] For younger applicants, compromised earning potential was tested more meticulously. This said, it is quite clear from pauper narratives and associated case files that a disease which made working and earning impossible could get a (younger) patient and his family suddenly and intensively into a persistently desperate situation, a common feature of all of the chapters in this volume. The speed with which the household economy could decline in the face of illness is amply demonstrated in a letter to the mayor of Bernkastel-Kues from the wife of Baptist Qu. on 30 August 1923 which noted that:

> My husband suffered a stroke 3 weeks ago, whereby his left arm and the right leg had become lame. In this way we got in a miserable state of affairs. Not only that because of the stroke the breadwinner of the family has become completely unable to work, through the medical treatment and provision of the patient with medicine we've got exorbitant costs we're not able to bear.[19]

Here, the material consequences of an inability to work were interlinked with the specific costs caused by a stroke in a way that had brought the family to the very edge of their dignity. More generally, when illness was the main reason for writing, applicants sought either long-term relief, especially when the physical condition was expected to be of long-term duration, or specifically requested that the direct expenses of the illness be reimbursed. The bills of the physician and the pharmacy had to be paid, in some cases therapeutic equipment and prosthesis like a hernia bandage, a surgical corset or glasses had to be acquired, and doctors often prescribed nourishing food like red wine or eggs the costs of which could hardly be sustained by poor families. It is clear from other chapters in this volume that such a range of 'acceptable' appeal and expenditure was common in most European welfare systems, and across the whole period of the long nineteenth century.

Narratives also often requested the reimbursement of indirect expenses. Thus, when a sick person had to be treated in a hospital or had to go away to a different, more healthful, environment to seek a cure, bills associated with travel or the acquisition of clothing or toiletries could often be pressing for poor labouring families. This was more especially so where the main breadwinner was the sick person in question. Moreover, for elderly people or the chronically sick nursing care in a home or with relatives had to be arranged and paid for. These costs often forced the sick person and their family to run into debt, especially in cases of long-term illness, exacerbating the material consequences of sickness and adding a psychological dimension of worry about one's reputation to the burdens of sickness. Alannah Tomkins explores this issue in more depth elsewhere in this volume. The narrative of Lukas K. to the head of the community of Zeltingen on 26 November 1909 provides a vivid impression of these observations:

> My and my children's complete recovery requires a very long time. Concerning my wife's recovery, no evaluation can be given for the present. Thus, I got into a very depressed situation, also because I had to give my cart [Fuhrwerk] into foreign hands. I possess almost no property and there are hardly any earnings from my cart. Also a horse of mine, worth 1100 Marks has perished recently, which I had to substitute through a new one, by what I had to run into debt, because my small savings didn't suffice by far. However, I could have overcome all this if only these diseases hadn't emerged. I'm not able to get the remedies for my recovery. I also made a claim on my kin far beyond their forces, so that I can't demand anything from them . . .[20]

This letter has many resonances with earlier narratives in other European states, emphasizing both the psychological and material consequences of illness, highlighting the fact that individual sickness was embedded in the surroundings of a family that was heavily burdened with the unexpected costs of illness, and suggesting the honourable intentions of the applicant towards his community evidenced by his essential desire to be independent were it not for extraordinary circumstances. Other letters illustrate that the monetary hardships as a consequence of illness (exhaustion of familial properties and the loss of the breadwinner) were exacerbated by the physical,

material and emotional costs of nursing the sick relative. Thus, and one of
many potential exemplars, Matthias W. wrote from Zeltingen to the Welfare
Administration of Bernkastel in July 1919 to say that:

> . . . My wife needed surgical treatment at the hospital in Bernkastel-Cues
> after a long duration of illness. She had been in agony over the past years
> and the medical treatment and the nursing of my wife did cost me a lot of
> money . . . The earnings of my two other daughters living with me aren't
> sufficient for our livelihood, particularly since last year one of both had
> to be permanently at home for nursing my wife. It is beyond our means
> to bear the costs of the operation and so I request the allocation of relief
> respectfully Matthias W.[21]

Here, then, the wife's loss of earnings was compounded by the fact that
her daughters had also had to give up work to provide nursing duties. This
was also the case when Amalie W. became sick: her sister had to look after
her. For the reimbursement not only of her loss of earnings but also of his
own, the sister's husband approached the poor relief council of the village
of Maring with the following explanatory statement:

> My sister-in-law Amalie W. called by my wife on December 7th 1905
> by telephone, because she was very ill and had no one to nurse her. In
> response to this call my wife drove immediately to her sister. At noon my
> eldest child called for me, I had to neglect my day-labouring in favour
> to prepare a meal for my children and to send them to school on time. I
> neglected 2 Mark 80 Pfennig daily wage and had to keep the house. My
> wife nursed her sister from December 7th to December 21st . . . Being an
> ironer she lost earnings amounting to 20 Mark, me as a day-labourer
> neglected 2 Mark 80 Pfenning per day, in fourteen days 39 Mark 20
> Pfennig. I'm a poor day-labourer and got nothing but my daily wage and
> my wife's earnings from ironing.[22]

Indeed, this theme of indirect inability to work because of family illness
pervades pauper letters for this period. It was at the core of one of the case
studies employed by Steven King and Alison Stringer in their contribution
to this volume. Especially in the case of sick mothers the older children had
to look after their younger brothers and sisters and therefore could not go
to school or work. In the worst case, other family members were physically
infected, as in the case of the aforementioned Lukas K., who reported that
'About four weeks ago both of my children came down with typhus and
about fourteen days ago I came down with typhus likewise. Because my
wife had a lot of efforts thereby, she now also is fallen ill . . .'[23] While his
wife had avoided typhus, the impact of nursing the whole family had in
turn brought her to sickness, exacerbating the family's already dire material
circumstances.

Sometimes sickness and its material consequences could create or worsen mental health, as Alannah Tomkins has already demonstrated in this volume. One applicant wrote about his wife:

> . . . For three years my wife has been suffering from sepsis on her whole body. After we've turned to the local physicians for help in vain, she was admitted to the surgical clinic in Bonn for 5 months at the recommendation of Dr Mayer in Bernkastel. Released unhealed, she stayed in Lieser for 2 months and was nursed by the Barmherzige Schwestern [Sisters of Mercy]. Since then, she's laid up in bed at home in nameless pain. For the purpose of better healing treatment under guidance (of Dr Wissemes – Mülheim) she should be nursed in the convent in Lieser again.[24]

The long duration of the illness, the fact that the physicians obviously were at a loss for an adequate therapy and 'being handed round' among various hospitals and physicians must have provoked – besides the physical pain – various fears within the woman affected and her family: She did not know how long the illness would last,[25] why certain therapies were ineffective, she may have lost confidence in her physician and been afraid of death. The phenomenon of illness and the weakening of the body must have often been experienced with great helplessness, ignorance concerning the reasons, symptoms and the course of disease and last but not least desperation. In this letter even the husband seems to have lost hope for recovery: he replaces the word 'healing' with 'treatment'. In turn, the onset of hopelessness is a common theme for paupers who wrote multiple letters seeking support, a point demonstrated well in most of the preceding chapters.

The risk of contagion was so high with some diseases that with the infection also came social isolation. Thus, disfigurement of the outward appearance is symptomatic of certain diseases like skin-tuberculosis and made contact with other people difficult or even impossible. A final, admittedly extreme, example to illustrate this aspect of illness is Phillipp K. The brothers of Philipp K. requested his hospitalization because their 'brother would be affected in such a way with rash on his face that nobody wanted to take him up for work'. The application was rejected by the municipal council not only because the brothers would be able to pay the hospital costs but also because 'it seems that the brothers wanted to get rid of their brother [Philipp] in easy ways, because his face is covered completely with rash in a repulsive way and therefore cohabitation is little pleasant'. Furthermore, the council argued, Philipp would be able to work. While upon detailed questioning the district physician suggested that the face would be disfigured in a way that would make it virtually impossible for Philipp K. to find any work, he also understood that the brothers did not want to live with Philipp because 'the suppurating abscesses exude such an odour that it can't be held against his brothers if they want to admit him to an adequate nursing home. The rash is also contagious.'[26]

As these narratives testify, illness could compromise the material circumstances of the individual and family, could become self-reinforcing as contagious disease shifted between family members and might affect mental health. These observations are perhaps familiar from other studies of sickness among the labouring poor, especially those relying on pauper narratives. However, this brief analysis has also suggested more diverse impacts: the impact of the need for nursing on wider familial engagement with the labour market, the impact of sickness and its physical and material costs on the nature and strength of familial relationships and the relationship between debt, sickness and psychological health.

Conclusion

Illness was one of the most important reasons for economic hardship, both in terms of lost earnings and the eating up of savings, and also because of the hefty indirect costs of sickness represented by a long stay in a hospital or the physician's treatment and medicine. In writing letters seeking relief from their local poor relief administration, the sick or their familial members and epistolary advocates tended to describe illnesses in only the vaguest ways, adopting terms such as 'illness' or 'suffering'. To some extent this is explicable by the communicative situation in which the pauper was engaged: the purpose of the narratives they wrote was not to recite the symptoms of their diseases as a pauper might in front of a physician, but to establish that the person concerned or about whom the letter reported detail was deserving of relief and to try and influence the scale and nature of that relief. Matters of shame or ignorance may have played an important role with some diseases. Unlike 'ego-documents' in the sense of the diary of Samuel Pepys, the letters examined here cannot provide explicit insight in what diseases really meant for the ill person. They described the consequences of illness which forced them to be in need of public support. This said, and as others have noted in this volume, pauper letters provide a strong rendering of what paupers thought poor relief authorities needed to know and what sickness conditions they thought were linked to entitlement. In this sense, a systematic and comparative study of European pauper narratives could tell us much about both differential understandings of disease and the ways in which paupers of different ethnicity, life-cycle stage and nationality exercised agency in their negotiations with authorities.

Notes

* This chapter develops a segment of my doctoral thesis 'Armut und Fürsorge auf dem Land. Vom Ende des 19. Jahrhunderts bis 1933.' (Göttingen, 2008).

1 Porter, R. (1985), 'The patient's view. Doing medical history from below', *Theory and Society*, 14, 167–74. Porter makes extensive use of the diary of Samuel Pepys. A presentation of Porter's work and the research agenda outlined in this article has been undertaken in Ernst, K. (1999), 'Patientengeschichte. Die kulturhistorische wende in der medizinhistoriographie', in Bröer, R. (ed.), *Eine Wissenschaft emanzipiert sich. Die Medizinhistoriographie von der Aufklärung bis zur Postmoderne*. Berlin: Pfaffenweiler, pp. 97–108. For other work, see Porter, R. (1992), 'The patient in England 1660–1800', in A. Wear (ed.), *Medicine in Society: Historical Essays*. Cambridge: Cambridge University Press, pp. 91–118; Gillis, J. (2006), 'The history of the patient since 1850', *Bulletin of the History of Medicine*, 80, 490–512; Wilde, S. (2009), 'Truth, trust and confidence in surgery, 1890–1910: Patient autonomy, communication and consent', *Bulletin of the History of Medicine*, 83, 302–30; White, P. (2006), 'Sympathy under the knife: Experimentation and emotion in late Victorian medicine', in Bound-Alberti, F. (ed.), *Medicine, Emotion and Disease, 1700–1950*. Basingstoke: Macmillan, pp. 100–24; Forster, E. (1980), 'From the patient's point of view. Illness and health in the letters of Liselotte von der Pfalz', *Bulletin of the History of Medicine*, 60, 297–320; and Ernst, K. (2003), *Krankheit und Heiligung. Die medikale Kultur württembergischer Pietisten im 18. Jahrhundert*. Stuttgart: Steiner.

2 For the difference between 'disease' and 'illness' – 'We can see disease as an undesirable physiological process or state. Illness, by contrast, can be depicted as the social and psychological phenomena that accompany these putative physiological problems.' – see Conrad, P. (1987), 'The experience of illness: recent and new directions', in Roth, J. A. and Conrad, P. (eds), *The Experience and Management of Chronic Illness*. Greenwich Connecticut: JAI Press, pp. 1–31, p. 2. Also Fitzpatrick, R. (1984), 'Lay concepts of illness', in Fitzpatrick, R. et al. (eds), *The Experience of Illness*. London: Tavistock, pp. 11–31.

3 For example, Sokoll, T. (2001), *Essex Pauper Letters, 1731–1837*. Oxford: Oxford University Press; Stollberg, G. (2002), 'Health and illness in German workers' autobiographies from the nineteenth and early twentieth centuries', *Social History of Medicine*, 6, 261–76; Risse, G. and Warner, J. (1992), 'Reconstructing clinical activities: patient records in medical history', *Social History of Medicine*, 5, 183–205; Hitchcock, T., King, P. and Sharpe, P. (eds) (1997), *Chronicling Poverty: The Voices and Strategies of the English Poor 1640–1840*. Basingstoke: Macmillan; Fontaine, L. and Schlümbohm, J. (eds) (2000), *Household Strategies for Survival 1600–2000*. Cambridge: Cambridge University Press; Sokoll, T. (2006), 'Writing for relief: rhetoric in English pauper letters 1800–34', in Gestrich, A., King, S. and Raphael, L. (eds), *Being Poor in Modern Europe: Historical Perspectives*. Frankfurt: Peter Lang, pp. 91–112. A contemporary report on health aspects of voices of the poor, the World Bank study of people's perspectives and experiences of poverty is *Dying for change – Poor peoples experience of health and ill health*, PDF–File on http://www.who.int/hdp/publications/ dying_change.pdf.

4 This sort of settlement is under-represented both in the general poverty literature and in the direct consideration of pauper narratives.

5 'In der Armut gedeiht keine gefestigte Gesundheit, wenn die Armut ein dauernder, aufreibender Kampf um die Existenz bedeutet.' Köhler, F. (1910) 'Die lungentuberkulose des proletariats. Sozial-medizinische und praktisch-soziale untersuchungen', *Preußische Jahrbücher*, 139, 19, cited after Blasius,

D. (1976) 'Geschichte und krankheit. Sozialgeschichtliche perspektiven der medizingeschichte', *Geschichte und Gesellschaft*, 2, 386–415.

6 Blasius, 'Geschichte', 397–402. See also Condrau, F. (2000), *Lungenheilanstalt und patientenschicksal. Sozialgeschichte der tuberkulose in Deutschland und England im späten 19. und frühen 20. jahrhundert*. Göttingen: Vandenhoeck & Ruprecht; Schwan, B. (1929), *Die Wohnungsnot und das Wohnungselend in Deutschland*. Berlin: Campus, p. 22. For later work, Hardy, A. (2003), 'Reframing disease: changing perceptions of tuberculosis in England and Wales 1938–70', *Historical Research*, 76, 535–56.

7 Landeshauptarchiv Koblenz (hereafter LHAK) Best. 655, 123 (Bürgermeisterei Zeltingen) Nr. 967 (Armenwesen, hiesige Ortsarme, 1898–1909): Jakob F., Zeltingen, to the mayor of Zeltingen, 22 December 1908. For the purposes of this chapter I tried to filter the letters that appeared to be written by the poor themselves by keeping an eye on the synchronicity of handwriting in the main body of the letter versus the straplines and signatures. The issue of collective writing of individual letters is considered in Snell, K. (forthcoming, 2012), 'Voices of the poor: 'home' and belonging, 'friends' and community', *Economic History Review*.

8 See Osten, P. (2004), Conference report on 'Krankheit Erzählen' – Anglo-Dutch-German Workshop on Illness Narratives, 8–10 July 2004, published on www.hsozkult.de, 27 July 2004. See also King, S. (2005), '"Stop this overwhelming torment of destiny": negotiating financial aid at times of sickness under the English Old Poor Law, 1800–40', *Bulletin of the History of Medicine*, 79, 228–60.

9 LHAK Best. 655, 213 (Bürgermeisterei Lieser) Nr. 190 (Ortsarmenverband Wehlen, 1905–20): Widow of Nikolaus J., Wehlen, to Head of Community Wehlen, 4 August 1910.

10 LHAK Best. 655, 213 Nr. 187 (Bürgermeisterei Lieser, Ortsarme, 1905–24): Widow of Richard V., Lieser, to the mayor of Lieser, 18 January 1914.

11 See Kreisarchiv Bernkastel-Wittlich (hereafter KAB-W) Nr. 2.0.343 (Beschwerden von Hülfsbedürftigen, 1910–14): Medical certificate of Relief physician (*Armenarzt*) Dr Köchling about the widow of Josef T., 28 February 1912. The widow would not be able to do hard work such as day-labouring, washing or cleaning. The physician also gave information about the unfavourable and unhygienic housing conditions: the widow and her daughter would sleep in one bed.

12 The connection between mental illness and social class cannot be further explored in this chapter, though it is dealt with in this volume by Cathy Smith. For the classic study on the matter, see Hollinghead, A. and Redlich, F. (1958), *Social Class and Mental Illness*. New York: Wiley. See also Suzuki, A. (2006), *Madness at Home*. Berkeley, University of California Press.

13 LHAK Best. 655, 213 Bgm. Lieser Nr. 188: Paul Qu., Maring to municipal council Maring-Noviand, 1. February 1913.

14 Herzlich, C. (1991), *Kranke gestern, Kranke heute. Die Gesellschaft und das Leiden*. München: Dotter, p. 9. A.

15 See Vanja, C. (2006), 'Arm und krank. Patientenbiographien im spiegel frühneuzeitlicher bittschriften', *BIOS*, 19, 26–35, p. 27, and King, "Stop this overwhelming torment of destiny". On the language of patients when describing

their illness to a physician, see Goltz, D. (1969), 'Krankheit und sprache', *Sudhoffs Archiv*, 53, 225–69.

16 For example, Castel, R. (2000), *Die metamorphosen der sozialen frage. Eine chronik der lohnarbeit*. Konstanz: Fayard. He defines as the three main components of 'indigence': impecuniousness, affiliation to the community and the inability to work. Also Dross, F. (1999), '"Der Kranke allein ist arm" – Die diskussion über den zusammenhang von krankheit und armut um 1800', *Vierteljahrschrift für Sozial- und Wirtschaftsgeschichte*, 12, 1–15, p. 12; Tomkins, A. (1999), 'Paupers and the infirmary in mid-eighteenth-century Shrewsbury', *Medical History*, 43, 208–27, and her chapter in this volume which deals specifically with the mental illness occasioned by unemployment.

17 For example, KAB-W 2.0.343: Mayor of Binsfeld to the *Landrat* of Wittlich, 13.10.1910: 'The widow of Peter A., 70 years old, but in physically healthy and lusty, is – from the point of view of the signatory – very well capable of earning what is necessary with peddling'

18 Thane, P. (2000), *Old Age in English History: Past Experiences, Present Issues*. Oxford: Oxford University Press. For a wider European survey, see King, S. and Stewart, J. (eds) (2007), *Welfare Peripheries: The Development of Welfare States in Nineteenth and Twentieth Century Europe*. Frankfurt: Peter Lang.

19 LHAK Best. 655, 213 Nr. 187: Protocol, Mayor of Bernkastel-Kues, Wife of Baptist Qu., Lieser, 30 August 1923.

20 LHAK Best. 655, 123 Nr. 967: Lukas K., Zeltingen, to head of community Zeltingen, 26 November 1909.

21 LHAK Best. 655, 123 Nr. 1040 (Armenwesen, hiesige Ortsarme, 1909–24): Matthias W., Zeltingen, to Welfare Administration Bernkastel, without date [receipt 17 July 1919].

22 LHAK Best. 655, 213: Bgm. Lieser Nr. 188: Friedrich St., Longkamp, to the mayor of Lieser, 13 September 1908.

23 LHAK 655, 123: Bgm. Zeltingen Nr. 967: Lukas K., Zeltingen, to head of community Zeltingen, 26 November 1909.

24 LHAK Best. 655, 123 Nr. 967: Georg N., Zeltingen, to mayor of Zeltingen, 24 December 1906

25 Ibid. He went on 'My wife has fallen very dangerously ill and I wasn't able to earn a single penny during the whole time and how long this illness will last is not to be foreseen.' On the sense that patients often had no idea how long illnesses would last, see Fissell, M. (1991), 'The disappearance of the patient narrative and the invention of hospital medicine', in French, R. and Wear, A. (eds), *British Medicine in an Age of Reform*. London: Routledge, pp. 92–109.

26 KAB-W Nr. 2.0.541 (Beschwerden von Hülfsbedürftigen, 1901–07): Mayor of Wittlich-Land to the *Landrat* of Wittlich, 14 November 1904.

11

Asking for the privilege to work: Applications for a peddling licence (Austria in the 1920s and 1930s)[1]

Sigrid Wadauer

Introduction

By the interwar period, a variety of forms of social insurance relating to old age, invalidity, illness or unemployment had been established in Austria.[2] Yet these new forms of social support excluded many people who relied on poor relief and often on precarious and highly disputed means of finding a livelihood. Besides job flexibility, geographic mobility was a basic feature of many such forms of earning one's bread. We might regard this mobility as merely compelled by poverty.[3] Yet in contemporary perceptions, these practices appeared to be quite ambiguous. There was a broad range of ways of being mobile in finding a livelihood, different institutional and legal contexts as well as different collective or individual representations. Indeed, we can find somewhat positive aspects of being 'on the road' in the most surprising contexts, such as the following letter from an unemployed wayfarer in 1932

> The provincial government! Beyond all pardoning. I want to address some lines to you. At Christmas I asked for the extension of entitlement to the Herbergen [relief for destitute wayfarers]. So I went around in

Carithia and Styria. 15 months I was wandering. That's enduring a lot! Sometimes you're too early, sometimes too late to stay overnight. Then the police asks for papers: 'Go back to your hometown'. Should you go where you've been made poor? (If I could only stay somewhere else later on.) A lot of people are having to work for longer, unemployment benefits – or wander. After a short-term job, the wayfarer hits the road again. And when you're not married. Have gone along the whole time with the war. If you are older, wandering is not so easy . . . Clothes full of lice and you don't have enough of them and not enough to chew on. I went to the hospital because of very little. If I could stay at the poor house . . . it would be cheaper. I want to find mercy. Prefer the unemployment benefit. I was interested in checking out different regions.[4]

This last remark is surprising yet not uncommon. Being on the move was doubtless hard, yet it still could be interesting. The mobility of young and skilled unemployed craftsmen in particular might show some relation to the traditional journeymen's years of wandering.[5] That this tradition persisted into the twentieth century was disputed and doubted by some contemporaries.[6] Tramping in search of employment did not seem clearly distinguishable from being a 'work-shy' vagrant or beggar; at the same time it was also not clearly distinguishable from tramping for leisure or in search of adventure and experience. By re-establishing *Herbergen* (relief places for unemployed male wayfarers willing and able to work) in the 1920s, the government aimed to institutionalize distinctions among wayfarers. Even within the context of an economic crisis and an increasingly strict policy against vagrants and beggars in the 1930s, the consensus was not to stop this tramping of the unemployed but rather to organize and control it more rigidly.[7]

Another established form of mobility in search of a livelihood was contemporaneously designated for the almost unemployable, that is older (and often sick or frail) people with greatly reduced employability: peddling. Of course, this does not mean that all who peddled were old and unemployable; this activity was actually always clearly distinguishable from other trades or unemployed drifting. Yet, in the eyes of the police peddling was suspected of being a disguised form of begging and vagrancy, especially if the goods offered for sale were worthless or if the person did not have legal permission to trade.[8] Indeed, legal regulations, bureaucracy, occupational organizations and various individuals tended towards the creation of a group with distinct features and a distinct image. Within the context of peddling (but also other sales occupations), one hardly finds any official and explicit references to the virtue of mobility – not in the context of the more respectable salesmen, market traders and the like and especially not in the context of peddling. Those who defended peddlers did so primarily by arguing for its necessity.[9] That is, mobility appears as something imposed by the requirements of survival, such that peddlers seem to prove the 'sedentarist'[10] assumption that people did not move until forced to do so. However, we cannot deduce from images produced by political debates and collective representations that individuals experienced the practice in such ways or with such motivations. Unlike others on the move, peddlers seldom left behind autobiographical accounts.[11] Those individual statements and self-descriptions available to us – in trade records, petitions or court cases – were produced in official contexts where it made perfect sense for an individual to present and justify his/her activity as a response to economic necessity. Peddling was of course part of an economy of makeshifts[12] and often perceived not only as a beggarly profession but as a disguised form of begging.[13] It was, however, also discussed in reference to 'real work' and to trades regarded as more valuable for the national economy. Nor was it clearly separated from 'decent trade'.[14]

Against this backdrop, the current chapter analyses letters written in order to obtain official permission to seek a livelihood as a peddler. The very existence of such letters challenges common assumptions that itinerant trades such as peddling declined in the late nineteenth century and disappeared with World War I.[15] Indeed, the assumption stands, as we will see, in striking contradiction to contemporaneous debates on the issue of migrant labour and to the abundance of records to be found in various regional archives of Austria. The first part of the chapter deals with legal regulation of peddling, particularly an act of 1922 regulating how licenses were to be issued and which generated the sources used in the rest of the chapter. The following section explores the rich documentation on a single peddler and demonstrates the intertwining of the economic fragility of the family economy, sickness and compromised employability as reasons for peddling, as well as the potentially harsh reactions of communities to the practice. The case also pinpoints the essence of the problem in using narratives: what was a truthful statement? How was information contestable? What part should competing priorities (the law, customs of manhood, disability, sickness) play in decision-making? And what was the genealogy of the language used by the various participants in each case? The final section of the chapter attempts to generalize aspects of the single case study, highlighting the considerable variability in narrative form and structure adopted by applicants in different circumstances and the frequent intertwining of narratives of poverty, sickness and under-employment in ways that have considerable resonance with narratives in England, Sweden or Denmark.

The legal regulation of peddling

Peddling was a contentious nineteenth-century practice.[16] After World War I, it was legally defined as unnecessary and anachronistic and the aim of a law of 1922 was to decisively restrict access to the trade.[17] From this date, peddling licences were only supposed to be given to Austrian citizens over the age of 30 who could prove a particular need and an inability to earn a living in other ways. These licences were preferably to be given to destitute war invalids and war dependents.[18] As in other trades, a good reputation (but also a certificate by a public health officer) was required. Proof was also needed of a restricted employability and that the applicant had no noxious or contagious diseases. Peddling should serve as a substitute for a pension or for sufficient poor relief, and indeed trade regulations aimed to restrict the economic efficiency of peddling so as to ensure a very small, not to say residual, income. Using carts or employing help required special permission from the provincial government. The licence had to be renewed once a year and the application was reviewed by the Trade Office and the Chambers of Commerce and of Labour. The available records on peddlers are thus often extraordinarily rich, since they will include a number of different perspectives on a single case. Furthermore, they contain context-bound self-descriptions by applicants for licences, that is, by people who were otherwise almost exclusively described by others. An application for a licence could be made in person at the trade office in the district where a person lived. In many cases, though, people sent in a letter written by themselves or others.

Dealing with a certain stock of records in the archives, we should not make the epistemological mistake of regarding the peddlers documented here – or people in other itinerate trades – as a clearly separated or homogeneous population. These are records of persons who successfully or unsuccessfully applied for a licence. Yet much peddling was conducted without permission or with other kinds of sales permissions.[19] In contrast to the legal definitions, a variety of selling practices could be regarded as peddling, often in a derogatory or defamatory perspective. In addition, holders of a peddling licence could conduct their trade in different ways and with varying dimensions. Records of those who applied for or received a peddling licence reveal quite a range of careers and situations. Any analysis must therefore examine this variety and the differences involved instead of aiming at describing a given population or the 'typical' peddler. The problems of interpretation, as well as the potentialities for history from below, represented by these trade records can be exemplified with a specific case from Salzburg.

The records on Karl Hasch

Thus, according to records, Karl Hasch was born in Vienna as an illegitimate child in 1878. His mother was a German national and died soon after his birth. Hasch was then fostered by two different travelling families in Hungary, both of them 'carneys'. Travelling with them, he did not get a regular school education and later he would have his own licences as a carney and a peddler. On the occasion of his military draft in 1903, it transpired that he had lost his German nationality due to his extended travels abroad. However, he served with the Austrian armed forces, took part in World War I and was severely injured, giving us a sense of how casual employment, poverty and sickness could intertwine. This is the (not unquestioned) background story told by Hasch,[20] who became the subject of a trade file in Salzburg in 1920, in the context of a complaint that reported:

> A certain Karl Hasch. is peddling within the city as a so-called 'Gottscheer'[21] in the inns and brings candies into circulation by gambling. Hasch is said to have lived earlier from begging; he pretends to be disabled war veteran, but he is not a war invalid. Presumably his licence was obtained by fraud.[22]

In turn, the complaint reflected the fact that peddling had been forbidden in the city of Salzburg since 1897; it was prohibited within an increasing number of cities and smaller communities during the interwar period. At the time he had a peddling licence issued from the city of Graz in 1921 but his permission for peddling *within* the city of Salzburg was apparently the result of a bureaucratic error. In the following inquiry, the organization of war invalids supported the applicant

> Comrade Hasch., who has been working in an altruistic way at the secretary of our organisation and beyond that is severely invalid, deserves from us just the best reputation. We therefore ask the right honourable municipality to benevolently approach the case and let Hasch., who is father of three underage children,[23] keep his livelihood.[24]

The intervention did not apparently help. In March 1921 Hasch received the final decision on the second appeal to the provincial government. It stated that his permission was not to be renewed. In any event, Hasch kept applying for a peddling licence in the city as a Gottscheer. He argued that as an invalid he had no other way to earn his daily bread. He intended 'nothing other' than to sell his candies and thereby earn his keep.[25] Due to his prosthesis, he felt unable to walk with dry goods and draperies in the countryside and therefore asked for an exemption from the law.[26] Moreover, Hasch argued that the ban on peddling in the city had not always existed. There had always been exceptions made, and 15 to 20 Gottscheers had been working in the city before the war. Because these Gottscheers were no longer there, he asked to have the ban suspended with respect to his person.[27] Furthermore, he had given up on a pension. Enclosed in the file is a letter from a local bakery confirming that he bought all his goods from them.

The Chamber of Commerce rejected this renewed application and stated 'that there is no reason to renew today the privilege' which had been granted for political reasons to a small circle of Austrian citizens with the lowest cultural status. Beside the economic reasons, the *Stadtmagistrat* also gave ethical ones against the approval of Hasch's request.'[28] The Chamber feared that many others would then demand similar privileges. Hasch's situation was, as the Chamber wrote, doubtlessly lamentable, but there was no proof that he actually was a war invalid. Even the Chamber of Labour, which usually supported these applicants, hesitated in this case and complained about lacking information. Not only was the origin of Hasch's invalidity in doubt – maybe it was obtained in his former occupation as a circus artist? – but 'indisputable' witnesses had also seen him 'running'.[29] The public health officer confirmed his stiff leg, but stated that since Hasch was not exclusively able to earn his bread as a peddler an occupation that permitted him to sit would be more convenient.[30]

In 1921 Hasch was *heimatlos* ('homeless', in the sense of stateless). He had no right of residence, and his nationality was unclear. Reports on Hasch's criminal record also varied. The local police reported initially that nothing negative could be found. The central criminal records unit in Vienna, on the other hand, reported that a Karl Hasch, a circus artist, was registered with three convictions: fraud in Vienna 1904, theft in Laibach (Ljubljana/Slovenia) 1906 and personal injury in an affray in Klagenfurt/ Carinthia 1911. There was, however, another person with a similar name – 'Carlo Has.', labourer – registered for a violation against the vagrancy act in Capodistria (Koper/Slovenia) in 1907. The issue of identity remained unclear.

Numerous requests and appeals were filed with the various authorities, right up to the Ministry of Trade and Commerce. Although Hasch was represented by a lawyer from 1923 onwards, he had no further success. In its decision of 1923, the Federal Ministry for Trade and Commerce stated that it was also bound to its own regulations and thus could not grant the exceptional permission requested.[31] Meanwhile, Hasch had registered as a travelling marketer, apparently without any problems.[32] His crime record, frequently held against him, was no obstacle here. In the same year, 1923, he received a further licence to sell roasted chestnuts in the streets of Salzburg.[33] Another application addressed by his lawyer completely lacks the emphasis of need: 'I intend now – since it is a common thing in Vienna, Linz, Graz and Innsbruck – to sell hot sausages in the evening; hence, as one would say it in Vienna, I wish to establish myself as a *Würstlmann* [sausage man]'.[34] This application was rejected because of 'insufficient local demand' and met stiff opposition from the innkeepers' official representation. They claimed that they feared not only 'real economic damage' to their business but also that passers-by would be annoyed. Finally, they also wrote that if the 'honourable municipality' did in fact acknowledge a local demand, there were still other more deserving citizens.[35] Hasch kept trying to obtain a peddling licence but now his other trades created a new obstacle, since peddling was not to be combined with any other licence.[36] His later applications added that he not only had to make a living for himself but also for his wife, who was severely ill.[37] In 1925, he received his *Heimatrecht* (right of residence) in Salzburg. A certificate from the police department in Vienna finally substantiated his military service from 1914 to 1918 and his battlefield injuries. A two-page file of a police interrogation presented further information on his identity and biography.[38] A local police officer confirmed the credibility of Hasch's statements and his war invalidity. By describing the course of events, Hasch convinced him that he too had taken part in battle in Gródek/Galicia.

With these impediments removed, from 1926 to 1930 Hasch received a peddling licence, despite the objections of the peddlers' organization which maintained that Hasch illegally worked as a Gottscheer and did not really peddle.[39] The Chamber of Commerce still pointed to his criminal record and his other options for making a livelihood,[40] but it had no more objections after 1929 and there is no evidence of Hasch's activities for some years hence. The next record derives from 1935, when Hasch tried to renew his licence.[41] According to his statements and correspondence, he had been ill and 'needed a change of air'.[42] He had spent the previous years in Italy with his sister-in-law, working in a different occupation, as the holder of a musician's licence. He indicated that his situation was 'now really in every respect sad'.[43] The application was rejected due to new restrictions on peddling (imposed in 1934) stating that it was not legally possible to accept new requests or applications which had not been renewed in time (and without any interruption).[44] In November 1935 Privy Councillor Dr A. Morsey, head of the *Österreichischer Heimatschutz*, wrote to *Landeshauptmann* (political position equivalent to a governor of an Austrian province) Dr Ernst Rehrl on Hasch's behalf to say:

> The severely invalided Karl Haf. [sic], who is highly recommended by Prince Franz-Josef Windisch-Graetz, adjutant of the *Bundesführer*, has asked the office of the *Bundesführer*, to support his petition for award of the Gottscheer-right for Salzburg at best. I warmly approve this application and thank you in advance for your friendly endeavours.[45]

In his answer *Landeshauptmann* Rehrl regretted that renewing the licence would be against the law,[46] though he did at least give Hasch 16 Schillings in December 1936.[47] In a petition to Federal Chancellor Schuschnigg dated 1936, Hasch asked for an act of mercy to regain his permission as a Gottscheer (*Gottscheer-Legitimation*) which – as he wrote – he had possessed from 1919 to 1930. He cited his war injuries and described himself as 75 per cent unemployable, but 'as a citizen and respected person' he wanted to make a living in his trade without burdening city or state. He hoped not to have approached the Chancellor in vain.[48] A further appeal addressed to the Federal Chancellor dates from April 1937. In this document, Hasch pointed out that he received no pension and the 17 Schillings of poor relief granted by his hometown of Salzburg was not enough to survive on. The letter includes a request for an audience, the chance to present his reasons in person.[49]

Enclosed in this file is a letter of recommendation by the *Vaterländische Front* (an organization funded 1933 by the Austro-Fascist regime) confirming his details.[50] The last available correspondence dates from December 1937: a letter to the *Landeshauptmann* of Salzburg, in which Hasch asked for a short private audience; he hoped it would be granted because it was about the existence of a sick businessmen.[51] He would, recorded the reply, receive notice when the *Landeshauptmann* was available again to hear his appeal.[52]

Problems of interpretation

This file represents a considerable effort to obtain a single peddler's licence! On the one hand, it seems amazing how much we can learn about one peddler; on the other, what we learn is frustratingly little. Hasch is a bureaucratic case not a person, and the story tells us about a bureaucratic process and not a life.[53] Everything we can learn derives from an official context and the records in question adhere to bureaucratic priorities. The authorities involved primarily gathered information relevant for their decisions. They expressed their opinions and conclusions according to conventions and legal requirements. But whether the applicant fulfilled the requirements of the law was still a matter for interpretation. What did a good reputation consist of? How long were previous convictions relevant and what kind of violations of the law really counted? How was poverty to be defined and to what degree was the applicant no longer employable? How much should sickness and disability of the applicant or his family count in the decision? Much that might be relevant for an actual bureaucratic decision, such as the impression made in a face-to-face encounter, was not usually mentioned.

On the other hand, the applicant statements were also not the result of 'authentic' self-expression,[54] but rather Hasch's more or less adequate sense of arguments and practices that would be useful for achieving the aims in that context. Indeed, and rather more widely than this particular case, the applicants' arguments were well adapted and indicate that people were familiar with the requirements for such a licence. Even the letters written were thus somehow standardized.

There were, however, different attitudes towards approaching the authorities and providing reasons for one's situation. Some arguments and attitudes appear to be inappropriate, irrational or even nonsensical in this context.[55] A person's attitudes, as Hasch's records indicate, might also vary according not only to personal situation but also to the kind of licence one sought. Furthermore, who actually spoke or wrote as an applicant? Are we really reading the language of the poor?[56] The handwriting of Hasch's letters varied and differed from his signature, which also varied on occasion. For a time, he had a lawyer, and on some occasions the letter was typewritten. His statements made verbally at the trade office were written down by a clerk.

This was not very likely done word-for-word and probably not with the same words the applicant used. And even if the clerk wrote them down, the question remains of where the applicants' arguments came from. Were these the statements made in front of a clerk when they were influenced by advice on what to say? Moreover, even barely legible handwriting or correctly recorded stammering do not allow us to observe feelings or thoughts. There is no way to empirically demonstrate the interrelation of representation, thinking and feelings, nor the extent of coherence or dissent.[57] There is also no way to decide what is true, adequate, overdrawn, a mistake or even a lie. Obviously, the records do not report unquestionable facts or describe a set reality. Data given by Hasch, but also by the authorities involved, vary and change over the years. Some data seem to have been accepted without question, such as for example the sex of the applicant. Other 'facts' – such as the three children alleged here – are not matter of dispute. For several years, however, the administration was not able to provide reliable information on Hasch's identity, nationality, military service, crime records and invalidity, matters crucial for obtaining a licence. Information finally acknowledged as truth was the result of dispute.

These problems should not, of course, be a reason to dismiss such records as source material, but to reconsider what they actually reveal. It seems more precise and adequate to regard them as evidence about interrelated practices of an applicant, all who supported him and all others involved (clerks, various authorities and institutions, associations, witnesses, etc.) in a certain situation that is not created by mere interaction but also by a broader historical context. The records represent the struggle of how to earn one's keep legally, often in the face of sickness and disability, as well as what peddling officially should be and who should have access to it. In order to understand these activities – the normal or extraordinary character of a particular case – it is necessary to compare it with other narratives, and this is the function of the rest of the chapter.[58]

Generalizing the case

Hasch's persistence might seem surprising. After all, asking took an effort and usually one had to pay a small fee for each application and appeal (unless one could prove destitution). Hasch, however, did not give up when his requests were rejected. Although he was on the move most of his life, there is no evidence indicating he was 'uprooted'.[59] He made good use of the opportunities and contacts available in Salzburg, producing letters of recommendation from the organization of war invalids and later on by the *Vaterländische Front*. A local bakery confirmed that he bought his goods there. Like a few other peddlers from Salzburg, he was represented by a lawyer (presumably by an *Armenanwalt*, i.e. an attorney for the poor who worked pro bono). The peddlers' organization, however, which aimed to protect its members from the competition of illegal and foreign workers, opposed his request.[60] Under interrogation by a police officer – a rather extraordinary document in this context – he managed to make his story plausible. Clearly, Hasch's mobile life caused troubles for the bureaucracy and made it difficult to provide reliable information on him. The effort made (and hence the volume of these records) was extensive; it was no easy case but then only a few people got such licences without problems. Indeed, the persistence demonstrated by Hasch was not uncommon. Numerous similar appeals addressed to provincial governments and the Federal Trade Ministry can be found. Many other applicants, however, tried once and then disappeared from the records. It is not possible to reconstruct why one person gave up and others did not, or which methods those unsuccessful applicants used to find a livelihood when they could not obtain another kind of licence to work.

Clearly there was a restrictive trade policy in Austria at the time. Yet access to different – though effectively similar – forms of itinerate trade was highly varied. Working as a travelling marketer, for example, was a 'free' trade and less encumbered, but one had to visit more remote marketplaces at certain times instead of offering goods door-to-door. Unlike peddling, such salesmen were not favoured with respect to taxes. As with Hasch, many of those rejected applied for other sales licences until they were able to obtain a peddlers' licence. Peddling without a licence was very common (in contemporary complaints at least), but such practice did violate trade law and this could subsequently create an obstacle in legalizing one's activities. By the same token, illegal peddling was not a violation of the vagrancy act (unlike begging) and was therefore punished with a fine and not with imprisonment.[61]

Applicants may have worked in a broad range of occupations before they tried to get a peddlers' licence, but among them the narrative archive reveals a considerable proportion of former itinerant traders, salesmen, marketers, rag-and-bone collectors and so forth. Working as a travelling artist, marketer, peddler and musician, Hasch seems to represent what might be called a modern type of 'nomad'.[62] Not all who tried to obtain a licence for itinerant trade show the same degree of mobility throughout their lives; some appear quite sedentary and did not change their place of residence that often. Indeed, working as peddler could include mobility in various respects, ranging from daily commuting within the surrounding of one's place of residence to seasonal or more enduring travel. Even in the case of Hasch, his desire to legally sell subtropical fruits in an itinerant way was coterminous with his desire to work and live in Salzburg. For obvious reasons, Hasch did not refer to his roots in the city as others in the narrative archive did. Instead, he pointed out his alleged ethnicity as a Gottscheer and that group's traditional privilege of peddling within the city. He asked for a licence 'as a Gottscheer', 'like a Gottscheer',[63] or 'like the former Gottscheer'.[64] Gottscheer referred both to a certain way of peddling and a German-speaking minority.

Belonging to this minority could mean something different than belonging to other ethnic or religious minorities with a traditionally high share of itinerant traders, such as Jews,[65] 'gypsies,[66] *Karrner* or *Jenische*.[67] Indeed, there were still some nostalgic depictions of street sellers, as somehow exotic figures who vanished with the 'good old days' of the monarchy.[68] German-speaking minorities outside the territory of Austria and Germany were also an object of political concern. And, in fact, unlike other foreign nationalities, Gottscheers managed get a peddler's licence once the trade agreement was made with the Kingdom of Serbs, Croats and Slovenes.[69] In this framework, it made sense to stress one's belonging to this minority, yet it could still be a reason for defamation, as the pejorative statement of the Chamber of Commerce in relation to Hasch illustrates.[70]

In general, arguments for continuity or tradition in this context could be effective, since in some respect the authorities accepted rights to trade granted earlier. For example, people who had had a peddling licence since 1914 were not subject to the new restrictions and usually acquired their licence without much fuss. Once obtained, licences for selling certain goods could also remain valid. Trade in lemons,[71] for example, was permitted within the monarchy, because lemons were regarded as native products. In the republic, these fruits were excluded from hawking as foreign products unless somebody already held a permission to sell them. Family tradition, however, was not acknowledged here. Unlike in other trades, a peddler's licence could not be transferred to a widow(er) or a child. Nevertheless, such a family tradition was emphasized by some applicants, as an argument for exceptional permissions, as in the case of Franziska Brand, a rag-and-bone collector born in 1900.[72] She repeatedly tried to obtain a peddler's licence in Salzburg between 1933 and 1936, arguing that she could not any longer make a living from her trade. Yet she was without success, writing in 1936:

> In our family, peddling has been a tradition for decades and so we didn't learn anything else from our father who had the peddler's licence, and we were only interested in peddling. After the death of my father, the licence was taken away from us and despite our requests not reapproved. This peddler's licence was for us – like for all other small businesspeople – a trade existence, for maintaining our whole family (and not just our parents). Because in this case it would be only a transfer from father to daughter, it is – in legal terms – only a transfer or signing over, not a new licence, and the statute of the law would not apply here. In addition, a negative decision affects the livelihood of our family (with many children), and one has to consider, in these economically hard times, whether I as a woman should not find a livelihood to support my family, that my request should be eliminated due to a rigid paragraph since as a good, patriotic [*vaterländisch*] woman I certainly don't deserve this. The business community will not be harmed by permitting the transfer of the licence; only the opposite can occur. Because the same goods from

the merchants will be offered in the most remote places and homes where there are not any stores. In addition, the state earns through sales taxes . . . and here the opposite is true: my family and I need support . . .[73]

The general political aim of restricting and reducing the incidence of peddling was often highlighted in the decisions rendered. Exceptions to the law were not made, whatever arguments were produced by applicants speaking in favour of them. If there was any official reason for a more favourable interpretation of a person's situation, it was primarily related to participation in World War I, as Hasch's case has already illustrated.

The crucial issues frequently under discussion in the wider sample of narratives were economic necessity and a lack of alternatives. Being out of work and poor through no fault of one's own was not, however, sufficient. This situation was common enough at the time. The decisive point was to make the addressee actually believe that such a licence was one's *sole* way to make a living. Applicants had to prove that they were more or less unemployable, and one significant way to do this was reference to disability, one's own sickness or caring duties for a family member who was sick. A higher degree of employability or the slight chance of making a living in other ways could be a reason for rejection, complaint or defamation, which is why applicants often highlighted their own or family sickness in their documentation. Thus, when Thekla Pru applied for a renewal of her peddler's licence in 1924, she stated that she was poor and had to care for her disabled husband, a request that had been accepted by the local trade association in 1923. She had lost two sons in the war. The local physician confirmed the disability. The local trade association wrote to the Chamber of Commerce in 1924 that a very meticulous investigation had revealed that:

> Mrs. Pru is a healthy person, almost powerful. Was an innkeeper in 1919 . . . marches great distances on foot and carries a heavy packet of textiles around all day long. I personally made an effort to check this distance on bicycle, 14 kilometres to 20 kilometres, almost every day. Well, one can't speak of unemployability. We can only say that Mr. Pru is a victim of inflation.[74]

Pointing out that they were having to pay plenty for welfare and taxes, the trade association definitively opposed the request. The state, it argued, should not damage the trade by allowing peddling. The fact that the application was made in a district of Lower Austria (Waidhofen/Thaya) that had a privilege for peddling with textiles in the monarchy[75] was not up for discussion.

Although the applicants usually pointed out that they were unwilling to burden the community, local shopkeepers – also struggling with economic crisis – demanded that the city prevent harm to their business and take care of the poor. Some applicants responded, like Hasch, that they would not be an economic threat but rather would be distributing local products. Some emphasized that they had always paid their taxes properly and certainly would do so in future. But with respect to legal requirements, peddling somehow represented a world of upside-down economics. Economic arguments of applicants were thus rather the exception in this context. A former shopkeeper from Vienna, for example, wrote:

> Because I have a clientele which I have acquired in almost 30 years of respectable conduct, and I only can serve them when my petition is approved; because otherwise my economic situation justifies it; because peddling intends to tickle out money from the most remote groups, thereby fulfilling its very designation as valuable asset of national wealth. It creates work and employment opportunities, which is sadly enough not appreciated adequately . . .[76]

Such arguments are also to be found in publications of the peddlers' organization. In the context of individual applications, however, it seemed to be more usual and also more promising to emphasize one's narrow limits, sickness and a very poor income, rather than refer to the business potential of this trade. Peddling was something to unburden the community, not to contribute to its welfare.

The narratives also, reveal, however, another aspect of the relationship between poverty, underemployment and sickness. Hence, being unemployable was a requirement, but being too sick or disabled also appears to have been an obstacle in many cases. Applicants thus raised suspicions of actually wishing to beg instead of to trade. One could even be *too* disabled for a licence as a begging musician, as in the case of Paul Juraso, 59 years old, who applied in 1931. Similar to peddlers, begging musicians or buskers were regarded as a considerable nuisance at the time. Legal permissions were rare:

> In view of the fact that I've been blind since childhood and thus can't hold down a job, I have permission to play harmonica in the courtyards. Since southern *Burgenland* is very inconvenient for me because of all the mountains, I ask you for a permit so I can play two or three months in your district in order for me to live a few more years. I am 59 years old and ask you politely for mercy. Almighty God shall reward you.[77]

Juraso's home town stated that he was receiving poor relief there. His provisions were sufficient and his activities were therefore unwelcome. Because he was blind, he would need a guide and thus bother not only his but also other communities.

Usually applicants stressed their and their families' poverty and desperation and their willingness to earn a living and fulfil their duties with respect to their relatives. Although they did not want to burden the local community, they probably would have to in case of rejection. This logic is common to pauper narratives across Europe, as we see in the other chapters in this volume, particularly those pertaining to England. Clearly, this was not welcome in every case. However, one's inability to earn a living otherwise in an honest way might also be regarded as a subtle threat towards the community. Few applicants made more explicit threats, for instance claiming that they would in case of rejection be forced to beg and steal. Some did, however, become more forceful. Thus, Rudolf Trie was born in 1887 in Upper Austria and was married with three children between the ages of two and six. In 1931, he lived in a caravan in Salzburg. According to his letter, he was 65 per cent invalid and had injuries to the head and his hand. In addition, he suffered from general neuropathy and was bedridden most of the time. He wrote:

> I am forced to reverse my *Option* [application for the Austrian citizenship] and don't want to be an Austrian because here one becomes a criminal just be trying to find a living . . . I now insist on three points. Either this way or that way: If I do not get documents to support my family and to have income, I will abandon my family, and the community will have to support them and take care of them. Or you give me a passport for Russia or France . . . I will abandon my family because I don't want to starve in Austria where it is not beautiful enough . . . I can't live without income as cripple . . . I expect an answer in 14 days.[78]

The protocol reported more moderately that the war invalid Rudolf Trie could not survive on his 19.50 Schilling pension and asked for urgent assistance. His repeated requests were rejected because, due to his criminal record, he did not meet the legal requirements.

Most letters were like Hasch's, rather straight and formal. He did not describe his situation in great detail. Nor did he explicitly and obediently ask for mercy. He did not utter threats. However, as pointed out above, style and arguments varied according to the situation, the kind of licence and the level of the appeal. Other applicants delivered more 'poetic' accounts of their situation. Josef Hub, for example, born in 1876, wrote in 1932:

> This is my first petition I have written in my life and the gentlemen may forgive me in advance if it is not written according to the rules of art. I am a green grocer, already without money and thus not able to survive. I therefore request the high gentlemen to award the peddling trade to me so that I may find a livelihood. Because I have to start something. I am not getting work because younger workers are preferred. I am ashamed to beg and I can't steal. What can I do? I have tried every possible thing to get back on my feet. Five times a week I went to the countryside to obtain goods and came home again to deliver them, and so on. I did this for years. Sometimes I thought I was making a little progress, but one

setback followed another and I was poorer than before . . . I live today a
life like a dog – whom I envy when I see it eating a bowl of soup . . . This
plea is written with the blood of my heart . . .[79]

Doubtless the vast majority of applicants were in very difficult situations.
However, it would be wrong exclusively to see the desperation described
in the last letter in all such attempts to find a livelihood. A decent wage or
unemployment benefits or a sufficient pension would have been preferable,
but peddling was nonetheless not just a subsistence vehicle. Some people,
particularly perhaps the sick and disabled, wished to peddle rather than
revert to other possibilities such as different trades, begging or the poor
house.[80] Peddling within legal restrictions did not provide an outlook of
prosperity, but it promised more income than poor relief, which according
to the applicants was seldom regarded as sufficient.[81] As described above,
efforts to achieve this particular possibility were often remarkable. Hence,
these records should not be seen not as mere manifestations of poverty
and distress but also as active attempts to deal with the situation. These
cases reveal more or less creativity in doing so, that is in finding adequate
arguments and support in to deal with legal requirements or attempt to
bend the rules.

Conclusion

The range of activities highlighted in this chapter ought to cast doubt on
the image of the unemployed as apathetic, depressed or passive, as depicted
in the famous contemporary study of those unemployed in Marienthal by
Jahoda, Lazarsfeld and Zeisl.[82] Inquiring why unemployment did not seem
to have a revolutionary effect on a community of former factory workers,
their study had little regard for activities that did not fit into the image
of a politically conscious, organized working class.[83] Attempts to simply
organize one's daily life by legal or illegal means were seen as undesirable
effects of unemployment. They did not fit into a narrow picture of work as
waged labour.

Beggarly forms of self-employment, particularly for the sick, seem instead
to fit more into common images of the 'underclass',[84] the 'Lumpenproletariat',
than those of the respectable working class even before the economic crisis.[85]
Many of the people making these attempts do not fit into the category of the
unemployed as defined by social insurance and labour market policy or even
in the broader sense found in political debates.[86] They had lost – or in many
cases never had – entitlement to unemployment benefits. They were simply
without income or means and more or less unemployable. Particularly at this
time of high unemployment and at times of sickness, the chances of finding
waged labour seemed minimal. As we have seen here, the character and
role of alternative economic activities was highly disputed, and narratives

coalescing around peddling reveal a struggle about the official character of work and the right (and obligation) to work.

Applicants for a peddling licence faced a somewhat paradoxical situation. The poor laws, the vagrancy law and also unemployment benefits all postulated a willingness to work and earn a living if possible. Precarious forms of self-employment could be an option, particularly if one had no financial means, no vocational training and no opportunity to get and hold a regular job. In this context, peddling appears as the very last career, an occupation with the lowest reputation. Access was highly restricted since this trade was regarded as a disguised form of begging and a threat to sedentary trades. Although it could unburden the local community from paying poor relief, it was regarded as of no value for the national economy and also as a threat to security. Peddling was an activity in between work and what nineteenth-century scholars called 'negative work'.[87] The administration contributed to this ambiguity. In the context of fundamental (yet for so many, particularly the sick and disabled, unavailable) social rights and in the context of new concepts of labour and vocation, the character of these occupations was even more disputed.

Notes

1   Research for this chapter was funded by the Austrian Science Fund (project number Y367-G14) and the ERC-Starting Grant 200918-production of work.

2   Tálos, E. and Wörister, K. (1994), *Soziale Sicherung im Sozialstaat Österreich. Entwicklung – Herausforderungen – Strukturen*. Baden-Baden: Nomos; Bruckmüller, E., Sandgruber, R. and Stekl, H. (1978), *Soziale Sicherheit im Nachziehverfahren, die Einbeziehung der Bauern, Landarbeiter, Gewerbetreibenden und Hausgehilfen in das System der österreichischen Sozialversicherung*. Salzburg: Neugebauer.

3   See, for example, Hufton, O. (1974), *The Poor of Eighteenth-Century France, 1750–1789*. Oxford: Oxford University Press, p. 68ff.; Jütte, R. (2000), *Arme, Bettler, Beutelschneider. Eine Sozialgeschichte der Armut in der Frühen Neuzeit. Weimar*: Böhlaus, p. 11.

4   Niederösterreichisches Landesarchiv (s.W.), Gruppe XI, Stammzahl 957/1932.

5   Wadauer, S. (2005), *Die Tour der Gesellen. Mobilität und Biographie im Handwerk vom 18. bis zum 20. Jahrhundert*. Frankfurt: Campus Verlaag; Wadauer, S. (2006), 'Journeymen's mobility and the guild system: a space of possibilities based on Central European cases', in Gadd, I. and Wallis, P. (eds), *Guilds and Association in Europe, 900–1900*. London: Centre for Metropolitan History, pp. 169–86. Similar ambivalence but with other referents can be found in narratives of hobos; see, for example, Tobias, F. (2003), *Higbie, Indispensable Outcasts. Hobo Workers and Community in the American Midwest 1880–1930*. Urbana: University of Illinois Press; Kusmer, K. (2002), *Down and Out on the Road. The Homeless in American History*. Oxford: Oxford University Press, particularly chapter 9.

6   See, for example, Wadauer, S. (2008), 'Vacierende gesellen und wandernde
    arbeitslose', in Buchner, T. , Steidl, A., Lausecker, W., Pinwinkler, A., Wadauer,
    S. and Zeitlhofer, H. (eds), *Übergänge. Beiträge zu Arbeit – Migration –*
    Demographie – Wissenschaft. Vienna: München, pp. 101–31.
7   Wadauer, S. (2997), 'Betteln – Arbeit – Arbeitsscheu (Wien 1918–1938)',
    in Althammer, B. (ed.), *Bettler in der Europäischen Stadt der Moderne.*
    Zwischen Barmherzigkeit, Repression und Sozialreform. Frankfurt: Peter Lang,
    pp. 257–300.
8   Börner, W. 'Problem des bettlerwesens (unter verwertung der ergebnisse
    einer umfrage)', in Das Bettlerwesen in Wien und seine Bekämpfung. Bericht
    über die am 19. Februar 1933 von der 'Ethischen Gemeinde' veranstaltete
    Konferenz. Vienna: PP, pp. 7–19 and 12.
9   See the periodicals of the peddlers' organizations such as the Wiener
    Hausierer-Zeitung (1906 ff); Allgemeine Hausierer-Zeitung. Offizielles Organ
    des seit 33 Jahren bestehenden Ersten österreichischen Rechtsschutzvereines
    für Hausierer. (1929 ff.); Der österreichische Globus, (1930 ff.); Der
    alpenländische 'Hausierer'. Fachblatt der vereinigten Rechtsschutzverbände
    für Hausierer von Ober-Österreich, Salzburg und die übrigen Alpenländer
    (1931 ff.).
10 Cresswell, T. (2006), *On the Move. Mobility in the Modern Western World*.
    London: Routledge, p. 26ff.
11 With rare exceptions such as, for example, Wattwil, F. B. (ed.) (2007), *Das*
    lange Leben eines Toggenburger Hausieres Gregorius Aemisegger 1815–1913.
    A few Roma describe their own or their families' memories before the NS-
    Regime, for example, Stojka, M. (2000), *Papierene Kinder. Glück, Zerstörung*
    und Neubeginn einer Roma-Familie in Österreich. Vienna: Molden. For this
    period in German, there seem to be no similar detailed descriptions to those
    Betty Naggar (1992) uses in her book *Jewish Pedlars and Hawkers 1740–1940*.
    Chamberly: Porphyrogenitus. The same applies to travelling salesmen. There
    are several novels but apparently not a great number of autobiographies to be
    found, unlike in the US context; see, for example, Friedman, W. (2004), *Birth*
    of a Salesman. The Transformation of Selling in America. Harvard: Harvard
    University Press.
12 King, S. and Tomkins, A. (2003), 'Introduction', in King, S. and Tomkins,
    A. (eds), *The Poor in England 1700–1850. An Economy of Makeshifts*.
    Manchester: Manchester University Press, pp. 1–38. Wadauer, S. (2008),
    'Ökonomie und notbehelfe in den 1920er und 1930er jahren', in Melichar, P.,
    Langthaler, E. and Eminger, S. (eds), *Niederösterreich im 20. Jahrhundert, vol.*
    2: Wirtschaft. Vienna: Böhlau, pp. 537–73.
13 Hitchcock, T. (2994), *Down and Out in Eighteenth-Century London*. London:
    Hambledon, p. 48.
14 Wadauer, S. (2007), 'Betteln und hausieren verboten?Ambulanter handel im
    Wien der Zwischenkriegszeit', *Jahrbuch für Wirtschaftsgeschichte/Economic*
    History Yearbook, 1, 181–203.
15 See, for example, Oberpenning, H. (1996), *Migration und Fernhandel im*
    'Tödden-System': Wanderhändler aus dem nördlichen Münsterland im
    mittleren und nördlichen Europa. Osnabrück: Universitätsverlag Rasch, p. 12;
    Fontaine, L. (1996), *History of Pedlars in Europe*. Padstow: Duke University

Press, pp. 3 and 140ff. Another perspective, which includes the different categories of sales, is Friedman, *Birth of a Salesman*. See also Wadauer, 'Betteln'.

16   See, for example (1899), *Untersuchungen über die Lage des Hausiergewerbes in Österreich*. Leipzig.

17   Bundesgesetz, 30 March 1922: betreffend die Ergänzung und Abänderung einiger Bestimmungen des Hausierpatentes und der Vorschriften über andere Wandergewerbe. Bundesgesetzblatt für die Republik Österreich, 1922, Nr. 204; Begründung zum Gesetzesentwurf betreffend die Ergänzung und Abänderung einiger Bestimmungen des Hausierpatentes und der Vorschriften über andere Wandergewerbe. 716 der Beilagen – Nationalrat, in: Protokoll des Nationalrates 1921, Beilagen 701–849.

18   Some 31.8 per cent of the 1,808 persons legally peddling in 1934 were women. Die Ergebnisse der österreichischen Volkszählung vom 22 March 1934. Bearbeitet vom Bundesamt für Statistik, Bundesstaat, Textheft. Wien 1935, (= Statistik des Bundesstaates Österreich, Heft 1), 167, 170.

19   Archiv der Wirtschaftskammer Wien (hereafter WIKA), Hausierverbot Allgemein S-Z 735/24: Hausierverbot für Wien.

20   Archiv der Stadt Salzburg (hereafter ASS), Gewerbeamt Ih 1926/4126, Hasch. Karl, Polizeidirektion Salzburg, Amtsvermerk 16752/5-25

21   The German-speaking minority of the Gottschee (located in the territory of the Habsburg province Carniola, nowadays Kočevsko in Slovenia) had a peddling privilege for centuries. After 1918 this region was not a part of the republic of Austria but of the Kingdom of Serbs, Croats and Slovenes. A trade agreement that would have allowed Gottscheers to conduct itinerant trade in Austria again had not been concluded at that time. In addition, Hasch was no actual Gottscheer but, as he maintained, the illegitimate son of a Gottscheer. Pickl, O. (1993), 'Die einstige Sprachinsel Gottschee/Kocevje (Slowenien) und ihre Wanderhändler', in Reininghaus, W. (ed.), *Wanderhandel in Europa. Beiträge zur wissenschaftlichen Tagung in Ibbenbüren, Mettingen, Recke und Hopsten vom 9.-11. Oktober 1992*. Hagen: Linnepe, pp. 91–9.

22   ASS, Gewerbeamt Ih 1920, Zl. 5649, Hasch. Karl.

23   These children are never mentioned again in the records. Nor are they listed on the residential registration form. Landesarchiv Salzburg (hereafter LAS), Meldezettel nach 1924, Karl Hasch.

24   ASS, Gewerbeamt Ih 1922, Zl 5649, Hasch. Karl, Alpenländischer Verband von Kriegsteilnehmer (Heimkehrer) der Jahre 1914–1918 an das Gewerbereferat des Stadtmagistrates der Stadt Salzburg, 16.12.1920.

25   ASS, Gewerbeamt Ih 1922, Zl 3051, Hasch. Karl, Verhandlungsschrift, 19.8.1922.

26   ASS, Gewerbeamt Ih 1923, Zl. 681 Hasch. Karl, Verhandlungsschrift, 31.1.1923.

27   ASS, Gewerbeamt Ih 1923, Zl 681, Hasch. Karl, Verhandlungsschrift vom 31.1.1923; Rekurs an das Bundesministerium für Handel, Industrie, Gewerbe und Bauten, 19.1.1924.

28   ASS, Gewerbeamt, Ih 1923, Zl. 681 Hasch. Karl; Kammer für Handel, Gewerbe und Industrie in Salzburg an den Stadtmagistrat (Gewerbeabteilung), Salzburg, 15.2.1923.

29 ASS, Gewerbeamt, Ih 1924 4710, Hasch., Karl, Amtsabtlg. F. Gewerbe an das Stadtphysikat, 21.1.1924.

30 ASS, Gewerbeamt, Ih 1924 4710, Hasch., Karl, Stadtphysikat Salzburg, 25.1.1924.

31 ASS, Gewerbeamt Ih 1923/681, Hasch. Karl, Stadtmagistrat Salzburg an Herrn Karl Hasch., Hausierer, 3.4.1923.

32 ASS, Gewerbeamt Ia1 1923/3103, Hasch. Karl.

33 ASS, Gewerbeamt Ia1 1923/4226, Hasch. Karl.

34 ASS, Gewerbeamt Ia1 1923/4710, Hasch. Karl.

35 ASS, Gewerbeamt Ia1 1923/4710, Hasch. Karl, Genossenschaft der Gast- und Schanksgewerbetreibenden der Stadt- Salzburg an die Stadt-Gemeindevorstehung Salzburg, 22.12.1923.

36 ASS, Gewerbeamt Ih 1924/623, Hasch. Karl.

37 ASS, Gewerbeamt Ih 1926/4126, Hasch. Karl, Karl Hasch. an das löbl. Stadtmagistrat Salzburg, 22.10.1925.

38 ASS, Gewerbeamt Ih 1926/4126, Hasch. Karl, Polizeidirektion Salzburg, Amtsvermerk 16752/5-25.

39 ASS, Gewerbeamt Ih 1927/117; Rechtschutzverein für Hausierer Salzburgs an die Kammer für Handel, Gewerbe und Industrie 12.2.1927; Ih 1929/120, Hasch. Karl.

40 ASS, Gewerbeamt Ih 1927/117, Kammer für Handel Gewerbe und Industrie in Salzburg an das Stadtmagistrat Salzburg, 15.2.1927.

41 ASS, Gewerbeamt Ih/Ib 1935.

42 Österreichisches Staatsarchiv (hereafter OST), Archiv der Republik, Bundesministerium für Handel und Verkehr 501r, Zl 144.065/1935, Karl Hasch. an Bundeskanzler Kurt Schuschnigg, 6.8.1936.

43 ASS, Gewerbeamt Ih/Ib 1935, Karl Hasch. an die Stadtgemeinde Salzburg, 6.11.1935.

44 Bundesgesetz vom 19. Oktober 1934 über die Abänderung der hausierrechtlichen Vorschriften. Bundesgesetzblatt für den Bundesstaat Österreich, Nr. 324, 1934.

45 LAS Rehrl Akten, Rehrlbriefe 1937/4517, Staatsrat Dr. A Morsey, Leiter der Interv. Abtlg. Österreichischer Heimatschutz an Landeshauptmann Dr. Ernst Rehrl, Wien, 26. November 1935.

46 LAS Rehrl Akten, Rehrlbriefe 1937/4517, Landeshauptmann Dr. Ernst Rehrl an Staatsrat Dr. Andreas Freiherr von Morsey, Salzburg am 4. Jänner 1936.

47 LAS Rehrl Akten, Rehrlbriefe 1937/4517, Brief des Herrn Landeshauptmannes an Herrn Karl Hasch., Salzburg am 5. Dezember 1936

48 OST, Archiv der Republik, Bundesministerium für Handel und Verkehr 501r, Zl 144.065/1935, Karl Hasch. an Bundeskanzler Kurt Schuschnigg, 6.8.1936.

49 OST, Archiv der Republik, Bundesministerium für Handel und Verkehr 501r, Zl 144.065/1935, Karl Hasch. an Bundeskanzler Kurt Schuschnigg, 5.4.1937.

50 Tálos, E. and Manoschek, W. (2005), 'Aspekte der politischen struktur des Austrofaschismus', in Tálos, E. and Neugebauer, W. (eds), *Austrofaschismus. Politik – Ökonomie – Kultur 1933–1938*. Vienna: Verlag fur Gesellschaftskritik, pp. 124–60, esp. 145–54.

51 LAS Rehrl Akten, Rehrlbriefe 1937/4517, Karl Hasch. an Landeshauptmann Dr. Franz Rehrl. Salzburg, am 7. Dez. 1937.

52 LAS Rehrl Akten, Rehrlbriefe 1937/4517, Schreiben des Herrn Regierungsvizedirektors an Herrn Karl Hasch. Maxglaner Hauptstraße 67, Salzburg, 14.12.1937.

53 Schulze, W. (ed.) (1996), *Ego-Dokumente. Annäherung an den Menschen in der Geschichte*. Berlin: Akademie.

54 Bräuer, H (2008), *Armenmentalität in Sachsen 1500 bis 1800*. Leipzig: Leipziger Universitätsverlag.

55 Similar questions can be found in Boltanski, L. (1987), 'Bezichtigung und selbstdarstellung: die kunst, ein normales ppfer zu sein', in Hahn, A. and Knapp, V. (eds), *Selbstthematisierung und Selbstzeugnis: Bekenntnis und Geständnis*. Frankfurt: Campus, pp. 149–69.

56 On this question, see, for example, Sokoll, T. (1996), 'Selbstverständliche armut. Armenbriefe in England 1750–1834', in Schulze, *Ego-Dokumente*, pp. 227–71, here p. 227ff., and Sokoll, T. (2006), 'Writing for relief: rhetoric in English pauper letters, 1800–1834', in Gestrich, A., King, S. and Raphael, L. (eds), *Being Poor in Modern Europe. Historical Perspectives 1800–1940*. Frankfurt: Peter Lang, pp. 91–111.

57 In this respect, I therefore partly disagree with Hitchcock, T., King, P. and Sharpe, P. (1997), 'Introduction', in Hitchcock, T., King, P. and Sharpe, P. (eds), *Chronicling Poverty. The Voices and Strategies of the English Poor, 1640–1840*. Basingstoke: Macmillan, pp. 1–17, here p. 4.

58 More cases are edited in the report of a pilot study by Sigrid Wadauer and Christa Putz, Reisende. Mobilität und Erwerb im Österreich der 1920er und 1930er Jahre, Manuscript Wien 2003 (= LBIHS Projektberichte Nr. 12).

59 Hufton, *The Poor*, p. 68.

60 Hausierer aus Jugoslawien dürfen in Oesterreich den Hausierhandel ausüben! in: Der österreichische 'Globus' No. 7 (1933), 5ff.

61 Gesetz vom 24. Mai 1885, womit strafrechtliche Bestimmungen in Betreff der Zulässigkeit der Anhaltung in Zwangsarbeits- oder Besserungsanstalten getroffen werden, Reichsgesetzblatt für die im Reichsrathe vertretenen Königreiche und Länder 89, 1885.

62 Ferdinand Tönnies, Soziologische Skizzen, in *Soziologische Studien und Kritiken*. Zweite Sammlung. Jena 1926, 1–62, here 26ff.

63 ASS, Gewerbeamt Ih 1922, Zl 3051, Hasch. Karl.

64 ASS, Gewerbeamt Ih 1923, Zl. 681 Hasch. Karl.

65 Roth, J. (1985), *Juden auf Wanderschaft*. Cologne: Verlag Die Schmiede, p. 42ff; Hoffmann-Holter, B. (1990), '*Abreisendmachung'. Jüdische Kriegsflüchtlinge in Wien 1914 bis 1923*. Vienna: Böhlau, p. 90.

66 See, for example, Lucassen, L, Willems, W. and Cottaar, A. (2001), *Gypsies and Other Itinerant Groups. A Socio-Historical Approach*. Basingstoke: Macmillan.; Gesellmann, G. (1989), *Die Zigeuner im Burgenland in der Zwischenkriegszeit. Die Geschichte einer Diskriminierung*. Vienna: Böhlau, p. 134; Freund, F. (2003), 'Zigeunerpolitik im 20. Jahrhundert', Unpublished Habilitation, University of Vienna, 2 vols.

67 Pescosta, T. (2003), *Die Tiroler Karrner: Vom Verschwinden des fahrenden Volkes der Jenischen*. Innsbruck: Tiroler Wirtschaftsstudien; Zagler, L. *Die Korrner: Grenzgänger zwischen Freiheit und Elend*. Bozen: Hecknort; Kronenwetter, J. (ed.), (2005), *Das Reisen im Blut. Über 100 Jahre Fichtenauer fahrende Leut*, Stödtlen-Niederroden.

68 Kaut, H. (1970), *Kaufrufe aus Wien. Volkstypen und Straßenszenen in der Wiener Graphik von 1775 bis 1914*. Vienna, Böhlau, p. 10; Wolf, H.-M. (2006), *Die Märkte Alt-Wiens. Geschichte und Geschichten*. Vienna: Pichler.

69 Zusatzabkommen zu dem am 3. September 1925 unterzeichneten Handelsvertrag zwischen der Republik Österreich und dem Königreiche der Serben, Kroaten und Slowenen. Bundesgesetzblatt für die Republik Österreich 3. Stück, 9/1929, Absatz 5 Artikel 16.

70 On anti-Semitism in debates on peddlers, see Wadauer, 'Betteln und hausieren' and Wadauer, 'Ökonomie und Notbehelfe'.

71 Beck, R. (2004), 'Lemonihändler. Welsche händler und die ausbreitung der zitrusfrüchte im frühneuzeitlichen Deutschland', *Jahrbuch für Wirtschaftsgeschichte*, 2, 97–123.

72 According to the *Meldeschein* (residential registration), she had worked before as a maid, LAS, Meldezettel nach 1924, Franziska Brand.

73 ASS, Gewerbeakten Ih/Ib 1936, Brand. Franziska.

74 Wirtschaftskammer Wien, Hausierbewilligungen 3231/23.

75 Kaiserliches Patent vom 4. September 1852, giltig für das gesammte Kaiserreich, mit Ausschluß der Militärgränze, wodurch ein neues Gesetz über den Hausierhandel erlassen wird, *Reichs-Gesetz- und Regierungsblatt für das Kaiserthum Oesterreich*, Nr. 252, §17 a).

76 Wiener Stadt- und Landesarchiv, Magistratisches Bezirksamt für den 20. Bezirk A25, C65/1935 Weintr. Chaim.

77 Niederösterreichisches Landesarchiv, BH Bruck an der Leitha 1931, XI– 296/1.

78 ASS, Gewerbemat ih 1932, Trie. Rudolf.

79 ASS, Gewerbeamt ih 1932, Hub. Josef.

80 Ehmer, J. (1990), *Sozialgeschichte des Alters*. Frankfurt: Suhrkamp, p. 115.

81 Gestrich, A., King, S. and Raphael, L. (2006), 'The experience of being poor in nineteenth- and early-twentieth-century Europe', in Gestrich, King and Raphael, *Being Poor*, pp. 17–40.

82 Jahoda, M., Lazarsfeld, P. and Zeisel, H. (1975), *Die Arbeitslosen von Marienthal. Ein soziographischer Versuch*. Frankfurt: Suhrkamp; Fleck, C. (1990), *Rund um 'Marienthal'. Von den Anfängen der Soziologie in Österreich bis zu ihrer Vertreibung*. Vienna: Verlaag für Gesellschaftskritik, pp. 171–8.

83 Warneken, B. (2006), *Die Ethnographie popularer Kulturen. Eine Einführung*. Vienna: Böhlau, p. 91ff.

84 See, for example, Welshman, J. (2006), *Underclass. A History of the Excluded, 1880–2000*. London: Hambledon; Mann, K. (1991), *The Making of an English 'Underclass'? The Social Divisions of Welfare and Labour*. Milton Keynes: Open University Press.

85 Burnett, J. (1994), *The Experiences of Unemployment 1790–1990*. London. Penguin, p. 160.

86   Stiefel, D. (1979), *Arbeitslosigkeit. Soziale, politische und wirtschaftliche Auswirkungen – am Beispiel Österreichs 1918–1938*. Berlin: Duncker & Humbolt; Zimmermann, B. (2006), *Arbeitslosigkeit in Deutschland. Zur Entstehung einer sozialen Kategorie*. Frankfurt: Campus; Garraty, J. (1978), *Unemployment in History. Economic Thought and Public Policy*. New York: Harper and Row; Evans, R. and Geary, D. (eds) (1987), *The German Unemployed. Experiences and Consequences of Mass Unemployment from the Weimar Republic to the Third Reich*. London: Croom Helm.

87   Die negative Arbeit, von Landesgerichtsdirektor Rotering zu Beuthen (Oberschlesien), in: *Zeitschrift für die gesamte Strafrechtswissenschaft* No.16 (1896), 198–223.

APPENDIX: NARRATIVES WRIT LARGE

Richard Dyson, Peter Wessel Hansen, Elizabeth Hurren and Steven King

The contributors to this volume use a variety of narrative sources by or about the poor. Some of the most compelling are letters (rather than simply petitions) written by paupers themselves. Our introductory chapter suggested the need for such letters to be read against multiple contexts (literacy levels, urbanization, age structure, etc.) and highlighted a clutch of potential problems associated with orthography, authorship, truth and representativeness. Even allowing for this backdrop, however, pauper letters and other narratives by or about the poor provide a unique route into understanding the linguistic competencies, concerns, feelings and agency of the poor themselves. In the rest of this appendix we therefore provide a sample of narratives transcribed from the original documents, as a resource for readers of the volume. While commentators such as Thomas Sokoll have highlighted the importance of preserving layout and providing supplementary detail (on the nature of paper, writing on the outside of envelopes etc), in this appendix we have sought to focus on the content of the narratives themselves. The spelling, punctuation and capitalization in the original documents have all been preserved. Original archival references follow each narrative rather than being confined to endnotes, and none of them has been previously published.

The sample begins with pauper letters (1–15) drawn from the Oxfordshire Record Office (hereafter ORO) for the small villages of Bampton, Finstock, Hook Norton, Rotherfield Greys, Shipton-under-Wychwood, Souldern, Wooton and the urban parishes of St Clements and St Giles, both in Oxford itself. Oxfordshire at this time was a heavily rural county dominated by the stagnating town of Oxford and with little by way of rapid urban growth outside of Banbury. It was, however, undergoing enclosure and agricultural improvement and had in the eighteenth and early nineteenth centuries witnessed sustained out-migration from rural areas. The letters themselves reflect such migration, with narratives sent from London, Kent, Sussex and other places but none at all from within Oxfordshire itself.

As with other samples of pauper letters, issues of sickness dominate the rationale for writing. Similar causation can be seen in the second tranche of letters (16–23) drawn from the Northamptonshire Record Office (hereafter NRO) and relating to the parish of Oxendon, on the Northamptonshire/ Leicestershire border. Both of these counties were experiencing urban and industrial/rural industrial development by the early nineteenth century. Oxendon itself, however, remained decidedly rural at the time the paupers whose narratives are reproduced here were writing. It is interesting, against this backdrop, that some paupers had managed to migrate as far as Manchester while the mobility of others only took them as far as Leicester. The letter set also includes some official and semi-official correspondence. Meanwhile, letters 24–7 take us into the late nineteenth century, though the focus on Northamptonshire is maintained, and letters written to the central authorities of the New Poor Law. Letters 24 and 25 must be read together, the first seeking the aid of the Central authorities after the pauper had been refused relief in his locality and the second constituting the draft reply from the same authorities and dispensing with the appeal. The extensive crossing out in the latter document demonstrates considerable thought on the part of London officials. Letter 26 comes from an entirely different source, written by a member of the 'shamefaced poor' to a Northamptonshire newspaper to remonstrate about the decision-making of local welfare officials. Meanwhile, letter 27 is written by an epistolary advocate, a son complaining about the fact that his aged and sick father had been denied relief, and typical of many thousands of such letters in British archives. Documents 28–32 change our focus completely to narratives about the poor, comprising articles on the shamefaced poor published in the later eighteenth-century *Copenhagen Evening Post*.

Collectively, the sources provide a flavour of the lived reality of poverty in the eighteenth and nineteenth centuries and also some of the potential and the potential problems of using narrative material.

1 To the Overseers of Bampton, Oxfordshire, from Eltham (Kent), 4 February 1818

Gentlemen, I am Sorry to be under the Nesesety of troubling you with this But bee Ashurd I am in destress at present as I am out off work and have had a Pore Afflicted Lad to maintain Many years and Cannot dow it any Longer with out your Astince iff you will Render me a triffell I will Endever to Get on Longer I should not have bee in this . . . had my Master Caried on busness aney Longer I served him 6 and twenty year I have been every ware after worke and Cannot get aney think to dow at present but am In oven [?] of some in a short time in I hope you will Comply with the above request Iff not wee must bee Brought home wich will bee Attended with more Expens you off Coarce [course] Now nothing off me at present this is to Informe you my name is James Stiles Son of Adam & mary Stiles pleas to direct for James Stiles Bricklayer Eltham Kent & pleas to Returne Answer By return off Post.

Source: ORO, Bampton, PAR 16/5/A11/8.

2 To the Acting Overseer of the Parish of Finstock near Charlbury, Oxfordshire, from Mortlake, Surrey, 17 December 1820

Gentlemen

Of this Parish of Finstock I am Sorry to Inform you that I Have a Family of 6 Children the Eldest not 12 years of Age – and my Wife Has Long Been Afflicted with a Rheumatic Complaint which Renders Her Unable at times even to Do for Her Family – and it has been my Misfortune not to Be in a Constant place of work for some time I Have made Application to Mortlake Parish for Relief – as I thought I was Parishoner Here by Renting – Part of a House – at Seven Pounds Ten Shillings A Year – and Likewise a House At the same time – at Six Guneas A Year Both Places was in my Possesion for Half a Quarter of a year – I gave up that which I paid £7-10s-0 for in Febry – and Have resided in the other ever since – I Have been Before a Bench of Justices – And Sworn to the Above Statement But they will not satisfy me whether I am A Parishioner or no – and Mortlake Parish tells me – if I come to them for Relief – they will pass me to Finstock – I expect to be out of work in the course of next week – and then I must Have Relief from somewhere – I Beg you will take my case into consideration – and write me an order as soon as possible – that I may know where my Parish is – And you will greatly oblige

Yr Most Obed^t Humble Servt

John Baylis

Please to direct from near the Church Mortlake Surry

Source: ORO, MSS. D.D. Par. Charlbury b.8/9, fol. 9.

3 To Mr. White, churchwarden of Hook Norton, Oxfordshire, from Louth, Lincolnshire, 29 December 1816

Mr Thos White I took this opertunety of Righting to you and to in form you that Mary Hyde is Bean Lying veary ill for the cors of thre wickes & is very much Deresede at this time and hase nothing to helpe here self and will be very much a Bleage to you if you will seande hir a Leetle mony to asest her at this time in hear Distres and you most Drect to Mr William Feanton.

James Street
Louth, Lincolnshire

Source: ORO, MSS. D.D. Par. Hook Norton b.12/10/9.

4 To Mr Rd Stawlwood, Rotherfield Greys, Oxfordshire, from Canterbury, 7 December 1812

Mr Stawlwood,

I take the liberty of writing to you requesting the favor through your intercession to the Parish of a trifle in order to pay my Rent. Has [sic] I have been in the Hospital the Main part of the Summer, and have never troubled you before. I have 5 Children, & my rent is 5 Guineas for the Twelvemont [sic]. Hope you will send it as soon as possible or else they will take Our Things and we must be obliged all to come home. Have the Goodness to remember me to my Brother John Collins & likewise my sister.

I Remain
Your Humble Servant
Robert Brookes

Source: ORO, MSS. D.D. Par. Rotherfield Greys c.11/13.

5 To Shipton under Wychwood, Oxfordshire, from Brighton (Ivory Place No 30, Sussex, 5 March 1832

Sir,

After receiving your letter last June things turned out better than I could have expected so that I did not answer it as I do not wish to trouble a Parish so long as I can provide for myself and Family, Respecting my belonging to Shipton I have gained a Settlement in two ways in the first place by having the Farm in my own possession more than Twenty years back & secondly by servitude to my Mother Now I must inform you that I am very much distressed at this time and it is quite out of my power to remain in Brighton without assistance provided I was help'd with the sum of Fiveteen pounds I make no doubt but I should get my Parish here as I have taken the House I am now in for a Twelvemonth for it is my wish & determination to do every thing to gain a settlement here, if I am not helped it will be utterly out of my power to remain here or gain a settlement, I expect my Wife to be confind in less time than two months which will be an expensive time and not the means to provide for her without help and at this time she is not able to do her own washing I am unfortunate for one of my children have [sic] been unwell sometime and myself so that I have not been able to saw any wood for this last two months as cutting wood is my employment at this time of the year which have [sic] been a great hurt to me and quite out of my power to go on any longer without help, if the Gentlemen of Shipton will allow me a weekly sum I might remain here but I should think it more advisable to allow the sum I mentioned as I may with that get a settlement here if not assisted their [sic] will be no alternative but my returning to Shipton an early Answer will much Oblige Sir.

Your most Obt & Hble Ser[t]

John Sharp

I hope Mr Hawkins & Family are well likewise our Shipton neighbours & c

Source: ORO, Shipton under Wychwood, PAR 236/5/A13/2/1.

6 To Shipton under Wychwood, Oxfordshire, from Brighton (Ivory Place No 30, Sussex, 27 March 1832

Sir,

I have been in daily expectation of hearing from you as it is now above three weeks since I wrote I must be under the necessity of applying here for relief if the Gentlemen of Shipton do not chuse to help me for it is quite out of my power to go on any longer without help my Wife is unwell now and not fit to be mov'd and I have no money to pay for a Docter or Nurse so that I shall compelld to apply here and that will be a heavy expence for a man that I know this parish allow'd him 15/- a week & paid is docter with but one child – it appears to me that they are afraid to trust me with a sum of money the[y] need not for it is my wish and determination to do evry thing to get settled here but without the sum I mention to you it will be no chance but with it I should be enabled to do it, so I shall leave it to their opinions to do as they like, my application put me in mind of the Boy & the Wolf I think they will drive it off like it is too late for me to get settled here which would cause them much greater expense and a continuance of it if I return which I must with out I am help'd and that without delay for we all know delay is dangerous, I have been nearly three quarters in this house so that if I am assisted I shall be able to get Quartly receipts but not without as I have had no receipt or settlement since I have been here I am as anxious as can be to get my parish here so they may depend on it I shall do all in my power to gain it but as I before mentiond with out the need [. . .] my plans will be quite frustrated and return I must for I have not got so easy a Landlord as I had last year an early answer will much oblige Sir

Your most Obt

& Hble Ser[t]

John Sharpe
I am compelled to apply for it is quite
out of my power to provide for my family myself

Source: ORO, Shipton under Wychwood, PAR 236/5/A13/2/3.

7 To Shipton under Wychwood, Oxfordshire, from Brighton (Ivory Place No 30, Sussex, 10 April 1832

Sir,

Your letter was brought to me Saturday Morn^g, but I could not take it in for want of money I met with a Friend yesterday afternoon who was so good as to lend me a shilling to pay for it, in yours you wish me to state the particulars of my gaining a Settlement I rented the Farm at Shipton of my Father for Twelvemonths from Lady day 1811 to Lady day 1812; I was hired by my Mother at Ten pounds a year in the way that servants generally are by her giving me a shilling earnest and sometimes two according as we agreed, The first hiring was the Michaelmas after Coombes gave up the Farm and continued being regular hired from year to year till the Farm was given up the last hiring being in 1826 I have never rented by the year allways weekly until I took the House I am now in, respecting what I mentiond about my old Landlord was that I have not so lenient a one as he was, I should be very much obliged to you to pay the Postage of the next letter and will be very much thankful to you to forward the Parish Officers answer as soon as possible for really I do not know how to get through the Week without assistance
I remain Sir
Your most Ob^t
& Hble Ser^t
John Sharpe

Source: ORO, Shipton under Wychwood, PAR 236/5/A13/2/4.

8 To Mr Boddington, Bearkhamstead, Hertfordshire, from a place unknown but relating to a pauper with settlement in Souldern, Oxfordshire, 6 November 1829

Dear Friend,

I am sorry to say I was out and could not rite the next morning to answare your letter I am very sorry to give you so much troble but had no one els to aply to now concerning owr parrish we are certain is it at Souldern and no ware els as we ware thare a 11 Months and had the whole years rent I taken the house of Mr Bailes and Mr Rogers togeather for one could not let it without the other so I am certain it is thear as we have had advice a bout it if the Gentlemen of Souldern dont think well of doing something more for me I must come to my parrish witch I should be sorry to do it but shall be oblegated so to do unless there is some thing done for us Mr Boddington you will much oblige me by giveing me a line as soon as you have seen your employers as my wife is worse again this week and oblige to keep the nurse on at present as she is in no ways likely to do for her self so I can drive it of no longer I am very much oblige to you for what you sent witch I do assure you was received very thankful give our best respects to Mrs Boddington and Jane and except [sic] the same your self

From your ever well wishes
John Fortnam

Source: ORO, MSS. D.D. Par. Souldern, c.7/i/7.

9 To Mr Randall, School master at Wooton, Oxfordshire, from Old Brentford, Middlesex, 6 January 1827

Sir,

I hope you will prevail on your Gent^n to forward me the Allowance that was due on 30th Dec last Am^tg to one Pound as the Season now has set in so severe I am much distressed for want of it I would not have solicited the favor of you but Mr Southam has stated I had better come home which should I do will quite put it out of my power of returning here again as I should lose the little employ I have & I trust at my time of Life 65 the Gent^n will not wish me to leave here as I am content with what they allow me.

& am Sir
Your hum Servt
Elizabeth Maunders

Source: ORO, Wooton P.C. IX/iv/9. Underlining in the original.

10 To the parish of St Clements, Oxford, from Camberwell, London, 29 June 1809

Sir I hope you will excuse the Liberty I take in sending Thess few lines to you my Husband having Distres^d and left me with my Children one of wich I have since Buried I wish to know of you, whether I can Claim this parish or if they can put me away as they threaten to do altho I have not hither to applied to them for releif, if Sir you think I belong to your parish I must beg the favour of a Certificate from you to indemnify me to this parish as I am willing to strive for a bit of bread and as this is my native place I think I am more likely to gain than any where else, sir I must [*page torn*]g the Favour of an, answer if no please and what you would advise me to I will abide by I remain your humble Servant

    Sarah parker
    please to direct for Sarah parker att
    Mr Howards
    Bower Lane
    Camberwell

Source: ORO, MSS. D.D. Par. Oxford St. Clements c.25.

11 To the parish of St Clements, Oxford, from Kingston, Surrey, 17 August 1831

Sur as the Time been up for me to Receive the money I wrote to you as I ham not at Kingston but my wife is I hope that you will [*page torn*] fail Sending at the Time as I have Allready Recived it to the Time for the Baicker Recives it at the post office and if I have not it He wont Lett my Wife Have aney Bread

    Thoˢ Pepall Cutler Kingston
    Surry

Source: ORO, MSS. D.D. Par. Oxford St. Clements c.25.

12 To the parish of St Clements, Oxford, from Kingston, Surrey, 19 January 1831

Sur I wrote to you for the Monney Due on the 8 of January Which I have not Received you Sayd that I should Received it in the Cours of to Days After now is A fortnight What Ham I for to Do I ham Summond by the Baicker and by my Landlord and Before I will go to Gale I will Lave my Wife & familey Chargable to the parish So Dont Be soprised at it if I Dough [Do] you may Depend of havin them again in St Clements if I have not the Monney in a few Days I will you may Depend on it 7 of us in family and I pay £7 16s 0d pr year I will have one of the Family With me and I will Leave my Master you may Depend on it if you Dont Send in a few Days for I never will come to Oxford I will Dround my Self furst you may Depend on

    Thos Pepall
    Cutler Kingston
    Surry

Source: ORO, MSS. D.D. Par. Oxford St. Clements c.25.

13 To the parish of St Clements, Oxford, from Kingston, Surrey, 26 March 1833

Gent[n]

I am truly sorry I am under the Necessity of writing to you again but tis now 13 Weeks since I received any thing from you – and I now assure you I am so distress'd I know not what to do – I have had but very little employment this Winter – indeed – and owing to your haveing taken off a Shilling pr week – I have been obliged to go into debt – and I fear I shall never be able to pay it unless you would please to consider my Situation and allow for the future the Shilling which has been taken off – I do assure you I have strove very hard and have felt more distress this Winter than ever I did in my Life – I am sorry to say I am now out of employ and my Girl can earn nothing – and I must beg to say that if I do not get more imployment than I have had – I must be obliged to come home for it can not be worse with me than it is now – Hopeing to hear from you as soon as possible I remain your obedient Servant

Eliz[h] Pepall

Source: ORO, MSS. D.D. Par. Oxford St. Clements c.25.

14 To the parish of St Clements, Oxford, from Kingston, Surrey, 28 March 1833

Gent[n]

It is now I believe a month since I wrote to you by the request of M[rs] Pepall – requesting you would send her some Money which she has nor receiv'd or heard any thing from you since – and I am now desired to write to you again on her behalf – and I assure you Gent[n] she is very much distressed indeed and is a great deal behind in her payments – so much so that nobody likes to credit her any further – my own Bill for Bread chiefly is £1-15-0 at present – and I do assure you I want my money verry Bad – I cannot go to any further lengths of Credit as I am oblidged to pay for my Bread Weekly – being only a Seller of it – and it don't pay me to give so long Credit – only I respect the poor woman – Knowing her to be a very honest principal – or I should not have given Credit at all – I fear your taking off the Shilling pr Week will be the means of obliding her to come home as she cannot support her self and Daughter upon her present allowance and she begs to say that she hopes you will write Directly and send her what you think proper for the Present – as she is intirely without money – and no one likes to give further Credit for her – I am Gent[n]

yours very Respectfully

B Handley

Source: ORO, MSS. D.D. Par. Oxford St. Clements c.25.

15 To the parish of St Giles, Oxford, from a place unknown. Undated note

Sir,

I hope you will excuse the liberty of my request for the sum of two shillings. I did not intend troubling you this week, had I not been disaponted [*sic*] by being unwell. I am now really in extreem [*sic*] pain and cannot get any thing this day. I hope it will be the last for some time."

Yr obedt Servt,

J.W. Penn

[N.b. in bottom left hand corner: 'John Bail']

Source: ORO, MSS. D.D. Oxford St Giles c.27, fol. 48 (no date).

16 To the parish of Oxendon, Leicestershire, from Manchester, Lancashire, 23 June 1831

I am sorry to have to say that the Depressed State of Trade again compels me to apply to you for assistance as we are 6 months in Arrears of Rent for which we are very strenuously pressed and threatened if not payed immediately which we have it not in our power to accomplish. We therefore humbly request that you will favour us with an Answer to this with your kind Relief by return of Post We have had no work of any consequence for the last 2 months and now we have not any at all more or less nor any sign of any therefore hope you will save the trouble of a second application which must inevitably follow if this be not immediately attended to for be assured We never trouble you untill Driven to the last extremity.

Yours respectfully

John Gunnell

Address

John Gunnell

No 60 Portugal Street

Oldham Road

Manchester

Source: NRO, 251p/98/1.

17 To the parish of Oxendon, Leicestershire, from Manchester, Lancashire, 25 March 1832

To the Overseer of Oxenden

I am sorry to have the necessity to trouble you again But the still low state of trade and Sickness together renders it impossible for me to pay my rent – I myself have been very poorly in health for a long time and my wife has be confined to her Bed of a Fever for 5 weeks but Thank God is by the Doctor pronounced out of Danger and in a fair way of recovery (if a relapse does not take place).

Under these circumstances I hope you will excuse my thus troubleing you which had it not been for illness I flattered myself I should have been able to have done without. In consequence of the above I am half a years rent behind.

I am your most obliged humble Servant
John Gunnell

Address
John Gunnell
No 60 Portugal Street
Oldham Road
Manchester

Source: NRO, 251p/98/2.

18 To the parish of Oxendon, Leicestershire, from Manchester, Lancashire, 19 August 1832

Sirs

I wrote a considerable time ago stating the depressed state of trade and Consequently our want of employ. I am sorry to say that after our waiting so long in expectation of some change for the better taking place things are Daily getting worse so that our situation is now become such that it is totally impossible for us to do any longer without Present[?] Relief and not that only but we have been so far back in rent that our Landlady's patience is wholy tired out. In fact to be candid and plain with you (which I hope you will excuse as I consider such conduct to be most improper) I have to say that if you do not remit me to the amount of 2 Pounds my goods must be sacrificed and we must come to you altogether and if that has to be the case it must be under a Sick order as neither myself nor my Wife are able through bad health and infirmities to come any other way.

Manchester is now become a Scene of Distress through the Violent raging of the Cholera it is this day stated that there has been 100 deaths this last week (God knows how soon it may be our lot) and it seems everyday to gain strength. A Neighbour 6 Doors below us was seized last Wednesday about 4 o'clock in the morning – Visited in the forenoon took to the Cholera Hospital about 2 in the Afternoon and died before 4 the same afternoon.

I hope what I have said will be sufficient to prevail upon you to favour me with an Immediate Answer as be Assured the above is a statement of real facts. I shall therefore Conclude and Subscribe myself
Your humble servant
John Gunnell

Address
John Gunnell
No 60 Portugal Street
Oldham Road
Manchester

Source: NRO, 251p/98/3.

19 To the parish of Oxendon, Leicestershire, from Manchester, Lancashire, 1 December 1833

Sir

I am sorry to have to write to you upon the present occasion of Distress I had the English Cholera in July last and in consequence of age and infirmity I have not been able to do anything since. I therefore hope you will have the Goodness to Relieve my Necessitous situation, I am considerably in Arrears of Rent, I hope Sir that what is said is sufficient and shall therefore humbly wait for your answer by return of post and
Am your most obliged
Humble servant
John Gunnell

117 Portugal Street
Oldham Road
Manchester
I am still in the same house but the Street is much enlarged and the number augmented from 60 to 117.

Source: NRO, 251p/98/4.

20 To the parish of Oxendon, Leicestershire, from Manchester, Lancashire, 6 January 1834

Sir

I wrote to you some time ago requesting your Assistance but have not gad any answer I therefore once more Repeat my Request nothing Doubting but it will be my last. I have for a long time been very ill, not able to do anything at all, and for a considerable time confined to my Bed with not the last hope or expectation of ever leaving it in this Vale of Tears but the Lord's will be Done I am Resigned to it and it alone for he alone knoweth best what to Do with his Children. With Desiring you to Answer this by return of post

I remain
Your much obliged servant
John Gunnell

117 Portugal Street
Oldham Road
Manchester

Source: NRO, 251p/98/5.

21 To the parish of Oxendon, Leicestershire, from Manchester, Lancashire, 22 January 1834

Gentlemen

About a fortnight ago my late husband wrote to you stating his and our Situation saying that he expected it would be his last time of troubling you which has been the case he Departed this transitory life on last Monday morning but one. We have not as yet received your answer I therefore write to inform you that I am left in a very precarious Situation as our Landlady has taken part of our Goods and I am in other Cases much embarrassed and in Respect to myself I am very Poorly in health and the worst is the loss of sight. I have long lost the sight of one Eye totally and have a Pearl far advancing upon the other. You will consider I am not able to provide for myself. Daughter Elizabeth is still at home but it is not in her power to support me but is willing to do her utmost if you will assist her I therefore hope you will have the Goodness to take our Situation into consideration and favour me with an immediate Answer as I must have assistance from some Quarter and would much rather have it from you than to have the trouble of applying to this town which you are confident I must Do if you do not prevent it by doing it yourselves. I hope I have sufficiently explained my situation and shall patiently wait for a few days or a Week for your (I hope favourable) Answer.

And remain
Your Obliged servant
Mary Gunnell

117 Portugal Street
Oldham Road
Manchester

Source: NRO, 251p/98/6.

22 To Richard Ward, overseer of the poor for Oxendon, Leicestershire, from Leicester, 24 July 1833

Mr Richard Ward
  Sir
  I am sorry I should be under the necessity of troubling you with this application I should not have done it but necessity compells me, My Wife is so unwell, that she is not able to do anything, And the times and all Business is so very bad, that I am not able to get work, sufficient to maintain my wife & self, & pay 2/6 per week for Rent, without you will assist me.
  I have stated my Case to my Landlord Mr William Harrison, who advised me to apply to you for assistance, otherwise I shall be forced and Obligated to bring her to the Parish. I will thank you to be so kind as to send me an answer as soon as possible, & you will oblige Sir,
  Your Distressed Humble servant
  Mark Illiff

  Orchard St
  Belgrave Gate
  Leicester

Source: NRO, 251p/99.

23 To Oxendon, Leicestershire, from Leicester, 2 July 1832

To the Overseers of the Poor of Oxen
  Gentlemen
  I think it duty incumbent on me to Inform you of the conduct of a man named James Harmstead & his wife who I am told receives Parochial weekly Pay from yr Parish while at the same time they are living in Drunkenness, Riot & Debauchery to t he great annoyance of the Neighbours. Hampstead [sic] is a stocking maker works for Josh Bec Wharf St, Bec pays him 9s & sometimes 10s pr week for his work in addition to which the wretched pair keeps a public Bawdy house in Barkby Lane in this Town it is also a Rendezvous for men of Bad character at all hours of the Night, and at present they have 5 Lewd women in the House. The above is a statement of facts that can be proved by the neighbours if required – I appeal to you as Parish officers expecting that you will investigate that matter before you pay any more Money to such undeserving People
  I am with Respect
  Your Very Humble servant

Thomas Derwin
Wharf St
Leicester
PS Mr Jonathan Wilson at the sign of the King's Dragoon Guards, Belgrave Gate can give you further information if call'd upon. He desired I should mention this. TD
Source: NRO, 251p/100.

24 Undated pauper letter, but pasted into 1871 central government file, from William Spokes, Holcot, Northamptonshire, to the Local Government Board

if you please your honer

i write to in form you i met the bord last Thursday for to get a paper for my wife for she is not well and i haven't not had any work for ten weeks only a day when i cold get sir i have had work to get a bit of Bread and i thought we should be next in the House being thy would not give me a paper for my wife for she is no time to count she was bad when i met the bord last Thursday last

We have wone child 11 months old i have no regular work the best of time i could not pay the doctor else sir it would sire but she must lay and die for i have done My best Sir

Source: The National Archives, MH12/8698, Local Government Board ref: No. 7281/71.

25 Draft reply to the above letter, dated 7 March 1871

State that ~~having~~ they have communicated with the Guardians of the Brixworth Union upon the subject of your complaint The Board are informed ~~to the effect that it came to the knowledge of the Guardians~~ that you had been offered work ~~but that you were not likely to accept it if you could avoid it~~ which you could have taken if you had felt disposed, and that having only one child they did not consider that you were in a position to require Medical Relief for your wife.

~~The Board can only observe that~~ it rests entirely with the Guardians to determine, ~~from their local knowledge of the circumstances of any case,~~ whether an applicant for relief is in a destitute condition which justifies ~~relief~~ its being afforded at the cost of Poor Rates ~~and that this~~ Board cannot

interfere to order relief in any individual case being expressly-prohibited by Law doing so I am
J. L. Hibbert
Secretary

Source: The National Archives, MH12/8698, Local Government Board ref: 9983A/1871.

26 Anonymous letter addressed to editor of the *Northampton Mercury* newspaper, 10 May 1873

Sir – I was glad to see the account of the Brixworth Board of Guardians in your paper on Saturday last and feel quite certain the ratepayers of the Union cannot wish the poor to be oppressed in the way they are now. The letter contained several cases of oppression, but from what one hears and knows, it is but a tenth of tithe of hard cases. Every one must regret to see one class set against another but what the guardians are now doing so most effectually. Why could their alterations not be made in the same way as in other Unions? It seems appointing a [medical relief] Committee and their report are the main causes of all the bother. One thing is quite certain – ratepayers should be very careful whom they entrust [with] the power to administer the rates; some Guardians know how to deal with the poor justly and firmly, whilst others don't care how the poor suffer as long as they can save their pockets. Trusting that the Leicestershire gentlemen are proud of their members doings
I remain – PAUPER on 1s 6d and LOAF
Source: Northampton Library Local Studies Room.

27 Letter from John Corby, The Mayorhold, Northampton, to the Local Government Board, 3 June 1873

Gentlemen
Robert Hollis aged 73 and Thomas Corby aged 75 both residing in this parish of Boughton near Northampton and having been for sometime in receipt of Parish relief, about a month since they were ordered to meet the Guardians of the Brixworth Union, two or three apparently unimportant questions being put and answered they were told the [outdoor medical] relief that had been receiving was stopped and without one word of previous warning or explanation given these two poor aged men were turned away penniless and foodless to live or die as the case might be.

A month has now elapsed and they have not received a farthing [cash] or a farthingsworth [in kind payment of medicine or food] of anything from the Board during that time and as far as can be seen there is no prospect of their doing so and during all that time they have been depending upon the charity of their fellow parishioners for subsistence getting a bit from one and a bit from another or none at all as the case might be.

Believing such an act of cruelty and oppression was never intended by the Legislature and would not be tolerated by the Commissioners [of the New Poor Law] in the hope and belief that they will cause enquiry to be made into the facts and circumstances of the case and see that justice is done to two poor Aged men who are unable to state their own case or defend themselves in any way and remain Most Respectfully, John Corby of Northampton, son of Thomas Corby

Source: The National Archives, MH12/8699, Local Government Board, memo no. 36, 433A/1873 and letter of complaint by paupers and their families.

28 The *Copenhagen Evening Post*, 20 June 1783

The News of the Shamefaced Poor.

When I speak of the shamefaced poor, I think of an honest widow, who went to see me the other day seeking my advice on my thoughts of her chances of being admitted to Vartou [Vartov Hospital], as she by reason of age and frailty couldn't endure for longer. I told her what I thought, first and foremost this would depend on if she had such friends and patrons, who could plead her cause, promote her, and get across with their recommendations. But she was totally unfamiliar with this and greatly poured out her troubles to me. I've, she said, since I was widowed, worked my way forward and lived by my diligence, without being a burden on anybody; but in a number of years strength entirely left me, and frailty entirely got the upper hand of me, so I can't go on. – Doesn't she have a family, who can take care of her? I asked. – No, nobody, she answered; now I have to draw on the remnants for the sake of my subsistence, and find help for my houseroom by means of some lodgers, whom I've taken in. – Doesn't she receive any social benefits or help from other high sources? – Not at all, she answered. I've hesitated to beg and strived to live by the work of my hands as long as possible; that's why I'm unknown. But now I can't go on anymore, now the need is present, and I'm not capable of getting anything for neither my recovery nor my refreshment. I've bemoaned my poverty for long, but in secrecy. Now it's getting too hard for me – At this point she shed a tear and I was moved. Among the needy, I thought, are however the fate of those who suffer in secrecy the most pitiful, especially when they are strangers to the beneficent of the world. I hope not to offend her by mentioning her, as I maybe could please the charitable among us, who prefer to know of the needy themselves, to whom they would distribute their gifts. In this way I didn't speak in vain for a widow of a customs official, who still suffers hardship; this time I will utter a secret wail of the widow of a poor journeyman barber-surgeon named Johanne Eggert, who lives in No. 91 Lavendel Lane, whose cumber I've witnessed, and for whose fate I would wish relief in her old age, which a diligent and hard-working woman deserves, when strength leaves her and shortage is near.

29 The *Copenhagen Evening Post*, 19 December 1783

The News of the Indigent.

The widow of the poor customs official in No. 202 Little Larsbjorn Lane, whose cumber I poured out in this paper in the beginning of this year, was back then lucky to be remembered by many generous benefactors, of both the high and the low estates, and at that time she was both comforted and soothed in her own and her children's pitiful condition. She did not alone get the strictly necessary for meat and drink, but also redeemed the necessities, which were pawned to get bread, and especially got her bed for the recreation of her weak and sick body. But now this pitiable mother again heaves profound sighs for the necessities of life! Her weakness doesn't allow her to work for her and her children's subsistence as she willingly would do, and she's bashful to put forward her wailings for a people, who have shown her so much good. Should I then be quiet, when I'm aware of her need? And when I feel it, and aren't able to relieve it? Heaven! How strange you lead the fate of man, and in how many ways you seek him to realize, that your hand only places happiness and blessing. This woman once smiled under more fortunate circumstances. There was a time when her husband owned both farms and estate. Back then, she was charitable towards others. Back then she couldn't have imagined that she would end up in a miserable attic, as a widow with two children and with a sickly body, which is the result of the grief of being unable to earn one's own bread. I suppose she feels her need double! Oh, who can rely on the circumstances in the world! But you, my wealthy fellow citizen! You, who in this minute are a stranger to hardships, pay her a visit in her home, when you pass by her door; and I'm sure her cumber will speak more clearly to your heart than my weak pen.

30 The *Copenhagen Evening Post*, 19 April 1784

The News of the Indigent.

A poor artisan called Ole Nielsen living in the back building of No. 82 Studi Lane, who with wife and two children is in the most pitiable state, in which destitution and sickness have brought them, has been visiting me and proven his misery. In order to pay rent and bread he has lost his poor belongings even his tools; misery and sorrow remain in their home. No relief of the cumber, no tools in his hands to earn the bread of which nature scream out for among old and young; no means to recollect the lost health; so the humanity cannot look into this home of destitution without being moved to tears. I recommend the need of this burgher for his fellow citizen's usual compassion for the needy among us. Maybe a small affectionate aid could support the need of this family, and mitigate their too bitter troubles; maybe a means of putting the idle hands of the man into work could be found, which he now downhearted carries owing to the lack of tools and support: And then we really perform a good deed!

31 The *Copenhagen Evening Post*, 11 February 1785

The News of the Indigent.

When we think of an honest and industrious burgher, who on account of sickness and unforeseen misfortune is succumbed to the tyranny of shortages; think of him looking at his wife and children with a greatly indebted heart, impecunious to provide for them, and homeless; and finally pursued by a severe creditor; what do we then feel in thinking about his unfortunate fate? The incapable sentient being, the poor tender-hearted being sighs and wishes: alas, if I could help, could rescue him. If the man is an honest and industrious man, if he is a competent burgher; if his wife is a loyal assistant to him, and if he is the father of dependent children; how fair, how civic and gently to come to his aid! – But what is the wealthy saying? I would gladly help my fellow citizen, when he hasn't brought ill-success on himself worsening his circumstances, when my assistance could rescue him and enable him to work for a better luck. – Oh, you righteous man! You, who increase your bliss by promoting others and are happy to see your suppressed fellow citizen with a cheerful face; then follow my direction to a middle-class family in this city, who haven't brought its fate on itself and haven't rendered itself unworthy of your helping hand. Ruin is at hand and many mouths shout: Rescue us! He won't beg for your gift but he will plead for a soft loan of 60 Rixdollars, which he will repay by dint of his trade. You and anybody needs his service; oh don't let him sigh for your assistance in vain, strengthen him by means of this loan to live and work for his family. You will receive the directions for his sad home in the ground floor front of No. 124 Mynter Street.

32 The *Copenhagen Evening Post*, 26 February 1790

An Intercession.

Could we indifferently hear the saddest account of a impoverished burgher family, who quite has lost its living, not because of dereliction of duties or misuse of the means for its care, but because of unavoidable incidents and failure of the trade, which lay upon their power to prevent; could we unfeelingly hear of the man who is cast to the sickbed because of grief, seeing that all strength to work for his family is lost, seeing the wife bowed down with sorrows and cumber for the sad change of her house, and the children moan about shortage of the necessary livelihood; well could we read our fellow citizens' testimonials of the fate of this man and hear how they pity him, who hasn't caused it themselves, and state that he and the wife are good and honest people, without being moved to compassion. Oh no! The Danish people couldn't act like that. The voice of humanity speaks too loud to its heart, that it could withhold concern of the hardships of the fellow citizen! – Surely my brothers! You my noble fellow citizens, who combine heart and ability with good deeds, unite and rescue our fellow citizen from his total fall. And if you couldn't raise him entirely, still help him with the aid you can do, so he may get back on his feet so far, that he supported by ye fellow brotherly hands can catch a glimpse of the hope by which he sees his way to recommence his interrupted trade. – Isn't a good and fair burgher worthwhile rescuing? His loss is great for the state, greater than we think at the first blush; for after all the state eventually will carry the burden of his destitution and pant from the consequences of his fall. Gladly I direct the benefactors to his home or receive what you contribute for his rescue. Em. [Emanuel] Balling, residing in No. 236 Admiral Street.

SELECT BIBLIOGRAPHY

Aarsleff, H. (1983), *The Study of Language in England 1780–1860*. Minneapolis: University of Minnesota Press.

Amelang, J. (1998), *The Flight of Icarus: Artisan Autobiographies in Early Modern Europe*. Stanford: Stanford University Press.

Baldwin, P. (1990), *The Politics of Social Solidarity and the Bourgeois Basis of the European Welfare State, 1875–1975*. Cambridge: Cambridge University Press.

Berringer, C. (1999), *Sozialpolitik in der Weltwirtschaftskrise: die Arbeitslosenversicherungspolitik in Deutschland und Großbritannien im Vergleich 1928–34*. Berlin: Duncker & Humbolt.

Bräuer, H. (2008), *Armenmentalität in Sachsen 1500 bis 1800*. Leipzig: Leipziger Universitätsverlag.

Bushaway, B. (2002), 'Things said or sung a thousand times: Customary society and oral culture in rural England, 1700–1900', in Fox, A. and Woolf, D. (eds), *The Spoken Word: Oral Culture in Britain 1500–1850*. Manchester: Manchester University Press, pp. 256–77.

Campbell, E. (ed) (2006), *Growing Old in Early Modern Europe: Cultural Representations*. Aldershot: Ashgate.

Crew, D. F. (1998), *Germans on Welfare. From Weimar to Hitler*. Oxford: Oxford University Press.

Cross, N. (1985), *The Common Writer: Life in Nineteenth-Century Grub Street*. Cambridge: Cambridge University Press.

Crossman, V. (2006), *Politics, Pauperism and Power in Late Nineteenth-Century Ireland*. Manchester: Manchester University Press.

Crossman, V. and Gray, P. (eds) (2011), *Poverty and Welfare in Ireland 1838–1948*. Dublin: Irish Academic Press.

Cunningham, H. and Innes, J. (eds) (1998), *Charity, Philanthropy and Reform: From the 1690s to 1850*. Basingstoke: Macmillan.

Dauphin, C. (2000), *Prête moi ta Plume ... Les manuels épistolaires au XIXe siècle*. Paris: Kimé.

Dekker, R. (2002), *Autobiographical Writing in its Social Context since the Middle Ages*. Hilversum: Veloren.

Delap, L., Griffin, B. and Wills, A. (eds) (2009), *The Politics of Domestic Authority in Britain since 1800*. Basingstoke: Palgrave.

Dinges, M. (2002), 'Men's bodies 'explained' on a daily basis in letters from patients to Samual Hahnemann (1830–35)', in Dinges, M. (ed.), *Patients in the History of Homeopathy*. Sheffield: European Association for the History of Medicine and Health Publications, pp. 85–118.

Dorwart, R. (1971), *The Prussian Welfare State before 1740*. Cambridge MA: Harvard University Press.

Earle, R. (ed) (1999), *Epistolary Selves: Letters and Letter Writers 1600–1945*. Aldershot: Ashgate.

Elspaß, S., Langer, N., Scharloth, J. and Vandenbussche, W. (eds) (2007), *Germanic Language Histories, from below' (1700–2000)*. Berlin: de Gruyter.

Fabre, D. (1993), *Ecritures Ordinaires*. Paris: POL.

Fahrmeir, A. (2000), *Citizens and Aliens: Foreigners and the Law in Britain and the German States, 1789–1870*. Oxford: Oxford University Press.

Fissell, M. (1991), 'The disappearance of the patient narrative and the invention of hospital medicine', in French, R. and Wear, A. (eds), *British Medicine in an Age of Reform*. London: Routledge, pp. 92–109.

Fontaine, L. and Schlumbohm, J. (eds) (2000), *Household Strategies for Survival 1600–2000*. Cambridge: Cambridge University Press.

Frohman, L. (2008), 'The break-up of the poor laws – German style: Progressivism and the origins of the welfare state, 1900–18', *Comparative Studies in Society and History*, 50, 981–1009.

Furger, C. (2010), *Briefsteller. Das Medium 'Brief' im 17. und 18. Jahrhundert*. Weimar: Böhlau.

Gagnier, R. (1991), *Subjectivities: A History of Self-Representation in Britain, 1832–1920*. Oxford: Oxford University Press.

Gerber, D. (2005), 'Acts of deceiving and withholding in immigrant letters: Personal identity and self-presentation in personal correspondence', *Journal of Social History*, 32, 315–30.

—(2006), *Authors of Their Lives: The Personal Correspondence of British Immigrants*. New York: New York University Press.

Gestrich, A. and Raphael, L. (eds) (2008), *Inklusion/Exklusion. Studien zu Fremdheit und Armut von der Antike bis zur Gegenwart*. Frankfurt: Peter Lang.

Gestrich, A., Raphael, L. and Uerlings, H. (eds) (2009), *Strangers and Poor People: Changing Patterns of Inclusion and Exclusion in Europe and the Mediterranean World from Classical Antiquity to the Present Day*. Frankfurt: Peter Lang.

Gillis, J. (2006), 'The history of the patient since 1850', *Bulletin of the History of Medicine*, 80, 490–512.

Gray, L. (2002), 'The experience of old age in the narratives of the rural poor in early modern Germany', in Ottaway, S., Botelho, L. and Kittredge, K. (eds), *Power and Poverty: Old Age in the Pre-Industrial Past*. Westport: Greenwood Press, pp. 107–23.

Grell, O., Cunningham, A. and Jütte, R. (eds) (2002), *Health Care and Poor Relief in 18th and 19th Century Northern Europe*. Aldershot: Ashgate.

Grell, O., Cunningham, A. and Roeck, B. (eds) (2005), *Health Care and Poor Relief in 18th and 19th Century Southern Europe*. Aldershot: Ashgate.

Harley, D. (1999), 'Rhetoric and the social construction of sickness and healing', *Social History of Medicine*, 12, 407–35.

Hennock, E. P. (1987), *British Social Reform and German Precedents*. Oxford: Clarendon Press.

—(2007), *The Origin of the Welfare State in England and Germany, 1850–1914: Social Policies Compared*. Cambridge: Cambridge University Press.

Hindle, S. (2004), *On the Parish? The Micro-Politics of Poor Relief in Rural England 1550–1750*. Oxford: Oxford University Press.

Hitchcock, T., King, P. and Sharpe, P. (eds) (1997), *Chronicling Poverty: The Voices and Strategies of the English Poor 1640–1840*. Basingstoke: Macmillan.

Hollen Lees, L. (1998), *The Solidarities of Strangers: The English Poor Laws and the People 1700–1948*. Cambridge: Cambridge University Press.

Hopkin, D. (2004), 'Storytelling, fairytales and autobiography: Some observations on eighteenth and nineteenth century French soldiers' and sailors' memoirs', *Social History*, 29, 186–98.

Hurren, E. (2007), *Protesting About Pauperism: Poverty, Politics and Poor Relief in Late-Victorian England, 1870–1900*. Woodbridge: Boydell.

Innes, J. (1999), 'The state and the poor: Eighteenth century England in European perspective', in Brewer, J. and Hellmuth, E. (eds), *Rethinking Leviathan: The Eighteenth Century State in Britain and Germany*. Oxford: Oxford University Press, pp. 225–80.

Joyce, P. (1991), 'The people's English: Language and class in England 1840–1920', in Burke, P. and Porter, R. (eds), *Language, Self and Society: A Social History of Language*. Cambridge: Polity, pp. 154–90.

Jütte, R. (1994), *Poverty and Deviance in Early Modern Europe*. Cambridge: Cambridge University Press.

—(1996), 'Syphilis and confinement: Hospitals in early modern Germany', in Finzsch, N. and Jütte, R. (eds), *Institutions of Confinement*. New York: Cambridge University Press, pp. 97–116.

—(2000), *Arme, Bettler, Beutelschneider. Eine Sozialgeschichte der Armut in der Frühen Neuzeit*. Weimar: Böhlau.

King, S. (2011), 'Welfare regimes and welfare regions in Britain and Europe, c.1750–1860', *Journal of Modern European History*, 9, 42–66.

Lachmund, J. and Stollberg, G. (1995), *Patientenwelten: Krankheit und Medizin vom späten 18. bis zum frühen 20. Jahrhundert im Spiegel von Autobiographien*. Opladen: Leske and Budrich.

Lawrence, C. (1994), *Medicine in the Making of Modern Britain*. London: Routledge.

Lawrence, P. (2000), 'Images of poverty and crime. Police memoirs in England and France at the end of the nineteenth century', *Crime, History and Societies*, 4, 63–82.

Leimgruber, M. (2008), *Solidarity Without the State? Business and the Shaping of the Swiss Welfare State, 1890–2000*.Cambridge: Cambridge University Press.

Lindemann, M. (1990), *Patriots and Paupers. Hamburg 1712–1830*. New York: Oxford University Press.

Lindert, P. (2004), *Growing Public: Social Spending and Economic Growth since the Eighteenth Century*. Cambridge: Cambridge University Press.

Lis, C. and Soly, H. (1979), *Poverty and Capitalism in Pre-Industrial Europe*. Brighton: Harvester.

Lyons, M. (ed) (2007), *Ordinary Writings, Personal Narratives: Writing Practice in 19th and early 20th Century Europe*. Frankfurt: Peter Lang.

Lyons, M. and Baggio, P. (2001), 'La culture littéraire des travailleurs. Autobiographies ouvrières dans l-Europe du XIXe siècle', *Annales, Histoire, Sciences Sociales*, 56, 927–46.

Martin, L., Gutman, H. and Hutton, P. (eds) (1988), *Technologies of the Self: A Seminar with Michel Foucault*. London: University of Massachusetts Press.

Mayer, T. and Woolf, D. (eds) (1995), *The Rhetorics of Life-Writing in Early Modern Europe. Forms of Biography from Cassandra Fedele to Louis XIV*. Ann Arbor: University of Michigan Press.

Métayer, C. (2000), *Au Tombeau des Secrets: Les écrivains Publics du Paris Populaire, Cimetière des Saints-Innocents XVIe–XVIIIe siècle*. Paris: Albin Michel.

Mommsen, W. (1981), *The Emergence of the Welfare State in Britain and Germany 1850–1950*. Newton Abbott: Croom Helm.

Poland, B. and Pedersen, A. (1998), 'Reading between the lines: Interpreting silences in qualitative research', *Qualitative Enquiry*, 4, 293–312.

Porter, R. (1985), 'The patient's view. Doing medical history from below', *Theory and Society*, 14, 167–74.

Porter, R. (ed.) (1985), *Patients and Practitioners*. Cambridge: Polity.

Porter, R. (1991), 'Expressing yourself ill: The language of sickness in Georgian England', in Burke, P. and Porter, R. (eds), *Language, Self and Society: A Social History of Language*. Cambridge: Polity, pp. 276–99.

Sachße, C. and Tennstedt, F. (1988), *Geschichte der Armenfürsorge in Deutschland, Fürsorge und Wohlfahrtspflege 1871 bis 1929*. Stuttgart: Kohlhammer.

Scheutz, M. (2003), *Ausgesperrt und gejagt, geduldet und versteckt: Bettlervisitationonen im Niederösterreich des 18. Jahrhunderts*. St Pölten: NÖ Institut für Landeskunde.

Schulze, W. (ed.) (1996), *Ego-Dokumente. Annäherung an den Menschen in der Geschichte*. Berlin: Akademie.

Sherman, S. (2001), *Imagining Poverty: Quantification and the Decline of Paternalism*. Columbus: Ohio University Press.

Smith, C. A. (2007), 'Parsimony, power and prescriptive legislation: The politics of pauper lunacy in Northamptonshire 1845–76', *Bulletin of the History of Medicine*, 81, 359–85.

Smith, T. (2003), *Creating the Welfare State in France 1880–1940*. Montreal: McGill-Queen's University Press.

Snell, K. D. M. (2006), *Parish and Belonging: Community Identity and Welfare in England and Wales 1700–1950*. Cambridge: Cambridge University Press.

Sokoll, T. (2001), *Essex Pauper Letters 1731–1837*. Oxford: Oxford University Press.

Stachura, P. (2003), 'Social policy and social welfare in Germany from the mid-nineteenth century to the present', in Ogilvie, S. and Overy, R. (eds), *Germany: A New Social and Economic History. Volume II: Since 1800*. Cheltenham: Edward Arnold, pp. 227–50.

Stollberg, G. (2002), 'Health and illness in German workers' autobiographies from the nineteenth and early twentieth centuries', *Social History of Medicine*, 6, 261–76.

Taylor, J. S. (1991), 'A different kind of Speenhamland: Nonresident relief in the Industrial Revolution', *Journal of British Studies*, 30, 183–208.

Tomkins, A. (2006), *The Experience of Urban Poverty 1723–82: Parish, Charity and Credit*. Manchester: Manchester University Press.

Vandenbussche, W. (2007), 'Lower class language in 19th century Flanders', *Multilingua*, 26, 279–90.

van Voss, L.-H. (ed) (2001), *Petitions in Social History*. Cambridge: Cambridge University Press.

Vincent, D. (1982), 'The decline of oral tradition in popular culture', in Storch, R. (ed.), *Popular Culture and Custom in Nineteenth-Century England*. Newton Abbott: Croom Helm, pp. 20–47.

von Kondratowitz, H.-J. (1991), 'The medicalization of old age: Continuity and change in Germany from the late eighteenth to the early twentieth century', in Pelling, M. and Smith, R. (eds), *Life, Death and the Elderly: Historical Perspectives*. London: Routledge, pp. 134–64.

Wannell, L. (2007), 'Patients' relatives and psychiatric doctors: Letter writing in the York Retreat, 1875–1910', *Social History of Medicine*, 20, 297–314.

Wertheimer, M.-M. (1997), *Listening to Their Voices: The Rhetorical Activities of Historical Women*. Columbia: University of South Carolina Press.

Whyman, S. (2009), *The Pen and the People: English Letter Writers 1660–1800*. Oxford: Oxford University Press.

Winter, A. (2008), 'Caught between law and practice: Migrants and settlement legislation in the southern Low Countries in a comparative perspective, c.1700–1900', *Rural History*, 19, 137–62.

Woolf, S. (1986), *The Poor in Western Europe in the Eighteenth and Nineteenth Centuries*. London: Methuen.

INDEX